Point-of-Care Technologies Enabling Next-Generation Healthcare Monitoring and Management

Sandeep Kumar Vashist • John H. T. Luong

Point-of-Care Technologies Enabling Next-Generation Healthcare Monitoring and Management

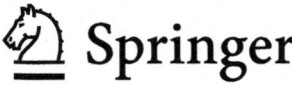 Springer

Sandeep Kumar Vashist
Labsystems Diagnostics Oy
Vantaa, Finland

John H. T. Luong
Innovative Chromatography Group,
Irish Separation Science Cluster (ISSC),
School of Chemistry and Analytical,
Biological Chemistry Research Facility
(ABCRF)
University College Cork
Cork, Ireland

ISBN 978-3-030-11415-2   ISBN 978-3-030-11416-9   (eBook)
https://doi.org/10.1007/978-3-030-11416-9

Library of Congress Control Number: 2018968020

This Springer imprint is published by the registered company Springer Nature Switzerland AG
The registered company address is: Gewerbestrasse 11, 6330 Cham, Switzerland

Preface

Together with physical assessment of signs and symptoms, testing before treatment is a prerequisite step for the diagnosis of diseases at a much earlier stage. Point-of-care (POC) testing tools (POCT) play a prominent role in healthcare to provide test results at or near the bedside within a couple minutes to a few hours with high sensitivity and selectivity. Consequently, healthcare professionals can start the treatment of their patients and take appropriate clinical decisions based on the POCT results, leading to better health outcomes and significant cost savings. The POCT market expands rapidly with a forecasting value of US$35 billion in 2024 (https://www.marketwatch.com/press-release/point-of-care-testing-poct-market-is-expected-to-be-worth-us-35-billion-by-2024-2018-06-06). Variants of emerging POC technologies are further pushing the limits of POCT by enabling rapid testing, employing minimal sample volumes, and better bioanalytical performance. They also employ minimal process steps, mobile healthcare technologies, automated assay formats, fully integrated platforms, and smart devices.

This book covers various emerging POC technologies that are leading to continuous advances and paving the way to next generation of healthcare monitoring and management. Smartphone-based tools together with the evolving trend toward mobile healthcare, smart technologies, and smart applications are acting as the trendsetters in the ongoing technological evolution of POC testing (POCT). Further, there is an extensive need for cost-effective assay formats, e.g., paper or lab-on-a-chip (LOC) platforms for the diagnostics in the remote settings or developing countries with limited healthcare infrastructure and resources; Ebola is a typical example for the need for POCT in isolation laboratories and field sites. These developments in POC technologies also facilitate the future trend toward personalized and integrated healthcare. Additionally, advanced complementary technologies, encompassing rapid assay concepts, novel biosensors, automated platforms, prolonged reagent storage strategies, and multiplex detection, foster the development of innovative POC technologies to revolutionize the healthcare management.

Objectives of the Book

This book aims to present the field of POC technologies, which are enabling next-regeneration healthcare monitoring and management. The emerging POC technologies are described in depth along with their characteristic features, advances, and applications in healthcare monitoring and management.

Scope of the Book

This book describes the emerging POC technologies, such as smartphone-based mobile healthcare technologies, commercial personalized technologies, paper-based IAs, LOC-based IAs, and multiplex IAs. Moreover, it provides insights into the POC diabetes management software and smart applications, determination of bioanalytical parameters, and future trends in POC technologies and personalized healthcare for chronic diseases.

Target Audience

This book provides a thorough understanding of the emerging POC technologies and next-generation healthcare monitoring and management to researchers, scientists, engineers, analysts, economists, policymakers, investors, software developers, and healthcare professionals. It serves as a very useful resource and teaching aid for professionals and researchers in healthcare monitoring and management, POC technologies, mobile healthcare, clinical diagnostics, medicine, bioengineering, diabetes, chronic diseases, wellness, and preventive healthcare.

Book Organization

This book describes the various emerging POC technologies that are leading to next-generation healthcare monitoring and management. The first chapter provides an overview of the various emerging POC technologies and the role that they are playing in the improved healthcare. The second chapter provides an expert insight into the wide range of smartphone (SP)-based POC technologies that have emerged during the last decade and significantly increased the outreach of healthcare and clinical diagnostics to the remote and decentralized settings. The commercial SP-based personalized mobile healthcare devices are comprehensively described in the third chapter. The fourth chapter describes the wide range of diabetes management software and smart applications, which are of great utility to the diabetics and significantly improving their healthcare. The fifth and sixth chapters provide the comprehensive information and expert insights into paper and lab-on-a-chip (LOC)-based POC immunoassays, respectively. Thereafter, the multiplex immunoassays, which are proving to be indispensable for the diagnosis of complex diseases, are discussed in the seventh chapter. The eighth chapter focuses on the determination of various bioanalytical parameters in immunoassays using appropriate statistical procedures along with the role that such parameters play in clinical diagnosis. The concluding chapter discusses the future trends for the next generation of personalized and integrated healthcare for chronic diseases.

We acknowledge the efforts devoted by the authors in drafting the outstanding book chapters, which serve as a valuable resource to professionals and students in the field of POCT and mobile healthcare. The knowledge and the expert insights provided in this book on the various emerging POC technologies will considerably improve the technical know-how of the professionals and students, which will lead to the development of superior POC technologies and make full use of the improved POC technologies for better healthcare monitoring and management. The information provided further empowers the general population with the detailed technical know-how on the emerging POC technologies and how they are shaping up the significantly improved healthcare to provide fast, reliable, and accurate results across a growing number of diseases at right to the point of care.

The guided insight and knowledge of POC technologies and varied aspects of healthcare monitoring and management provided in this book will act as a potential resource for professionals, researchers, and students, who are working or would like to work in the field of POCT. The demand for point-of-care testing is growing worldwide to reflect the increased need for testing in emergency management, biomarkers for various diseases, antimicrobial resistance, and infectious outbreaks.

Vantaa, Finland   Sandeep Kumar Vashist
Cork, Ireland   John H. T. Luong

Contents

Contributors

Sandeep Kumar Vashist Labsystems Diagnostics Oy, Vantaa, Finland

John H. T. Luong Innovative Chromatography Group, Irish Separation Science Cluster (ISSC), School of Chemistry and Analytical, Biological Chemistry Research Facility (ABCRF), University College Cork, Cork, Ireland

Lionel G. G. Djoko Immunodiagnostics Systems SA, Liege, Belgium

Stuart Blincko Immunodiagnostics Systems SA, Liege, Belgium

Chapter 1
An Overview of Point-of-Care Technologies Enabling Next-Generation Healthcare Monitoring and Management

Sandeep Kumar Vashist and John H. T. Luong

Contents

1.1 Introduction

POC technologies empower the POC testing (POCT), just near to the site of patient care, where medical care is critically needed for the diagnosis, monitoring, and management of diseases [1–3]. POCT devices offer the cost-effective rapid

© Springer Nature Switzerland AG 2019
S. K. Vashist, J. H. T. Luong, *Point-of-Care Technologies Enabling
Next-Generation Healthcare Monitoring and Management*,
https://doi.org/10.1007/978-3-030-11416-9_1

detection of clinical analytes, using minimal sample volumes and portable instruments, at the patient's bedside or in a physician's office lab (POL), paramedical support vehicles, secondary and tertiary care settings, or home [4]. The distinct feature is its capability to provide the results of the analysis for a patient sample matrix (blood, urine, plasma, serum, etc.) in just a few minutes. POCT devices employ single-use cartridges/strips for qualitative/quantitative analysis via an inbuilt reader. Multiple-use cartridges together with portable benchtop readout instruments offer precise quantitation.

POCT plays a critical role in healthcare as the precise early-stage detection of analytes is an essential requirement for the effective diagnosis, monitoring, and management of the patients' health. Consequently, the treatment of patients can be implemented at an early stage, resulting in remarkable healthcare cost savings and improved health outcomes. The current trend is strongly inclined toward the next-generation POCT for personalized mobile healthcare, i.e., the general population can monitor and manage their own health.

The global POCT market estimated US$23.16 billion in 2016 is expected to grow to US$36.96 billion in 2021 with a compound annual growth rate (CAGR) of 9.8% [5]. North America enjoys the most predominant share, followed by Europe and Asia-Pacific. The trend also indicates that the POCT market is expected to grow at the CAGR of 14.2% in Asia-Pacific [5]. The estimated global blood glucose monitoring is $12.2 billion in 2017 [6], mainly shared by Roche, LifeScan, Bayer, Abbott, and Alere. It accounts for the largest market share of POCT followed by the pregnancy test and care tests for various diseases and genetic disorders.

Among different POC technologies [7], the most prospective POC technologies are based on SP, LOC, paper, microfluidics, biosensors, and/or novel assay formats [7]. The complementary technologies, such as system integration, device automation, prolonged sample storage strategies, and signal readout, are further providing a significant support for the continuous developments in POC technologies.

As the prevalence of chronic and infectious diseases is increasing at a rapid pace worldwide, there is a growing need for low-cost POCT, especially in India and China with a substantial increase in such diseases. An ideal POCT method would apply a simple, sensitive, and specific assay procedure with a short turnaround time (TAT). It would simply process unrefrigerated assay reagents to detect analytes accurately and precisely by portable low-cost devices.

The present 425 million diabetics in the world will increase to 629 million in 2045 [8]. In the past, the World Health Organization underestimated the increasing number of diabetics: 171 million in 2000 to 366 million in 2030 [9]. In reality, the number of diabetics was confirmed as 382 million in 2013. This is a wake-up call for all nations as diabetes is increased at an unprecedented pace. It signifies an urgent plan to take immediate measures and build up international strategies and an action plan to tackle this global epidemic.

The WHO [10] also estimates over 1 million people are acquiring sexually transmitted infections (STIs) daily due to their exposure to more than 30 different bacteria, viruses, and parasites. There are also ~357 million persons infected with STIs every year due to chlamydia, gonorrhea, syphilis, and trichomoniasis. Over 500 million people have genital infection with herpes simplex virus (HSV), while over 290 million women have an infection with human papillomavirus (HPV). Some STIs such as HSV type 2 and syphilis can increase the risk of HIV acquisition over threefold, while others can lead to serious reproductive health consequences. The most dangerous is the fact that most STIs have no or only mild symptoms or warning signs, which makes them hard to be identified.

The number of fatalities due to cardiovascular diseases (CVDs) is the topmost cause of death globally [11], 17.7 million people died from CVDs in 2015, or 31% of all global deaths. Another critical healthcare concern is tuberculosis (TB) with10.4 million infected people in 2016 [12]. This communicable disease could be easily transmitted from the infected individual to others by air. About 1.7 million died from TB in 2016, which accounts for over 95% TB deaths in low- and middle-income countries. TB is also the leading killer of HIV-positive people accounting for about 40% of HIV deaths. The critical health security threat is the growing incidence of drug-resistant TB. The WHO estimated about 600,000 new cases of drug resistance to rifampicin, one of the most effective first-line drugs against TB. Out of these, 490,000 were observed to have multidrug-resistant TB (MDR-TB).

Cancer is the second leading cause of death globally with 8.8 million fatalities in 2015 [13], i.e., 70% of cancer deaths in low- and middle-income countries. There were 14 million new cancer cases in 2012 with the incidence expected to increase 70% over the next two decades [13]. Cancer has a huge economic impact as the estimated annual economic cost of cancer is about US$1.16 trillion in 2010 [13]. Similarly, malaria is another healthcare threat as evident from estimated 216 million cases and 445,000 deaths in 2016 [14]. Malaria is a preventable and curable life-threatening disease that is caused by the bites of infected female *Anopheles* mosquitoes.

The most "somewhat" surprising is the depression, which has been recognized as a hidden burden by the WHO. At least 300 million people were living with depression in 2013 [15], whereas over 450 million were suffering from mental disorders mainly due to psychological stress, who are more prone to depression in the near future. About 800,000 depressed people die by committing suicide every year [15]. Therefore, the incidence of depression is similar to that of diabetes.

This chapter provides an overview of POC technologies emphasizing the growing need for POCT, an overview of POC technologies, challenges involved, and the emerging trend toward next-generation healthcare monitoring and management.

1.2   Need for Point-of-Care (POC) Technologies

POCT is needed in intensive care units, emergencies, and clinical facilities dealing with infectious diseases, to offer the assay turnaround time (TAT) of a few minutes so that the medical intervention is started immediately and the spread of infectious diseases is prevented. Similarly, POCT can be deployed in case of epidemics so that the desired steps could be taken in time to curtail the spreading. The incidence of some chronic diseases has increased much more than expected, which makes it impossible for the healthcare to monitor each affected individual. In such cases, POC technologies have facilitated the effective healthcare monitoring and management. An ideal example is diabetes, where the POC devices for the monitoring of blood glucose are being used by few hundred million diabetics every day [16–19]. Similarly, there is a new trend toward the monitoring of glycated hemoglobin (HbA1c) as it provides the long-term average of blood glucose [18]. Similarly, there has been a rapid increase in sedentary behavior [20–22], which is attributed to the rapid increase in obesity, cardiovascular diseases, cancer, diabetes, and other metabolic disorders. The POC devices for monitoring the basic healthcare parameters are contributing significantly by motivating the subjects to break down their sedentary behavior and live an active lifestyle. During the last decade, several POC tests have emerged for clinically relevant analytes such as electrolytes, C-reactive protein, etc., which need to be monitored very frequently in most patients. However, there is still a need to develop POC tests for a large number of other analytes. Of urgent need is the development of clinical score-based multiplex analyte detection assays to diagnose diabetes, depression, and cancer at a much earlier stage.

There is an emerging trend toward digital health [23], which is facilitated by the rapid developments in mH, smart applications, portal services, and Cloud computing. It is empowering the healthcare personnel and patients to effectively monitor and manage their health. In some cases, the growing use of mH-equipped POC devices in ambulances and by primary healthcare workers and patients is enabling the doctors in taking better clinical decision-making and providing better healthcare, leading to favorable clinical outcomes.

The developments in POC and complementary technologies would lead to advanced POC clinical analyzers with diversified features and increased functionality. During the recent years, several prospective benchtop models and handheld POC analyzers have been commercialized by Roche, Abbott, Siemens, etc.

Apart from the clinical settings, POC technologies for analyte detection in food, environment, and security are also needed. POC tests are required for detecting harmful chemicals (like pesticides, mercury, arsenic, etc.), toxins (like botulinum), pathogens (such as *E. coli* O157:H7, *Salmonella*, *Campylobacter*), or biowarfare agents (such as anthrax spores) in food products, water supply, soil, and other media. The early-stage detection of these analytes is essential to avoid epidemics. There were many outbreaks of *E. coli* O157:H7 [24, 25], botulinum toxin [26, 27], and other pathogens such as *Salmonella* [28, 29] and *Campylobacter* [30] in food products. There is also a growing need to test the food products for allergens [31], one of the main concerns in the Western society.

There is a requirement for POC tests for STIs considering the phenomenal increase of persons acquiring STIs every day. Although syphilis and HIV POC tests are being widely used [32], they must be overhauled for all STIs for personal and clinical use. According to WHO, about 36.7 million people were living with HIV in 2016, while 1.8 million people were newly infected with HIV in 2016 [33]. Therefore, improved POC tests for HIV are of uttermost importance. Improved

POC tests for the early diagnosis of CVDs are required so that the life-saving medical therapeutic intervention can start at the earliest possible. CVDs are the leading cause of mortality worldwide that accounts for over 75% of all deaths in low- and middle-income countries [11]. Of significance is the early diagnosis of cancer by developing POC tests for the detection of new cancer biomarkers with improved predictability. Similarly, it is essential to detect TB an early stage via POC tests so that the infected individuals can be treated immediately. Other possibilities are POC tests for the resistance to drugs such as those used for the TB treatment with aspirin as an example. Lastly, there is a necessity to develop POC tests for the clinical and personalized monitoring and management of depression, which is a hidden epidemic with an incidence similar to that of diabetes. The diagnosis of depression is challenging considering the lack of the specificity of involved biomarkers. Nevertheless, the better understanding of physiological mechanisms and biomarkers involved in depression might lead to the desired POC tests in near future.

1.3 Target Analytes for Point-of-Care Testing (POCT)

1.3.1 Small Molecules

Most POCT devices, such as those from Roche, Abbott, and Siemens, measure the clinically relevant target analytes, i.e., electrolytes, small molecules, and glucose employing electrochemical or optical detection technologies [34]. Blood glucose testing (BGT) accounts for the predominant market share of the POCT market taking into account the exponentially increasing number of diabetics worldwide and the need for the frequent monitoring of blood glucose. Blood glucose monitoring is an essential part of diabetic management [18, 19], which enables diabetics to maintain their blood glucose levels within the normal physiological range by lifestyle/nutritional/therapeutic intervention. Consequently, the diabetics continue enjoying a healthy lifestyle, avoiding costly and life-threatening diabetic complications of diabetic retinopathy, kidney damage, heart diseases, stroke, neuropathy, and/or birth defects.

Most POCT devices for BGT employ glucose dehydrogenase that is oxygen-independent and provides accurate results for all blood specimen types [35]. Such devices, however, are susceptible to interference by maltose. Most previous generation and some current BGT devices are still based on glucose oxidase (GOD), which is oxygen-dependent and thus not recommended for blood glucose measurements during shock, diabetic coma, and dehydration. Electroanalysis of H_2O_2, a by-product of GOD, is susceptible to interferences from electroactive several drugs and their metabolites [36]. Several noninvasive glucose measurement techniques have been demonstrated during the last decade [16], but they still lack the desired accuracy and precision as required for diabetic healthcare monitoring. The painless glucose monitoring demonstrated by Abbott's FreeStyle Libre is of interest [37] as it is based on a pioneering technology that is a major step toward continuous glucose monitoring (CGM) with a potential market of US$783.9 million in 2019 [38].

1.3.2   Cardiac and Cancer Biomarkers

POC tests are also available for the determination of cardiac injury biomarkers: myoglobin and creatine kinase isoenzyme MB (CKMB). In particular, the cardiac troponins (cTnI and cTnT) are the most widely used and the best validated cardiac biomarkers, which are determined by several POC tests. The determination of cTnT and cTnI facilitates the effective screening of cardiac patients, which provides tremendous cost savings and lower hospitalization rates [39]. Other POC tests target different cardiac biomarkers consisting of copeptin, fatty acid-binding protein, B-type natriuretic peptide, ischemia-modified albumin, glycogen phosphorylase isoenzyme BB, and myeloperoxidase [40, 41]. Similarly, POC tests become available for cancer biomarkers such as prostate-specific antigen, platelet factor 4, and carcinoembryonic antigen.

1.3.3   Cells

POC tests have been developed for the determination of complete blood cell counts for the diagnosis and monitoring of various disease conditions, such as anemia and human immunodeficiency virus (HIV)/acquired immune deficiency syndrome (AIDS). The most widely used POC test for cells is the CD4+ T-lymphocyte counting in HIV-infected patients to monitor the progression of HIV/AIDS and evaluate the progress of antiretroviral therapy. However, the POC tests need to be considerably improved to match the performance of flow cytometry, which is the widely used clinical technique for the counting of cells.

1.3.4   Other Analytes

Several POC tests have been developed for the detection of HIV antibodies, influenza virus, *P. falciparum*, *Streptococcus*, *Treponema pallidum*, *Chlamydia trachomatis*, rotavirus, and *Trichomonas*. The prospective analytes for the development of new POC tests would be galectin-3 or β-galactoside-binding protein (for fibrosis), copeptin (for myocardial infarction), neutrophil gelatinase-associated lipocalin (for acute renal failure), and endoglin, placental growth factor, and tyrosine kinase (for preeclampsia).

1.3.5   Future Target Analytes

The potential future target analytes for POC tests are growth hormone, adrenocorticotrophic hormone, parathyroid hormone, sepsis biomarkers, stroke biomarkers, tuberculosis biomarkers, malaria pathogen/biomarkers, diarrhea pathogen,

pathogen for STDs, immunosuppressants and related metabolites, deoxyribonucleic acid (DNA), and pathogens (air-, water-, or foodborne) responsible for disease outbreaks and epidemics.

1.4   Point-of-Care Technologies

1.4.1   Clinical POC Technologies

Various automated POC analyzers have been developed by all major IVD companies. They are widely used in the clinical settings for the determination of analytes. Roche Diagnostics has developed several prospective POC analyzers. Cobas b221 [42] is the first FDA-cleared blood gas analyzer, a benchtop system, for pleural fluid pH testing with fast TAT for 1 min. It employs zero-maintenance electrodes, load-and-go reagents with smart chips, barcode scanner, LCD touch screen, and AutoQC module. It has five modules for the measurement of blood gases (pH, pCO_2, pO_2), electrolytes (Na^+, K^+, Ca^{2+}, Cl^-, Hct), hemoglobin (tHb, sO_2), metabolites (glucose, lactic acid, and urea), and CO-oximetry (tHb-COOX, O_2Hb, HHb, COHb, MetHb, SO_2 COOX, bilirubin (neonatal), barometric pressure). Cobas u411 [43] is a compact semiautomatic urine analyzer that employs urine test strips for the measurement of various urine parameters: pH, glucose, nitrite, leukocytes, protein, glucose, ketones, urobilinogen, bilirubin, specific gravity, color, and blood (erythrocytes, hemoglobin). Cobas LIAT PCR system [44] is a POC system for performing real-time PCR in less than 20 min using an innovative lab-in-a-tube technology. It is used for the diagnosis of infectious diseases such as Influenza A/B, Strep A, and respiratory syncytial virus (RSV), based on the amplification and detection of DNA or RNA. A portable handheld POC device developed for systematic anticoagulation management is CoaguChek XS [45], which measures the prothrombin time and international normalized ratio (PT/INR) using a simple procedure that involves inserting a test strip into the POC device, pricking the finger with a lancing device, placing a drop of blood on the strip, and reading the result on the device's display in a minute. PT/INR testing is essential for the monitoring of anticoagulation therapy with warfarin. Accutrend Plus [46] is another portable handheld POC device for the total cholesterol and glucose in the blood sample using a similar measurement procedure.

   Siemens also offers similar POC analyzers and devices [47] such as RAPIDLab 1200 and 500 systems for blood gas analysis, Stratus CS for cardiac care, Xprecia Stride Coagulation Analyzer for PT/INR testing, DCA Vantage Analyzer for the measurement of HbA1c and microalbumin products, and CLINITEK Advantus Urine Chemistry Analyzer for strip test-based analysis of various analytes in urine. Similarly, various IVD companies, such as Abbott, Alere, EKF Diagnostics, HemoCue AB, etc., have developed several POC analyzers, devices, and tests.

   The i-STAT handheld analyzer [48] by Abbott determines analytes in whole blood in just a few minutes using single-use i-STAT test cartridges. The POCT procedure employs four steps: (1) inserting 2–3 drops of blood into the test cartridge; (2) closing the test cartridge and inserting it into the i-STAT handheld analyzer; (3) viewing the results of the test on the i-STAT handheld screen in a few minutes; and (4) uploading the test information automatically into the lab or hospital information system. The test results are delivered wirelessly with the i-STAT Wireless or directly when the i-STAT handheld is placed in a downloader. The i-STAT system features a wide range of test cartridges for the measurement of cardiac biomarkers (cTnI, CK-MB, BNP), endocrinology (beta human chorionic gonadotropin), electrolytes and chemistries (Na, K, Cl, TCO_2, anion gap, ionized Ca, glucose, urea nitrogen/urea, creatinine, lactate), blood gases (pH, pCO_2, pO_2, TCO_2, HCO_3, base excess, sO_2), hematology parameters (hematocrit, hemoglobin), and coagulation parameters (ACT, PT/INR).

The POCT application and analytical performances of selected commercial POC devices are shown in Table 1.1.

1.4.2 Smartphone-Based POC Technologies

A large number of SP-based devices and smart applications for personalized mH monitoring and management have been developed [49] and commercialized successfully by iHealth Labs Inc., Runtastic GmbH, Cellmic Inc., AliveCor Inc., Apple Inc., Samsung, and Fitbit. These include SP-based devices for the measurement of general healthcare parameters such as heart activity, pulse rate, blood pressure, physical activity, weight, blood oxygen saturation, and sleep. During the last 4 years, three generations of Apple Watch were launched with continuously increased capabilities and features. Most of these smart devices equipped with advanced mH tools have now become an integral part of our lives. They are empowering the strong emerging trend toward personalized digital health (Table 1.2), resulting in decreasing healthcare costs and better healthcare outcomes.

Apart from general healthcare, SP-based technologies become available for a wide range of bioanalytical applications [50–52], based on colorimetric [53–56], fluorescent [57, 58], luminescent [59–61], surface plasmon resonance (SPR) [62, 63], electrochemical [64–68], and Mie scattering [69] signals in assays. Compact optomechanical attachment-based diagnostic test readers were launched by Cellmic for the readout of colorimetric and fluorometric lateral flow assays (LFA) [70] (Fig. 1.1). The iHealth Align is the smallest Food and Drug Administration (FDA)-approved blood glucose meter developed by iHealth Labs [71] (Fig. 1.2).

An SP-based flow cytometer based on optofluidic fluorescent imaging can be used for screening of pathogens in whole blood and water [72]. Moreover, SP-based microscopes for bright-field, fluorescence, dark-field, transmission, and polarized microscopy [73–75] are applicable for the imaging of blood cells, platelets, and waterborne parasites [76] and fluorescent imaging of single nanoparticles (NPs) and human cytomegaloviruses [77]. An SP dongle detected HIV, syphilis, and active syphilis infection in just 15 min [78], while an SP-based fluorimeter measured the full emission spectrum of light emitters [79].

Table 1.1 POCT applications and analytical performance of selected commercial POC devices

A. Current and emerging uses of POCT
(see: http://wwwn.cdc.gov/cliac/pdf/addenda/cliac0207/addendumf.pdf)

POCT	Analytes
Routine	Glucose, lactate, pO$_2$, pCO$_2$, electrolytes (Na$^+$, K$^+$, Ca^{++}, Cl$^-$) Activated clotting time Occult blood, hemoglobin, *Streptococcus*, and other bacteria Urine dipsticks, including that for pregnancy testing
Variable	Cardiac markers, heparin, drug/toxicology, lactate, INR, coagulation for hemostasis, assessment (TEG), heparin D dimer for thromboembolism, magnesium Transcutaneous bilirubin, lipids, hemoglobin A1c, microalbumin, enzymes (amylase, alkaline phosphatase, CK, AST, ALT, c-GT), creatinine HIV, influenza, *Helicobacter pylori*, and other bacteria
Emerging	Complete blood count, white blood cell count, platelet function testing, platelet function testing Coagulation for transfusion algorithms, transfusion needs

B. Analytical performance of some selected commercial POCT devices [34]

Manufacturer/ instrument	Type	Sample volume (μL)	Analysis time (s)	Target analytes
Abbott Diagnostics • I-Stat	H	65–95	90–140	pO$_2$, pCO$_2$, pH, electrolytes, Hct, urea nitrogen, glucose, lactate, creatinine
AVL Scientific Corp.				
• AVL OMNI	T	40–161	60–90	pO$_2$, pCO$_2$, pH, electrolytes, Hct, Hb, urea nitrogen, glucose, lactate, creatinine
• AVL OPTI	P	125	<120	pO$_2$, pCO$_2$, pH, electrolytes, Hct, Hb
Agilent Technologies • IRMA SL (series 2000)	P	125	90	pO$_2$, pCO$_2$, pH, Na$^+$, K$^+$, Ca^{++}, Hct
Bayer Diagnostics • RAPIDLab 800 series	T	140–175	85	pO$_2$, pCO$_2$, pH, electrolytes, glucose, lactate
HemoCue AB • HemoCue B-Hemoglobin	P	10	45–60	Hb
Instrumentation Laboratory • Gem Premier 3000, 3001	P	135	<120	pO$_2$, pCO$_2$, pH, Na$^+$, K$^+$, Ca^{++}, Hct, glucose, lactate
Nova Biomedical Corp.				
• Nova series 16	T	385	85	Electrolytes, Hct, urea nitrogen, glucose, creatinine
• Stat profile M/ M7.	T	85–190	78–108	pO$_2$, pCO$_2$, pH, SO$_2$%, electrolytes, Hct, urea nitrogen, glucose, lactate, creatinine
• Stat profile pHOx	T	40–70	45	pO$_2$, pCO$_2$, pH, sO$_2$%, Hct, Hb

(continued)

Table 1.1 (continued)

B. Analytical performance of some selected commercial POCT devices [34]				
Manufacturer/ instrument	Type	Sample volume (μL)	Analysis time (s)	Target analytes
Radiometer America Inc.				
• ABL 70 series	P	<180	<60	pO_2, pCO_2, pH, Na^+, K^+, Ca^{++}, Hct
• ABL 700 series	T	55–195	80–135	pO_2, pCO_2, pH, electrolytes, glucose, lactate

Reproduced with permission from Cell Press [7]
Electrolytes: Na^+, K^+, Ca^{++}, Cl^-

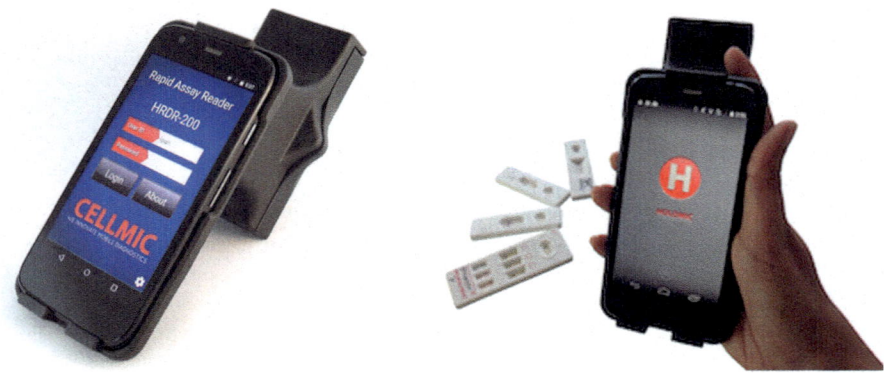

Fig. 1.1 A holomic rapid diagnostic reader (HRDR) for the readout of lateral flow immunoassays. Left: HRDR-200. Right: HRDR-300. Reproduced with permission from Cellmic, USA

Fig. 1.2 iHealth Align, the smartphone-based blood glucose meter developed by iHealth Labs. Reproduced with permission from iHealth Labs

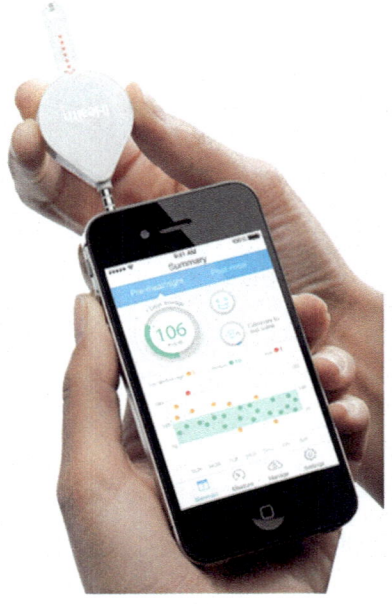

Table 1.2 The conceptual potential of emerging technologies for next-generation POCT

Parameters	CP (1)	PBA (2)	LOC (3)	Next-generation POCT[a] (1 + 2 + 3)
Performance:				
Suitability for POCT	(High)	(High)	(High)	(High)
Technology penetration	(High)	(Low)	(Low)	N.A.[b]
Utility in epidemics and emergencies	(High)	(High)	(Medium)	(High)
Prerequisite of *prolonged storage of reagents*	✓	✓	✓	✓
Prerequisite of *rapid assay*	✓	✓	✓	✓
Portability	(High)	(High)	(Medium)	(High)
Cost-effectiveness of consumables	(High)	(High)	(Medium)	(High)
Overall cost-effectiveness	(High)	(High)	(Medium)	(High)
Quantitative	✓	✗	✓	✓
Sensitivity	(High)	(Low)	(Medium)	(High)
Specificity	(High)	(Medium)	(Medium)	(High)
Throughput	(High)	(High)	(Medium)	(High)
Precision	(High)	(Low)	(High)	(High)
Reproducibility	(High)	(Low)	(Medium)	(High)
Capable of mass production	✓	✓	✓	✓
Compliance with regulatory guidelines	✓	✗	✓	✓
Ease of Operation:				
Ease of operation	(High)	(High)	(High)	(High)
Labor intensiveness	(Medium)	(Low)	(Low)	(Low)
Need for power supply	✗	✓	✓	✗
Need for readout instruments	✗[c]	✗	✓	✗[c]
Standalone analysis	✓	✓	✓	✓
Personalized	✓	✗	✗	✓
Accessibility of POCT results anytime anywhere	✓	✗	✗	✓
Basic skillset required for operation	✓	✓	✗	✓
Connectivity:				
Connectivity to cloud	✓	✗	✗	✓
Smart applications and portal services	✓	✗	✗	✓
Test history and data patterns	✓	✗	✓ (Limited)	✓
Spatio-temporal mapping	✓	✗	✗	✓
Demographic data and statistics	✓	✗	✗	✓
Telemedicine support	✓	✗	✗	✓
Text alerts	✓	✗	✗	✓
Preventive healthcare tools	✓	✗	✗	✓

CP, PBA, LOC, and POCT stand for cellphone, paper-based assay, lab-on-a-chip, and point-of-care testing, respectively. Reproduced with permission from Cell Press [7]

(High ●; Medium ●; Low ●)

[a]This column has been computed conceptually taking into account the characteristics of the component technologies

[b]N.A. not applicable

[c]A smartphone attachment or interfaced instrument would be required for nonoptical signal detection such as in case of electrochemical readout

1.4.3   Paper-Based Assays (PBA)

PBA is the most cost-effective format and well suited for diagnostics in the developing countries and remote settings (Table 1.2). Various types of PBA formats have emerged comprising lateral flow assay (LFA), dipstick assays, and microfluidic paper-based analytical devices (μPADs) [80, 81] (Fig. 1.3). Nitrocellulose membrane, filter paper, chromatography paper, and paper/polymer or paper/nanomaterial composites [82] are the most commonly used substrates for PBA. The surface chemistry, porosity, and optical properties of these materials [83] are critical for the diagnostic applications of PBA. Nitrocellulose membranes are still the most widely used substrate for PBA as they have a broad distribution of pore sizes (0.05–12 μm). However, they are difficult to handle at low humidity due to the accumulation of static electricity [84].

Colorimetric PBA can be read qualitatively via the naked eye only by comparing against a predetermined score chart [85]. Cameras, scanners, commercial test strip readers, and handheld colorimeters are added for the precise determination of color intensity. The current trend is the highly precise quantitative determination via image analysis using a CP-based rapid diagnostic test reader [70].

The most widely used PBA format is the LFA [86], which has been extensively used for the testing of pregnancy based on the detection of hormone human chorionic gonadotropin (hCG) in urine. LFA become available for cancer biomarkers [87], HIV diagnosis [88], and nucleic acid testing [89]. LFA usually employ a nitrocellulose membrane test strip along which the sample flows laterally via capillary forces provided by the absorbent pad. The sample dispensed onto a sample pad flows laterally over a conjugate pad where the target analyte binds conjugate particles (e.g., gold nanoparticles (AuNPs)).

Two-dimensional (2D) or three-dimensional (3D) μPADs [90, 91] are prepared by the patterning of paper. The 3D μPADs are usually obtained by stacking layers of 2D patterned paper that are well-suited for multiplexing [92]. The μPADs have been used for sandwich ELISA [93, 94]. The microfluidic paper-based electrochemical devices (μPEDs), fabricated by printing the electrodes on paper, have been attempted for the detection of alcohol, uric acid, nucleic acid, lactate, glucose, and cholesterol [95, 96].

To date, the sensitivity of the PBA needs to be critically improved by signal enhancement strategies [97, 98] as it is inappropriate for diagnostic applications. There is still a need to devise strategies to circumvent the poor reproducibility, nonuniformity, and variable accuracy of PBA. The current efforts focus on the multiplex analyte detection [99, 100] and development of fully integrated platforms [101].

1.4.4   Lab-On-A-Chip Platforms

LOC platforms have been widely used in POCT due to their simplicity and ease of operation (Table 1.2). The most prominent LOC platform is used in the blood glucose sensing strip, which accounts for the predominant share of POCT market [18, 19, 104]. A wide range of LOC platforms has emerged during the last two decades

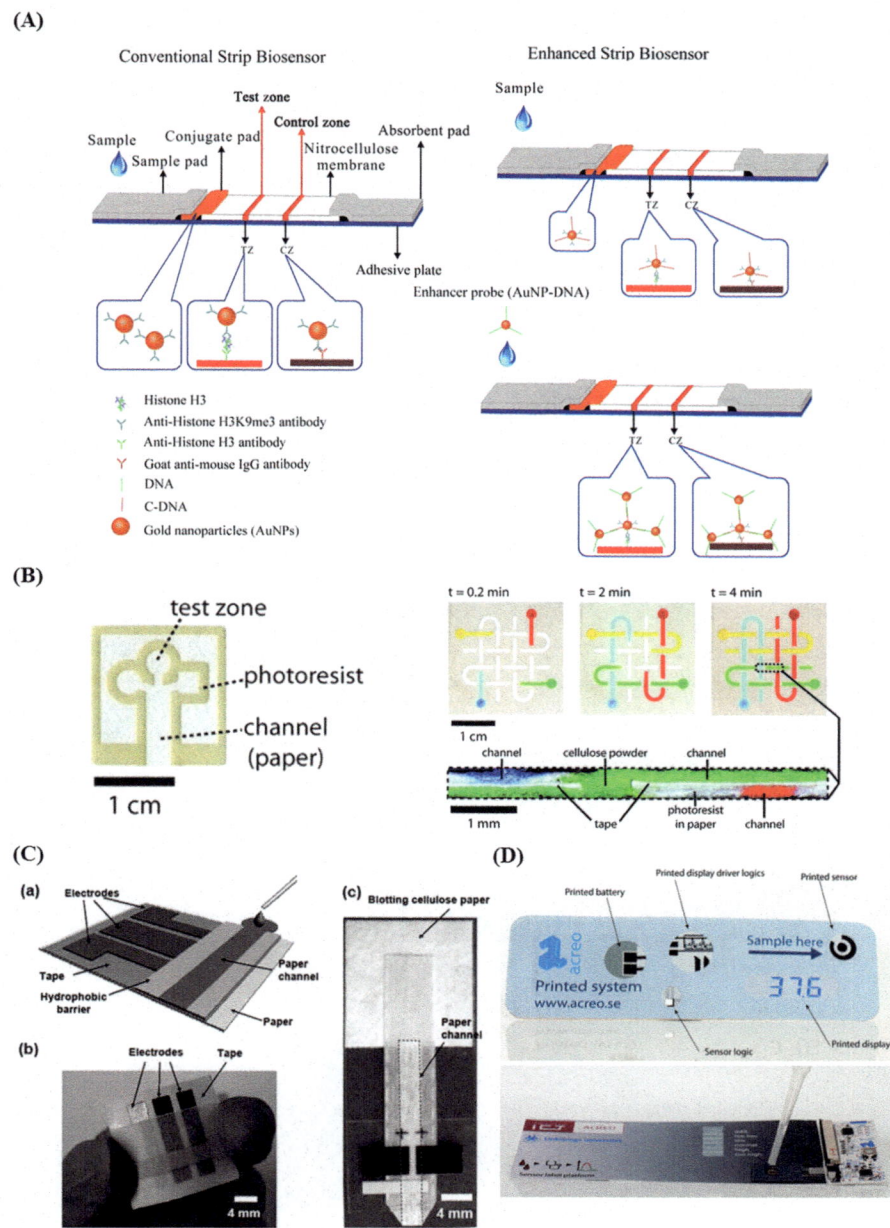

Fig. 1.3 Paper-based technologies for POCT. (**A**) Conventional and enhanced LFIA for the visual detection of trimethylated lysine 9 of histone H3 (H3K9me3) in histone extract from HeLa cells [102]. (**B**) A typical 2D [91] (left) and 3D [92] (right) microfluidic paper-based analytical device (μPAD). (**C**) Microfluidic paper-based electrochemical devices (μPEDs) [103]. (**D**) Conceptual rendering (top) and image (bottom) of a completely printed paper-based amperometric biosensor [104]. Reproduced with permission from the Cell Press [7]

using various microfluidic operations, sample storage concepts, sample treatment procedures, and biosensor principles. They can be fabricated from polymers, paper, silicon, glass, ceramics, cloth, and composites using conventional or emerging fabrication techniques.

Among the most prominent LOC platform-based assays and analyzers [106, 107], the centrifugal microfluidics-based LabDisk platform (Abaxis Inc.) can simultaneously monitor 14 tests on a single LabDisk. It provides several Clinical Laboratory Improvement Amendments (CLIA) waived multi-analyte tests and other tests. The company employs its portable Piccolo Xpress™ whole blood chemistry analyzer [105] (Fig. 1.4A) for the running and readout of their LabDisk assays. Similarly, the centrifugal microfluidics-based LabDisk platforms and analyzers of Gyros AB [106] (Fig. 1.4B–C) are widely used by the pharmaceutical industry to develop fully automated IAs with broader dynamic ranges, shorter assay times, and reduced reagent volumes compared to conventional ELISA assays. The LabDisk platform-based assays have also been targeted for biomarkers, nucleic acids, pathogens, toxins, and other potential analytes [107].

(A)

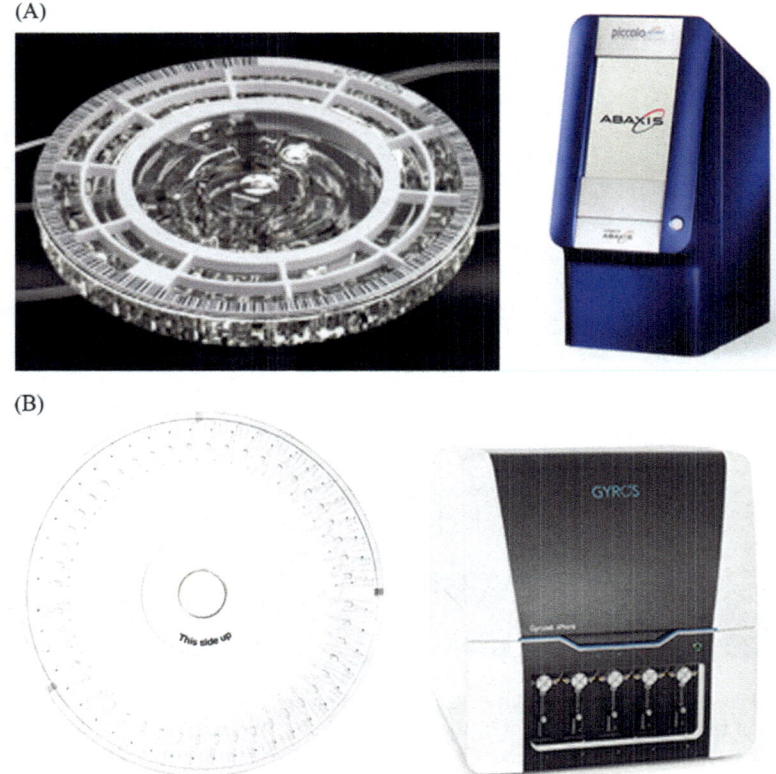

(B)

Fig. 1.4 (**A**) Centrifugal microfluidics-based LabDisk platform and POC analyzer for fully automated immunoassays by (**B**) Abaxis Inc., USA, and (**C**) Gyros AB, Sweden. Reproduced with permission from Abaxis Inc. and Gyros AB

1.4.5   Complementary Technologies

The drastic advances in the complementary technologies and the continuous improvements might play a key role in the development of next-generation POC technologies. The novel assay formats and prolonged storage of assay reagents are the critical complementary technologies that would definitely play a key role in the development of prospective POC technologies.

1.4.5.1   Novel Assay Formats

There is a requirement for novel assay formats having high analytical performance, ease of operation, and cost-effectiveness. Several prominent assay formats have been developed during the last decade that would be highly prospective for POCT. The AlphaLISA® [108] from PerkinElmer is a truly innovative assay format, which involves the interaction of streptavidin-coated alpha donor beads with anti-analyte Ab-conjugated AlphaLISA® acceptor beads. The formation of a sandwich immune complex in the presence of analyte leads to the generation of a chemiluminescence signal. The **cobas®** lab-in-a-tube (LIAT) assay format [44] from Roche Diagnostics is a compact polymerase chain reaction (PCR) assay. It employs a small benchtop analyzer and a sealed-tube design for sample and reagent storage in multiple vertical chambers, with a typical analysis time below 20 min. It is widely used in POCT for **cobas®** Influenza A/B, **cobas®** Influenza A/B and RSV, and **cobas®** Strep A assays, while the assays for several infectious diseases are under development.

Another prospective assay format is the Optimiser™ ELISA [109] from Siloam Biosciences Inc., based on an innovative microfluidic microtiter plate with a simple microfluidic assay procedure with minimal process steps. The format requires minimal assay reagents' volumes and offers a turnaround time of just a few minutes. The electrochemiluminescent ELISA from Meso Scale Diagnostics LLC [110] offers highly sensitive wash-free sandwich immunoassays in complex sample matrices. The assay format employs carbon electrode surface-based microwell plates and SULFO-TAG™-labeled detection antibody that emits light upon electrochemical stimulation. The most interesting feature of this assay is the multiplex analyte detection in the same microwell, which makes it a high-throughput format. Various SP-based EasyELISA platforms for rapid immunoassays [111] and highly simplified and rapid one-step kinetics-based immunoassay procedures [53, 54, 112] have been reported.

1.4.5.2   Prolonged Assay Reagents Storage Strategies

The ability to prolong the storage of assay reagents without losing their functional activity constitutes one of the prerequisites for POCT because this factor significantly affects the bioanalytical assay performance. In particular, the reagents need to withstand anticipated harsh environmental conditions during storage, shipping, and testing [113]. Various prolonged storage strategies have emerged, which involve the use of stabilizers, sugars, sugars with transition metal ions, sugar alcohols, sugar alcohols with cationic polymers or zinc ions, freeze-drying, lyophilization, and reagent pouches. Pullulan is a nonionic natural polysaccharide produced by *Aureobasidium pullulans* that forms an oxygen impermeable solid upon drying. This enables the storage of labile biomolecules in the form of water-soluble pellets [114], which can be stored at room temperature for months without any decrease in their functional activity due to thermal denaturation and chemical modification. Another prospective approach is the long-term dry storage of reagents used in ELISA by drying them onto a glass fiber pad together with horseradish peroxidase-conjugated antibody and its colorimetric substrate [115]. The procedure was developed by the customization of a previously patented procedure, which involves the freeze-drying of peroxidases in glass tubes in the presence of polyvalent ions with stability for prolonged storage at 37 °C [116].

1.5   Challenges

Despite significant advances in POC technologies, there are still numerous challenges that need to be tackled so that they could be employed for next-generation healthcare monitoring and management. The technical issues associated with POC devices are summarized in Table 1.3, while the challenges are discussed further in this section.

Table 1.3 Various issues associated with POCT

Major issues	Remarks
Interference due to endogenous substances in the sample can affect result	- Inaccuracy and imprecision can be caused by endogenous substances in the test samples, poorly controlled environments, and degradation of reagents and controls
Result is operator dependent	- Inadequate operator training - Device is prone to instrument malfunction or operator error
Narrower measurement ranges for some analytes or variability in results	- Measured glucose level is slightly higher than venous blood - Potential interference from hematocrit, pO_2, temperature, and humidity when glucose oxidase is used; not recommended for shock, diabetic coma, and dehydration
Higher cost of POCT compared to laboratory testing	- Costs can, however, be partially offset by processing small sample volumes on-site with resulting short therapeutic turnaround times to minimize the overall hospital cost
An extra step is required to integrate test results with hospital or laboratory information system	- Lack of connectivity between device and central hospital system; and this implementation step is still formidable and expensive

Reproduced with permission from Cell Press [7]

1.5.1 Compliance with Regulatory Guidelines and Healthcare Requirements

The compliance of developed POC technology with the regulatory guidelines and healthcare requirements is the most stringent challenge that must be met before the technology could be used in healthcare. The POC technology should have the requisite bioanalytical performance, robustness, reproducibility, and stability as specified by the US Food and Drug Administration [117] and other regulatory agencies [118]. The sensitivity, specificity, precision, accuracy, and recovery of the developed POC technology should be comparable to that of accepted clinical technologies. The technology should be able to precisely and reproducibly quantify the analyte in a large number of patient samples without incurring any interference from potential non-specific physiological and pharmacological substances. Although LOC platforms and established POC technologies are complying with most of these criteria, the batch-to-batch variability is still a challenge for PBA [119, 120]. In contrast, the frequently changing specifications of SPs are a limitation for ubiquitous applications and regulatory compliance as they could significantly impact the bioanalytical performance of SP-based POC test.

1.5.2 Need for Fully Integrated Bioanalytical Platforms

The bioanalytical platforms used in POC technologies need to be fully integrated so that they can be used for POCT at remote and decentralized settings without any requirement for refrigeration or ancillary equipment for upstream microfluidic actuation (sample dilution, dispensing, preparation, pre-concentration and mixing or biomolecule/cell manipulation, etc.) and downstream detection [7]. The advances in SP-based detection have circumvented the need for bench-scale detection equipment (e.g., lasers, microscopes, etc.) and hence allow for integration with microfluidic devices that carry out the assay. Passive capillary transport obviates the need for large bench-scale syringe pumps or electronic equipment such as signal generators and amplifiers. However, it is inadequate in some cases when on-chip mixing or biomolecule/cell manipulation steps are required to speed up the assay or to increase the detection sensitivity and selectivity. In addition, there remains considerable difficulty in miniaturization of the components needed for active microfluidic transport, which involves the application of external fields. As such, most recent technology developments remain unviable for true POCT functionality and portability considering the requirement for large, cumbersome, and expensive bench-scale ancillary equipment that cannot be miniaturized and integrated with the chip-based assays. Further, there is a need to integrate the prospective strategies for long-term reagent storage [7]. Doubtlessly, the advances in complementary technologies could address these limitations in the coming years.

1.5.3 Material Safety

The increasing popularity of incorporating nanomaterials and nanocomposites into assays, given reports on their propensity to enhance sensitivity and analytical performance, has led to growing concerns about their safety due to their potential cytotoxicity [121, 122]. The problem is compounded by the lack of standard overarching guidelines for analyzing the toxicity of nanomaterials and nanocomposites, which has resulted in conflicting results for the same set of nanoscale materials. Therefore, there is a need for extensive toxicity testing guided by a rigorous regulatory framework or set of guidelines that govern the use of nanomaterials and nanocomposites.

1.5.4 Data Security

The widespread use and communication of electronic data and the advent of Cloud computing via Bluetooth and wireless networks have raised concerns about the data security and ownership [123–125]. This is especially pertinent in the upcoming and next-generation POC devices geared for mobile healthcare provisions in which a patient's test data is envisaged to be stored on the device or on a network and/or transmitted to the certified healthcare personnel such as patient's medical practitioner. Therefore, there is a need to maintain the ownership of confidential data such as the patient's personal health records by securing it using advanced encryption algorithms [126]. The recorded data must be synchronized to necessitate bidirectional communication between POCT instruments at all sites and the central data storage server of the healthcare information network.

Many countries have imposed legal restrictions and requirements pertaining to the physical storage or transmission of data within their national boundaries, requiring compliance by network and service providers (e.g., Amazon Web Services and Google). Efforts are also being devoted to establishing an international Cloud computing standard, e.g., the creation of EuroCloud and Google Data Liberation Front [49]. Addressing and complying with the above requirements impose additional design considerations and costs in the development of POC devices.

1.5.5 Economic Evidence, End Users' Perspective, and Reimbursement Policy

The rate of success associated with the translation of a technology into a commercial POC device does not always correlate strongly with the level of its novelty and technical capability. Many breakthrough POC devices have failed along the commercialization pipeline as many other factors play a role in its commercial and clinical viability [127], the most obvious being the economic feasibility, the existence of competing technology, and the benefits to and the embrace of the POC device by end users. A rigorous cost vs. benefit analysis is, therefore, a useful and often prudent in the assessment of a technology for its commercial viability and certainly expected by investors in startup ventures.

Extensive consultation with potential end users forms a critical part of this exercise to identify and address potential hurdles in the uptake of the technology. For example, the technical benefits of a device may be immediately obvious to users and practitioners but may not always be appreciated by the administrators responsible for procuring instrumentation in the case of organizational equipment acquisition. Testing requirements can also play a significant factor in these decisions as many organizations intentionally limit their acquisitions to POCT programs that have waived testing requirements. There can also be considerable inertia to embracing new and unfamiliar technology, particularly if there has been a considerable investment in existing equipment to carry out similar tasks. Complex instrumentation involving multiple cartridges and multiplex operations require extensive and costly training as well as competency assessment, which neither practitioners nor healthcare organizations may be able to afford or are willing to undertake.

Another overlooked factor is the role of the health insurance industry [128]. The potential market size of a POC device or test is critically dependent on its affordability, which, in turn, can be influenced by the reimbursement covered by health insurance policies for the test or equipment. Consultation and involvement of the health insurance industry are therefore crucial in the early stages of commercial POC development.

1.6 Conclusions and Prospects

The tremendous advances made in POC technologies to date and the trend toward smart POC technologies equipped with mH capabilities are paving the way to next-generation healthcare monitoring and management. The recent years have witnessed many smart applications for personalized mH, which collect the general healthcare parameters of the subjects via Bluetooth and synchronize the data in the device to the web portal via wireless connectivity and Cloud computing. Moreover, several healthcare frameworks such as iHealth Pro have further enabled the doctors and healthcare providers to keep track of their patients in real time. It links the direct communication between the doctors and the patients, thereby enabling the effective monitoring and management of the patients. The upcoming digital health revolution would empower the general population to manage and keep track of their health effective. The most prospective POC technologies for personalized digital health would be based on SP thanks to their tremendous outreach, advanced features, continuously increasing specifications, connectivity, and affordability. SP would play an instrumental role in healthcare as they are equipped with all the desired features for mH and telemedicine. Several LOC and paper-based assays would also be transduced successfully to SP, which has already been the trend during the last few years. However, the central laboratory-based POC technologies and instruments would also be equally relevant for POCT in hospitals. A wide range of novel assay formats and developments in complementary technologies would drive the future developments in POC technologies together with the increasing number of POC tests for future target analytes. These developments would drastically reduce the healthcare costs and lead to improved health outcomes in addition to counteracting the pending challenges in POCT. The next few years would witness the digital health revolution, which would change the landscape of healthcare and would lead to critically improved next-generation healthcare monitoring and management.

References

1. Kost GJ. Guidelines for point-of-care testing. Improving patient outcomes. Am J Clin Pathol. 1995;104(4 Suppl 1):S111–27.
2. Yager P, Domingo GJ, Gerdes J. Point-of-care diagnostics for global health. Annu Rev Biomed Eng. 2008;10:107–44.
3. Gubala V, Harris LF, Ricco AJ, Tan MX, Williams DE. Point of care diagnostics: status and future. Anal Chem. 2012;84(2):487–515.
4. Luppa PB, Müller C, Schlichtiger A, Schlebusch H. Point-of-care testing (POCT): current techniques and future perspectives. Trends Anal Chem. 2011;30(6):887–98.
5. Point-of-Care Diagnostics Market. https://www.marketsandmarkets.com/Market-Reports/point-of-care-diagnostic-market-106829185.html. Accessed 30 Dec 2017.
6. Blood glucose monitoring devices (Meters, test strips, lancets) - Global pipeline analysis, competitive landscape and market forecasts to 2017. https://www.businesswire.com/news/home/20120111006216/en/Research-Markets-Blood-Glucose-Test-Strips-Market#.Vdw5LPTIDCs. Accessed 30 Dec 2017.
7. Vashist SK, Luppa PB, Yeo LY, Ozcan A, Luong JHT. Emerging technologies for next-generation point-of-care testing. Trends Biotechnol. 2015;33(11):692–705.
8. International Diabetes Federation (IDF). Diabetes atlas. 8th ed. http://www.diabetesatlas.org/across-the-globe.html. Accessed 30 Dec 2017.
9. Wild SH, Roglic G, Green A, Sicree R, King H. Global prevalence of diabetes: estimates for the year 2000 and projections for 2030: response to Rathman and Giani. Diabetes Care. 2004;27(10):2568–9.
10. Sexually Transmitted Infections (STIs). http://www.who.int/mediacentre/factsheets/fs110/en/. Accessed 30 Dec 2017.
11. Cardiovascular diseases (CVDs). http://www.who.int/mediacentre/factsheets/fs317/en/. Accessed 30 Dec 2017.
12. Tuberculosis. http://www.who.int/mediacentre/factsheets/fs104/en/. Accessed 30 Dec 2017.
13. Cancer. http://www.who.int/mediacentre/factsheets/fs297/en/. Accessed 30 Dec 2017.
14. Malaria. http://www.who.int/mediacentre/factsheets/fs094/en/. Accessed 30 Dec 2017.
15. Depression. http://www.who.int/mediacentre/factsheets/fs369/en/. Accessed 30 Dec 2017.
16. Vashist SK. Non-invasive glucose monitoring technology in diabetes management: a review. Anal Chim Acta. 2012;750:16–27.
17. Vashist SK. Continuous glucose monitoring systems: a review. Diagnostics. 2013;3(4):385–412.
18. Vashist SK, Luong JHT. Point-of-care glucose detection for diabetic monitoring and management. Boca Raton: CRC Press; 2017.

19. Vashist SK, Zheng D, Al-Rubeaan K, Luong JHT, Sheu FS. Technology behind commercial devices for blood glucose monitoring in diabetes management: a review. Anal Chim Acta. 2011;703(2):124–36.
20. Owen N, Sparling PB, Healy GN, Dunstan DW, Matthews CE, editors. Sedentary behavior: emerging evidence for a new health risk. Mayo Clin Proc. 2010;85(12):1138–41.
21. Owen N, Healy GN, Matthews CE, Dunstan DW. Too much sitting: the population health science of sedentary behavior. Exerc Sport Sci Rev. 2010;38(3):105–13.
22. Vashist SK. Too much sitting: a potential health hazard and a global call to action. Aust J Basic Appl Sci. 2015;11:131–5.
23. Brownstein JS, Freifeld CC, Madoff LC. Digital disease detection—harnessing the web for public health surveillance. N Engl J Med. 2009;360(21):2153–7.
24. Ostroff SM, Griffin PM, Tauxe RV, Shipman LD, Greene KD, Wells JG, et al. A statewide outbreak of *Escherichia coli* O157: H7 infections in Washington state. Am J Epidemiol. 1990;132(2):239–47.
25. Davis B, Brogan R. A widespread community outbreak of *E coli* O157 infection in Scotland. Public Health. 1995;109(5):381–8.
26. Arnon SS, Schechter R, Inglesby TV, Henderson DA, Bartlett JG, Ascher MS, et al. Botulinum toxin as a biological weapon: medical and public health management. JAMA. 2001;285(8):1059–70.
27. Wein LM, Liu Y. Analyzing a bioterror attack on the food supply: the case of botulinum toxin in milk. Proc Natl Acad Sci. 2005;102(28):9984–9.
28. Hennessy TW, Hedberg CW, Slutsker L, White KE, Besser-Wiek JM, Moen ME, et al. A national outbreak of *Salmonella enteritidis* infections from ice cream. The investigation team. N Engl J Med. 1996;334(20):1281–6.
29. De Buyser ML, Dufour B, Maire M, Lafarge V. Implication of milk and milk products in food-borne diseases in France and in different industrialised countries. Int J Food Microbiol. 2001;67(1–2):1–17.
30. Zhao C, Ge B, De Villena J, Sudler R, Yeh E, Zhao S, et al. Prevalence of campylobacter spp., *Escherichia coli*, and *Salmonella serovars* in retail chicken, turkey, pork, and beef from the greater Washington, DC, area. Appl Environ Microbiol. 2001;67(12):5431–6.
31. Taylor SL, Nordlee JA, Niemann LM, Lambrecht DM. Allergen immunoassays—considerations for use of naturally incurred standards. Anal Bioanal Chem. 2009;395(1):83–92.
32. Tucker JD, Bien CH, Peeling RW. Point-of-care testing for sexually transmitted infections: recent advances and implications for disease control. Curr Opin Infect Dis. 2013;26(1):73–9.
33. Global estimates by WHO region. http://www.who.int/hiv/data/epi_plhiv_2016_regions. png?ua=1. Accessed 30 Dec 2017.
34. Boonlert W, Lolekha PH, Kost GJ, Lolekha S. Comparison of the performance of point-of-care and device analyzers to hospital laboratory instruments. Point of Care. 2003;2(3):172–8.
35. Kost GJ, Vu HT, Lee JH, Bourgeois P, Kiechle FL, Martin C, et al. Multicenter study of oxygen-insensitive handheld glucose point-of-care testing in critical care/hospital/ambulatory patients in the United States and Canada. Crit Care Med. 1998;26(3):581–90.
36. Young DS. Effects of drugs on clinical laboratory tests. Ann Clin Biochem. 1997;34(6):579–81.
37. FreeStyle Libre. https://www.freestylelibre.co.uk/libre/. Accessed 30 Dec 2017.
38. Continuous Glucose Monitoring (CGM): Technologies and Global Markets. https://www.bccresearch.com/market-research/healthcare/continuous-glucose-monitoring-cgm-technology-markets-report-hlc102b.html?utm_source=hs_email&utm_medium=email&utm_content=15754702&_hsenc=p2ANqtz-91CFptaehTf6Rxg-Jo3B2Tn9ZAE0_vGdJE8768hWOwA6YJiIhKHcHW5me__5CSA7gH1rbKhSV t2J_SudLnPgmLXeAZsYSjaYhan35UuWEqK1c4gCU8&_hsmi=15754702. Accessed 30 Dec 2017.
39. Kost GJ, Tran NK. Point-of-care testing and cardiac biomarkers: the standard of care and vision for chest pain centers. Cardiol Clin. 2005;23(4):467–90.. vi

40. Floriano PN, Christodoulides N, Miller CS, Ebersole JL, Spertus J, Rose BG, et al. Use of saliva-based nano-biochip tests for acute myocardial infarction at the point of care: a feasibility study. Clin Chem. 2009;55(8):1530–8.
41. Jaffe AS, Babuin L, Apple FS. Biomarkers in acute cardiac disease: the present and the future. J Am Coll Cardiol. 2006;48(1):1–11.
42. Cobas b221 Blood Gas System. https://usdiagnostics.roche.com/en/point-of-care-testing/poc-testing/blood-gas-and-electrolytes/cobas-b221.html. Accessed 30 Dec 2017.
43. Cobas u441 Analyzer. https://usdiagnostics.roche.com/en/core_laboratory/instrument/cobas-u-411-analyzer.html. Accessed 30 Dec 2017.
44. Cobas Liat PCR System. https://usdiagnostics.roche.com/en/point-of-care-testing/poc-testing/infectious-disease/cobas-liat-pcr-system.html. Accessed 30 Dec 2017.
45. CoaguChek XS System. http://www.coaguchek-usa.com/coaguchek_hcp/en_US/home/coaguchek-products/coaguchek-xs-system.html. Accessed 30 Dec 2017.
46. Accutrend Plus System. https://usdiagnostics.roche.com/en/point-of-care-testing/poc-testing/cholesterol/accutrend-plus.html. Accessed 30 Dec 2017.
47. Siemens Healthcare GmbH. Point-of-Care Testing. https://www.healthcare.siemens.com/point-of-care-testing. Accessed 30 Dec 2017.
48. i-STAT Handheld. https://www.pointofcare.abbott/us/en/offerings/istat/istat-handheld. Accessed 30 Dec 2017.
49. Vashist SK, Schneider EM, Luong JHT. Commercial smartphone-based devices and smart applications for personalized healthcare monitoring and management. Diagnostics. 2014;4(3):104–28.
50. Vashist SK, Mudanyali O, Schneider EM, Zengerle R, Ozcan A. Cellphone-based devices for bioanalytical sciences. Anal Bioanal Chem. 2014;406(14):3263–77.
51. Ozcan A. Mobile phones democratize and cultivate next-generation imaging, diagnostics and measurement tools. Lab Chip. 2014;14(17):3187–94.
52. Vashist SK, Luong JHT. Handbook of immunoassay technologies: approaches, performances, and applications. 1st ed. Cambridge, MA: Academic Press; 2018.
53. Vashist SK, Marion Schneider E, Zengerle R, von Stetten F, Luong JHT. Graphene-based rapid and highly-sensitive immunoassay for C-reactive protein using a smartphone-based colorimetric reader. Biosens Bioelectron. 2015;66(0):169–76.
54. Vashist SK, van Oordt T, Schneider EM, Zengerle R, von Stetten F, Luong JHT. A smartphone-based colorimetric reader for bioanalytical applications using the screen-based bottom illumination provided by gadgets. Biosens Bioelectron. 2015;67:248–55.
55. Coskun AF, Wong J, Khodadadi D, Nagi R, Tey A, Ozcan A. A personalized food allergen testing platform on a cellphone. Lab Chip. 2013;13(4):636–40.
56. Wei Q, Nagi R, Sadeghi K, Feng S, Yan E, Ki SJ, et al. Detection and spatial mapping of mercury contamination in water samples using a smart-phone. ACS Nano. 2014;8(2):1121–9.
57. Rajendran VK, Bakthavathsalam P, Ali BMJ. Smartphone based bacterial detection using biofunctionalized fluorescent nanoparticles. Microchim Acta. 2014;181(15–16):1815–21.
58. Walker FM, Ahmad KM, Eisenstein M, Soh HT. Transformation of personal computers and mobile phones into genetic diagnostic systems. Anal Chem. 2014;86(18):9236–41.
59. Zangheri M, Cevenini L, Anfossi L, Baggiani C, Simoni P, Di Nardo F, et al. A simple and compact smartphone accessory for quantitative chemiluminescence-based lateral flow immunoassay for salivary cortisol detection. Biosens Bioelectron. 2015;64:63–8.
60. Roda A, Michelini E, Cevenini L, Calabria D, Calabretta MM, Simoni P. Integrating biochemiluminescence detection on smartphones: mobile chemistry platform for point-of-need analysis. Anal Chem. 2014;86(15):7299–304.
61. Petryayeva E, Algar WR. Multiplexed homogeneous assays of proteolytic activity using a smartphone and quantum dots. Anal Chem. 2014;86(6):3195–202.
62. Preechaburana P, Gonzalez MC, Suska A, Filippini D. Surface plasmon resonance chemical sensing on cell phones. Angew Chem Int Ed Eng. 2012;51(46):11585–8.

63. Coskun AF, Cetin AE, Galarreta BC, Alvarez DA, Altug H, Ozcan A. Lensfree optofluidic plasmonic sensor for real-time and label-free monitoring of molecular binding events over a wide field-of-view. Sci Rep. 2014;4:6789.
64. Lillehoj PB, Huang MC, Truong N, Ho CM. Rapid electrochemical detection on a mobile phone. Lab Chip. 2013;13(15):2950–5.
65. Wang X, Gartia MR, Jiang J, Chang T-W, Qian J, Liu Y, et al. Audio jack based miniaturized mobile phone electrochemical sensing platform. Sensors Actuators B Chem. 2015;209:677–85.
66. Sun A, Wambach T, Venkatesh A, Hall DA, editors. A multitechnique reconfigurable electrochemical biosensor for integration into mobile technologies. Biomedical Circuits and Systems Conference (BioCAS), 2015 IEEE; DOI: 10.1109/BioCAS.2015.7348314.
67. Sun AC, Yao C, Venkatesh AG, Hall DA. An efficient power harvesting Mobile phone-based electrochemical biosensor for point-of-care health monitoring. Sensors Actuators B: Chemical. 2016;235:126–35.
68. Sun A, Wambach T, Venkatesh A, Hall DA, editors. A low-cost smartphone-based electrochemical biosensor for point-of-care diagnostics. Biomedical Circuits and Systems Conference (BioCAS), 2014 IEEE; DOI: 10.1109/BioCAS.2014.6981725.
69. You DJ, San Park T, Yoon J-Y. Cell-phone-based measurement of TSH using Mie scatter optimized lateral flow assays. Biosens Bioelectron. 2013;40(1):180–5.
70. Mudanyali O, Dimitrov S, Sikora U, Padmanabhan S, Navruz I, Ozcan A. Integrated rapid-diagnostic-test reader platform on a cellphone. Lab Chip. 2012;12(15):2678–86.
71. iHealth Align. https://ihealthlabs.com/glucometer/ihealth-align/. Accessed 30 Dec 2017.
72. Zhu H, Mavandadi S, Coskun AF, Yaglidere O, Ozcan A. Optofluidic fluorescent imaging cytometry on a cell phone. Anal Chem. 2011;83(17):6641–7.
73. Smith ZJ, Chu K, Espenson AR, Rahimzadeh M, Gryshuk A, Molinaro M, et al. Cell-phone-based platform for biomedical device development and education applications. PLoS One. 2011;6(3):e17150.
74. Breslauer DN, Maamari RN, Switz NA, Lam WA, Fletcher DA. Mobile phone based clinical microscopy for global health applications. PLoS One. 2009;4(7):e6320.
75. Zhu H, Yaglidere O, Su TW, Tseng D, Ozcan A. Cost-effective and compact wide-field fluorescent imaging on a cell-phone. Lab Chip. 2011;11(2):315–22.
76. Tseng D, Mudanyali O, Oztoprak C, Isikman SO, Sencan I, Yaglidere O, et al. Lensfree microscopy on a cellphone. Lab Chip. 2010;10(14):1787–92.
77. Wei Q, Qi H, Luo W, Tseng D, Ki SJ, Wan Z, et al. Fluorescent imaging of single nanoparticles and viruses on a smart phone. ACS Nano. 2013;7(10):9147–55.
78. Laksanasopin T, Guo TW, Nayak S, Sridhara AA, Xie S, Olowookere OO, et al. A smartphone dongle for diagnosis of infectious diseases at the point of care. Sci Transl Med. 2015;7(273):273re1-re1.
79. Yu H, Tan Y, Cunningham BT. Smartphone fluorescence spectroscopy. Anal Chem. 2014;86(17):8805–13.
80. Mao X, Huang TJ. Microfluidic diagnostics for the developing world. Lab Chip. 2012;12(8):1412–6.
81. Li X, Ballerini DR, Shen W. A perspective on paper-based microfluidics: current status and future trends. Biomicrofluidics. 2012;6(1):11301–1130113.
82. Hu J, Wang S, Wang L, Li F, Pingguan-Murphy B, Lu TJ, et al. Advances in paper-based point-of-care diagnostics. Biosens Bioelectron. 2014;54:585–97.
83. Pelton R. Bioactive paper provides a low-cost platform for diagnostics. Trends Anal Chem. 2009;28(8):925–42.
84. Fernandez-Sanchez C, McNeil CJ, Rawson K, Nilsson O, Leung HY, Gnanapragasam V. One-step immunostrip test for the simultaneous detection of free and total prostate specific antigen in serum. J Immunol Methods. 2005;307(1–2):1–12.
85. Dineva MA, Candotti D, Fletcher-Brown F, Allain JP, Lee H. Simultaneous visual detection of multiple viral amplicons by dipstick assay. J Clin Microbiol. 2005;43(8):4015–21.

86. Posthuma-Trumpie GA, Korf J, van Amerongen A. Lateral flow (immuno)assay: its strengths, weaknesses, opportunities and threats. A literature survey. Anal Bioanal Chem. 2009;393(2):569–82.

87. Yang Q, Gong X, Song T, Yang J, Zhu S, Li Y, et al. Quantum dot-based immunochromatography test strip for rapid, quantitative and sensitive detection of alpha fetoprotein. Biosens Bioelectron. 2011;30(1):145–50.

88. van den Berk GE, Frissen PH, Regez RM, Rietra PJ. Evaluation of the rapid immunoassay determine HIV 1/2 for detection of antibodies to human immunodeficiency virus types 1 and 2. J Clin Microbiol. 2003;41(8):3868–9.

89. Mao X, Ma Y, Zhang A, Zhang L, Zeng L, Liu G. Disposable nucleic acid biosensors based on gold nanoparticle probes and lateral flow strip. Anal Chem. 2009;81(4):1660–8.

90. Nilghaz A, Wicaksono DH, Gustiono D, Majid FAA, Supriyanto E, Kadir MRA. Flexible microfluidic cloth-based analytical devices using a low-cost wax patterning technique. Lab Chip. 2012;12(1):209–18.

91. Martinez AW, Phillips ST, Whitesides GM, Carrilho E. Diagnostics for the developing world: microfluidic paper-based analytical devices. Anal Chem. 2009;82(1):3–10.

92. Martinez AW, Phillips ST, Whitesides GM. Three-dimensional microfluidic devices fabricated in layered paper and tape. Proc Natl Acad Sci. 2008;105(50):19606–11.

93. Cheng CM, Martinez AW, Gong J, Mace CR, Phillips ST, Carrilho E, et al. Paper-based ELISA. Angew Chem Int Ed Eng. 2010;49(28):4771–4.

94. Apilux A, Ukita Y, Chikae M, Chailapakul O, Takamura Y. Development of automated paper-based devices for sequential multistep sandwich enzyme-linked immunosorbent assays using inkjet printing. Lab Chip. 2013;13(1):126–35.

95. Nie Z, Deiss F, Liu X, Akbulut O, Whitesides GM. Integration of paper-based microfluidic devices with commercial electrochemical readers. Lab Chip. 2010;10(22):3163–9.

96. Lu J, Ge S, Ge L, Yan M, Yu J. Electrochemical DNA sensor based on three-dimensional folding paper device for specific and sensitive point-of-care testing. Electrochim Acta. 2012;80:334–41.

97. Parolo C, de la Escosura-Muniz A, Merkoci A. Enhanced lateral flow immunoassay using gold nanoparticles loaded with enzymes. Biosens Bioelectron. 2013;40(1):412–6.

98. Hu J, Wang L, Li F, Han YL, Lin M, Lu TJ, et al. Oligonucleotide-linked gold nanoparticle aggregates for enhanced sensitivity in lateral flow assays. Lab Chip. 2013;13(22):4352–7.

99. Vella SJ, Beattie P, Cademartiri R, Laromaine A, Martinez AW, Phillips ST, et al. Measuring markers of liver function using a micropatterned paper device designed for blood from a fingerstick. Anal Chem. 2012;84(6):2883–91.

100. Pollock NR, Rolland JP, Kumar S, Beattie PD, Jain S, Noubary F, et al. A paper-based multiplexed transaminase test for low-cost, point-of-care liver function testing. Sci Transl Med. 2012;4(152):152ra29.

101. Yang X, Forouzan O, Brown TP, Shevkoplyas SS. Integrated separation of blood plasma from whole blood for microfluidic paper-based analytical devices. Lab Chip. 2012;12(2):274–80.

102. Ge C, Yu L, Fang Z, Zeng L. An enhanced strip biosensor for rapid and sensitive detection of histone methylation. Anal Chem. 2013;85(19):9343–9.

103. Nie Z, Nijhuis CA, Gong J, Chen X, Kumachev A, Martinez AW, et al. Electrochemical sensing in paper-based microfluidic devices. Lab Chip. 2010;10(4):477–83.

104. Turner AP. Biosensors: sense and sensibility. Chem Soc Rev. 2013;42(8):3184–96.

105. Piccolo Xpress. http://www.abaxis.com/medical/piccolo-xpress. Accessed 30 Dec 2017.

106. https://www.gyrosproteintechnologies.com/gyrolab-immunoassay-products. Accessed 30 Dec 2017.

107. Gorkin R, Park J, Siegrist J, Amasia M, Lee BS, Park JM, et al. Centrifugal microfluidics for biomedical applications. Lab Chip. 2010;10(14):1758–73.

108. Beaudet L, Rodriguez-Suarez R, Venne M-H, Caron M, Bédard J, Brechler V, et al. AlphaLISA immunoassays: the no-wash alternative to ELISAs for research and drug discovery. Nat Methods. 2008;5(12).

109. Kai J, Puntambekar A, Santiago N, Lee SH, Sehy DW, Moore V, et al. A novel microfluidic microplate as the next generation assay platform for enzyme linked immunoassays (ELISA). Lab Chip. 2012;12(21):4257–62.
110. MSD Technology Platform. https://www.mesoscale.com/~/media/files/brochures/techbrochure.pdf. Accessed 30 Dec 2017.
111. Vashist SK, Czilwik G, Venkatesh AG. Elisa system and related methods. WIPO Patent Pub No WO/2014/198836.
112. Vashist SK, Czilwik G, van Oordt T, von Stetten F, Zengerle R, Marion Schneider E, et al. One-step kinetics-based immunoassay for the highly sensitive detection of C-reactive protein in less than 30min. Anal Biochem. 2014;456:32–7.
113. Then WL, Garnier G. Paper diagnostics in biomedicine. Rev Anal Chem. 2013;32(4):269–94.
114. Jahanshahi-Anbuhi S, Pennings K, Leung V, Liu M, Carrasquilla C, Kannan B, et al. Pullulan encapsulation of labile biomolecules to give stable bioassay tablets. Angew Chem Int Ed Eng. 2014;53(24):6155–8.
115. Ramachandran S, Fu E, Lutz B, Yager P. Long-term dry storage of an enzyme-based reagent system for ELISA in point-of-care devices. Analyst. 2014;139(6):1456–62.
116. Dawson EC, Homan JD, Van Weemen BK. Stabilization of peroxidase. US Patent 4331761.
117. Bioanalytical Method Validation. https://www.fda.gov/downloads/drugs/guidances/ucm368107.pdf. Accessed 30 Dec 2017.
118. Guideline on Bioanalytical Method Validation. http://www.ema.europa.eu/docs/en_GB/document_library/Scientific_guideline/2011/08/WC500109686.pdf. Accessed 30 Dec 2017.
119. Abe K, Kotera K, Suzuki K, Citterio D. Inkjet-printed paperfluidic immuno-chemical sensing device. Anal Bioanal Chem. 2010;398(2):885–93.
120. Li CZ, Vandenberg K, Prabhulkar S, Zhu X, Schneper L, Methee K, et al. Paper based point-of-care testing disc for multiplex whole cell bacteria analysis. Biosens Bioelectron. 2011;26(11):4342–8.
121. Vashist SK, Venkatesh A, Mitsakakis K, Czilwik G, Roth G, von Stetten F, et al. Nanotechnology-based biosensors and diagnostics: technology push versus industrial/healthcare requirements. Bionanoscience. 2012;2(3):115–26.
122. Sharifi S, Behzadi S, Laurent S, Forrest ML, Stroeve P, Mahmoudi M. Toxicity of nanomaterials. Chem Soc Rev. 2012;41(6):2323–43.
123. Pearson S, Benameur A, editors. Privacy, security and trust issues arising from cloud computing. IEEE Sec Int Conf Cloud Comput Technol Sci (CloudCom). 2010;2010:693–702. https://doi.org/10.1109/CloudCom.2010.66.
124. Subashini S, Kavitha V. A survey on security issues in service delivery models of cloud computing. JNCA. 2011;34(1):1–11.
125. Chen D, Zhao H, editors. Data security and privacy protection issues in cloud computing. Int Conf Comp Sci Electron Eng. 2012;2012:647–51. https://doi.org/10.1109/ICCSEE.2012.193.
126. Yu S, Wang C, Ren K, Lou W, editors. Achieving secure, scalable, and fine-grained data access control in cloud computing. Proc IEEE Infocom. 2010;2010:1–9. https://doi.org/10.1109/INFCOM.2010.5462174.
127. Junker R, Schlebusch H, Luppa PB. Point-of-care testing in hospitals and primary care. Dtsch Arztebl Int. 2010;107(33):561–7.
128. Weisbrod BA. The health care quadrilemma: an essay on technological change, insurance, quality of care, and cost containment. J Econ Lit. 1991;29(2):523–52.

Chapter 2
Smartphone-Based Point-of-Care Technologies for Mobile Healthcare

Sandeep Kumar Vashist and John H. T. Luong

Contents

2.1 Introduction

Smartphones (SPs) have become a communication tool of 6.8 billion cell phone subscribers or 94% of the world population [1] with over 70% from developing countries. The current generation of SPs is equipped with advanced processors, increased memory, high-resolution camera, high-end security via fingerprinting, numerous smart applications, and a variety of built-in sensors. Therefore, SPs have been transformed into a prospective personalized IVD system to deliver mobile healthcare (mH) to remote, resource-deficient, private, and public settings [2–4]. Individuals can perform several important diagnostics at their personalized settings and receive the real-time feedback from healthcare professionals. SP-IVD data are tagged with spatiotemporal information to greatly facilitate the monitoring and management of epidemics and emergency scenarios [5]. Significant advances have

© Springer Nature Switzerland AG 2019
S. K. Vashist, J. H. T. Luong, *Point-of-Care Technologies Enabling
Next-Generation Healthcare Monitoring and Management*,
https://doi.org/10.1007/978-3-030-11416-9_2

been made to improve signal response, robustness, and cost-effectiveness, while considerable efforts are well underway to reshape the landscape of healthcare and bioanalytical sciences [6].

There are substantial efforts in the development of SP-IVD based on lateral flow assays (LFA) [7–11], microscopy [12–16], electrochemical sensing [17–20], immunoassays (IA) [21–24], surface plasmon resonance-based biosensing [25, 26], flow cytometry [14, 27], and optical detection [28–31]. Several companies have emerged, and most of the healthcare and diagnostic giants and SP manufacturers are also participating in this competitive and emerging field [32]. Consequently, numerous SP-based devices for general healthcare and fitness are commercially available from iHealth, AliveCor, GENTAG, Mobile Assay, CellScope, Holomic, Runtastic, Nonin, etc., which are being used by millions of customers worldwide [33]. The current trends indicate the forthcoming SP-based mH era will revolutionize personalized healthcare monitoring and management via highly efficient and cost-effective SP-IVDs. This chapter provides a critical overview of SP-IVD together with the technical challenges, the trends, and future possibilities for the next generation of personalized mH devices.

2.2   Smartphone-Based Point-of-Care Technologies for Mobile Healthcare

The SP's high-resolution rear camera, ranging from a few megapixels (MP) to 41 MP, can be transformed into a potential POC reader to detect colorimetric, fluorescence, luminescence, SPR, and other optical signals. The last decade has witnessed the emergence of numerous low-cost and compact SP-based readers that could be deployed at POC settings for several bioanalytical applications.

2.2.1   Colorimetric Detection

Colorimetric detection-based SP-IVD uses an optically opaque attachment, consisting of light-emitting diodes (LEDs) and diffusers for uniform illumination, apertures for the desired imaging field of view (FOV), and a sample chamber [22, 34]. The FOV is enhanced by placing a plano-convex lens in front of the camera [34]. Table 2.1 provides a summary of SP-based POC colorimetric detection of various analytes.

The CP-based colorimetric imaging was pioneered for quantitative analysis of high-sensitivity C-reactive protein (hsCRP) [24], where the colorimetric product obtained in the sandwich enzyme-linked immunosorbent assay (ELISA) after the enzyme-substrate reaction in a 96-well microtiter plate (MTP) was imaged by the CP. The procedure simply placed an MTP on a white paper and the use of a desk lamp with a 40 W bulb inclined at an angle of 50° to the benchtop surface. The white paper provides a uniform white background, the bulb reduces the shadowing effects, and the CP placed at ~12 cm above the MTP captures the colorimetric images of 96-well MTP. Custom

Table 2.1 SP-based POC colorimetric detection

Analytes detected	Bioanalytical application	Refs.
Peanut	Detects 1–25 ppm of peanut within 20 min using a commercial food allergy test kit and an SP testing platform	[22]
25-Hydroxyvitamin D	AuNP-based IA detects 25-hydroxyvitamin D [15–110 nM]	[41]
CRP	Detects CRP [0.035–0.182 µg/mL] with a LOD of 0.026 µg/mL using a conventional sandwich IA	[24]
CRP	Detects CRP [0.3–81 ng/mL] with a LOD of 0.4 ng/mL using a rapid one-step kinetics-based IA	[30]
CRP	Graphene nanoplatelet-based signal-enhanced rapid IA detects CRP [0.03–81 ng/mL] with a LOD of 0.07 ng/mL using a rapid one-step kinetics-based IA	[29]
Cholesterol	Detects total cholesterol level in blood in the relevant physiological range of 140–400 mg/dL within 60 s using standard test strip-based assay	[31]
Proteases	A QD-based multiplex assay for the activity of trypsin, chymotrypsin, and enterokinase [pM–nM]	[42]
Cocaine	AuNP and aptamer-based assay for cocaine [0.2–0.8 mg/mL]	[43]
HE4	Microchip ELISA for HE4 in urine with the linearity of 19.5–1250 ng/mL and a LOD of 19.5 ng mL^{-1}	[37]
Hg	Plasmonic AuNP and aptamer-based assay for Hg^{2+} with a LOD of ~3.5 ppb	[34]
Hg(II)	Colorimetric sensory polymer membrane detects Hg(II) in aqueous media with sensitivity in the range of mM–nM with a response time of less than 25 min	[44]
Hg^{2+}	An aptamer-based biosensor detects Hg^{2+} in the linear detection range of 1–32 ng/mL in 20 min	[45]
Chlorine	Detects 0.02–2.0 ppm of chlorine in water based on its chemical reaction with an o-tolidine solution	[46]
Chlorine	Detects 0.3–1.0 ppm of chlorine in water using a chemical reaction between potassium-starch solution and chlorine	[47]
BDE-47	Detects BDE-47 [10^{-3}–10^4 µg/L] by microfluidic ELISA	[48]
Explosives (TATP, HMTD, 4A2NP, NB, PA)	Detects explosives as low as 0.2 µg using a disposable paper array and chemometric approach	[49]
Human IgG	AuNP-labeled microfluidic IA for the detection of human IgG	[21]
pH	Detection of pH in sweat and saliva	[50]
pH	Detects pH using a novel calibration technique that enables accurate measurements under varying ambient conditions	[28]
Cocaine	Detects 1 mg/mL cocaine using an aptamer-AuNP conjugate-based assay	[43]
Multiple analytes (ascorbic acid, leucocyte, glucose, protein, ketones, urobilinogen, bilirubin, RBC)	Developed an SP application for the colorimetric readout of multi-analyte paper-based sensing arrays	[51]

(continued)

Table 2.1 (continued)

Analytes detected	Bioanalytical application	Refs.
KSHV nucleic acid	Detection of KHSV nucleic acids down to 1 nM using a microfluidic cartridge-based colorimetric nanoparticle assay	[52]
KSHV and Bartonella DNA	Multiplex detection of KSHV and Bartonella DNA with sensitivity [1–20 nM] using AuNP- and AgNP-based aggregation reactions with a multicolor-change system	[53]
K	Measurement of the K concentration [0.31 μM–0.1 M] with a LOD of 0.31 μM	[54]
Cr	DMSA-functionalized AuNPs for the detection of Cr^{3+} and $Cr_2O_7^{2-}$ in soil with linearity in the range of 10–500 nM	[55]
Fe^{2+} and Cu^{2+}	A paper-based microfluidic IA detects Fe^{2+} and Cu^{2+} in the linear detection range of 100–400 μg/mL	[56]
BCA and CCK8	Conventional BCA protein assay and cell counting kit (CCK8) assay with high precision and sensitivity	[57]
Organophosphate pesticides	A paper-based analytical device detects the presence of organophosphate pesticides based on the inhibition of immobilized acetylcholinesterase	[39]
Tetracycline	Detects tetracycline in bovine milk [0.5–10 μg/mL] with LOD and LOQ of 0.5 μg/mL and 1.5 μg/mL, respectively	[58]
UDG	Detects UDG [0.008–0.2 U/mL] with a LOD of 0.008 U/mL based on the target-triggered formation of the G-quadruplex	[59]
Glucose and protein	Paper-based microfluidic assays detect glucose and protein in artificial urine samples	[60]
CD4 cells	Micro-a-fluidic ELISA determines rapid CD4 cell count at POC settings in fully automated fashion	[61]
Cu(II), Ni(II), Cd(II), Cr(VI)	3D paper-based microfluidic assay detects Cu(II), Ni(II), Cd(II), Cr(VI) with LODs of 0.29 ppm, 0.33 ppm, 0.19 ppm, and 0.35 ppm, respectively	[62]
pH, protein, and glucose	SP application algorithm with interphone repeatability was used for the detection of pH, protein, and glucose with linearity of 5.0–9.0, 0–100 mg/dL, and 0–300 mg/dL, respectively	[63]
HIV antibody, *Treponema* antibody, and non-*Treponema* antibody	Lab-on-a-chip-based microfluidic IA detects HIV antibody, *Treponema* antibody for syphilis, and non-*Treponema* antibody for active syphilis infection with good sensitivity and specificity in less than 15 min	[64]
Human IgG	AuNP-labeled microfluidic IA detects human IgG in the concentration range of ng/mL with a good correlation with conventional IA	[21]
Mumps IgG, Measles IgG, and HSV IgGs (HSV-1 and HSV-2)	SP detection-based conventional IAs detected Mumps IgG, Measles IgG, and HSV IgGs (HSV-1 and HSV-2) with accuracies of 99.6%, 98.6%, 99.4%, and 99.4%, respectively	[40]

(continued)

Table 2.1 (continued)

Analytes detected	Bioanalytical application	Refs.
Soil color	An Android SP application for the detection of the soil color under controlled illumination	[65]
Phosphorous in soil	A standard assay for the available phosphorous content in soil [0.0–1.0 mg/pL] with a LOD of 0.01 mg/pL	[66]
Chlorophyll content of corn leaves	An Android application was used to determine the chlorophyll content of corn leaves by direct contact imaging via SP back camera	[67]
Rice leaf color	An Android application was employed to determine the rice leaf color level, which enabled the estimation of the needed amount of nitrogen fertilizer	[68]
BChE	Detects BChE with accuracy equivalent to standard Ellman's assay using paper strips soaked with indoxylacetate	[69]
Glucose and BUN	Determines glucose and BUN using Vitros® glucose and BUN colorimetric assays with results in agreement with clinical chemistry gold standard assay	[70]
Dengue antibody IgG	Determines dengue antibody IgG concentration in samples using a lab-on-a-compact disc platform with 95% sensitivity and 100% specificity	[71]
Fe	Determines the Fe content in zeolites [0–1.2% (w/w)]	[72]
Fluorine	Detects fluorine in water using zirconium-xylenol orange reagent [0–2 mg/L]	[73]
Hg^{2+}	Detected Hg^{2+} with a LOD of 80 nM using nitrogen-doped carbon nanodots	[74]
Glucose and lactate	A paper-based analytical device detects glucose and lactate, 0.3–8 mM and 0.02–0.50 mM, respectively	[75]
Creatinine	A paper-based sensor detected creatinine in the linear range of 20–140 ppm with a LOD of 8.02 ppm	[76]
STX and OA	Detects STX and OA with linearity of 0.02–0.32 ppb and 0.2–5 ppb	[77]
Gallic acid	Image-based Folin-Ciocalteu assay for the detection of gallic acid in the linear range of 0–20 mg/L	[78]
Formaldehyde	Colorimetric assay based on G-quadruplex halves of formaldehyde in the linear range of 1–600 μM	[79]
Thiram	An upconversion paper sensor detects thiram in the linear range of 0.1 μM–1 mM with a LOD of 0.1 μM	[80]
Glucose and human cTnI	Colorimetric assay detected glucose [0.8–20 mM] and human cTnI [500 ng/mL–2 μg/mL]	[81]
Dengue IgM and IgG antibodies	Multivariate image analysis-based assay on laser printed microzones discriminates infected and non-infected dengue patients based on the detection of IgM and IgG antibodies in serum	[82]
Cortisol and CRP	SP diagnostic unit detects CRP and cortisol in the range of 0–100 ng/mL	[83]

(continued)

Table 2.1 (continued)

Analytes detected	Bioanalytical application	Refs.
CRP and PCT	A biochemical-immunological hybrid biosensor based on two-dimensional chromatography detects CRP, PCT, and lactate in the dynamic ranges of 0.01–100 µg/mL, 0.01–10 ng/mL, and 9–72 mg/dL, respectively	[84]
AChE	AChE inhibitors assay involving the immobilization of AChE on commercial pH strips detects AChE inhibitors, i.e., galanthamine and donepezil with LODs of 149 nM and 22.3 nM, respectively	[85]
Aging of bloodstain	Determines the age of a bloodstain from the brightness of the image	[86]
Mycobacterium tuberculosis	A point-of-need enzyme-linked aptamer assay for *Mycobacterium tuberculosis* with a LOD of 10^4 CFU/mL within 5 h	[87]
Blood hematocrit	Determination of blood hematocrit levels from 10% to 60% with a LOD of 0.1% using a disposable microfluidic device	[88]
L-lactate	Multilayer paper reflectometry is used for the detection of L-lactate in oral fluid with a LOD of 0.1 mM	[89]
Ammonia	Localized surface plasmon resonance of AgNPs detects ammonia in the range of 10–1000 mg/L with a LOD of 200 mg/L and a response time of 20 s	[90]
OTA, AFB1, and DON	Multiplexed capillary microfluidic IA detects OTA, AFB1, and DON within 10 min with sensitivities of <40 ng/mL, 0.1–0.2 ng/mL, and <10 ng/mL, respectively	[91]
OA	Cell viability biosensor detects OA in the linear detection range of 10–800 µg/L using HepG2 cells	[92]
Streptomycin	Aptamer-conjugated AuNPs detect streptomycin with a LOD of 12.3 nM	[93]

BDE-47 2,2′,4,4′-tetrabromodiphenyl ether, *TATP* triacetone triperoxide, *HMTD* hexamethylene triperoxide diamine, *4A2NP* 4-amino-2-nitrophenol, *NB* nitrobenzene, *PA* picric acid, *KSHV* Kaposi's sarcoma-associated herpesvirus, *DMSA* meso-2,3-dimercaptosuccinic acid, *BCA* bicinchoninic acid, *UDG* uracil-DNA glycosylase, *HSV* herpes simplex virus, *BChE* butyrylcholinesterase, *BUN* blood urea nitrogen, *STX* saxitonin, *OA* okadaic acid, *cTnI* cardiac troponin I, *CRP* C-reactive protein, *PCT* procalcitonin T, *AChE* acetylcholinesterase, *OTA* ochratoxin A, *AFB1* aflatoxin B1, *DON* deoxynivalenol

MATLAB software on a PC transforms the CP-captured images from native RGB to normalized RGB color space to minimize the effects of variations in illumination intensity. Thereafter, the normalized blue channel image and 121 pixels (11×11-pixel region) from each MTP well are employed for the quantitative determination of hsCRP with a limit of detection (LOD) of 0.026 ± 0.002 µg/mL. Another demonstration of CP-based colorimetric analysis is the quantitative detection of human IgG concentrations in plasma via gold nanoparticle (AuNP)-enabled microfluidic IA [21].

A CP-based method for the POC quantitative analysis of colorimetric paper test strips, i.e., commercially available urine test strips and pH paper tests, was also demonstrated [28]. It employs the chromaticity values of CP captured images for the quantitative determination of an analyte and compensates partially the variations in ambient light.

An SP-based colorimetric reader (SBCR) was developed for the readout of immunoassays and biochemical assays. The bottom illumination of a 96-well microtiter plate (MTP) is provided by the illuminated screensaver on the gadgets' screen [30, 35] (Fig. 2.1). The SBCR comprises an SP (Samsung Galaxy SIII mini, back camera 5 MP resolution), a gadget (iPad mini, iPAD4, or iPhone 5s), and a custom-made dark hood and base holder assembly (made up of polyamide). Initially, the gadget with an illuminated screensaver is put on top of the base holder. The 96- or 24-well MTP is then positioned on the gadget's screensaver, which provides white light-based bottom illumination only in the MTP's wells. Thereafter, the dark hood is put on top of the base holder followed by the alignment of the SP back camera by putting the SP into the SP containment at the top of the dark hood. The containment with an aperture of 1.5 cm diameter is aligned with the SP back camera. The distance of the SP back camera from the gadget's screen is 30 cm for iPad4- and iPad mini-based SBCRs, while it is 15 cm for iPhone 5s-based SBCR. Finally, the images are captured by the SP, and their pixel intensity is determined by an image processing algorithm using image J 1.48v. The SBCR matches the superior bioanalytical performance of the commercial MTP reader for the human CRP sandwich ELISA, HRP direct ELISA, and bicinchoninic acid (BCA) protein estimation assay. The design has a particular advantage of not requiring any external power supply as the illumination and detection of the colorimetric assay solution are done by the gadget and SP, respectively, which could run on an internal battery for the desired POC applications.

A compact (22 mm × 67 mm × 75 mm) and lightweight (40 g) 3D-printed optomechanical SP attachment (termed iTube) for SP-based colorimetric readout detects varying amounts (1–25 part per million, ppm) of peanut concentrations in commercially available cookies [22] (Fig. 2.2). The developed method detects peanut concentration with a LOD of ~1 ppm in less than 20 min. The iTube is attached mechanically to the SP back camera, followed by the insertion of test and control tubes from the side. The tube cross sections (8 mm × 12 mm) are vertically illuminated by two separate but interchangeable LEDs (650 nm peak wavelength) using two diffusers between the tubes and the LEDs for uniform illumination. The transmission images through each tube via two circular apertures (1.5 mm diameter) are captured by the SP back camera (Samsung Galaxy S II, 8 MP back camera with F/2.65 aperture, and 4 mm focal length lens) using a plano-convex lens (focal length 28 mm) in front of the SP camera. The use of the plano-convex lens is essential for fitting both the tubes into the FOV of the SP camera to provide an optical demagnification of the tube cross section by sevenfold. The images are then processed in less than 1 s using the smart application running on the SP to estimate the peanut concentration in the sample. The test results could then be uploaded to secure servers. The food allergen IA including sample preparation and incubation requires about 20 min.

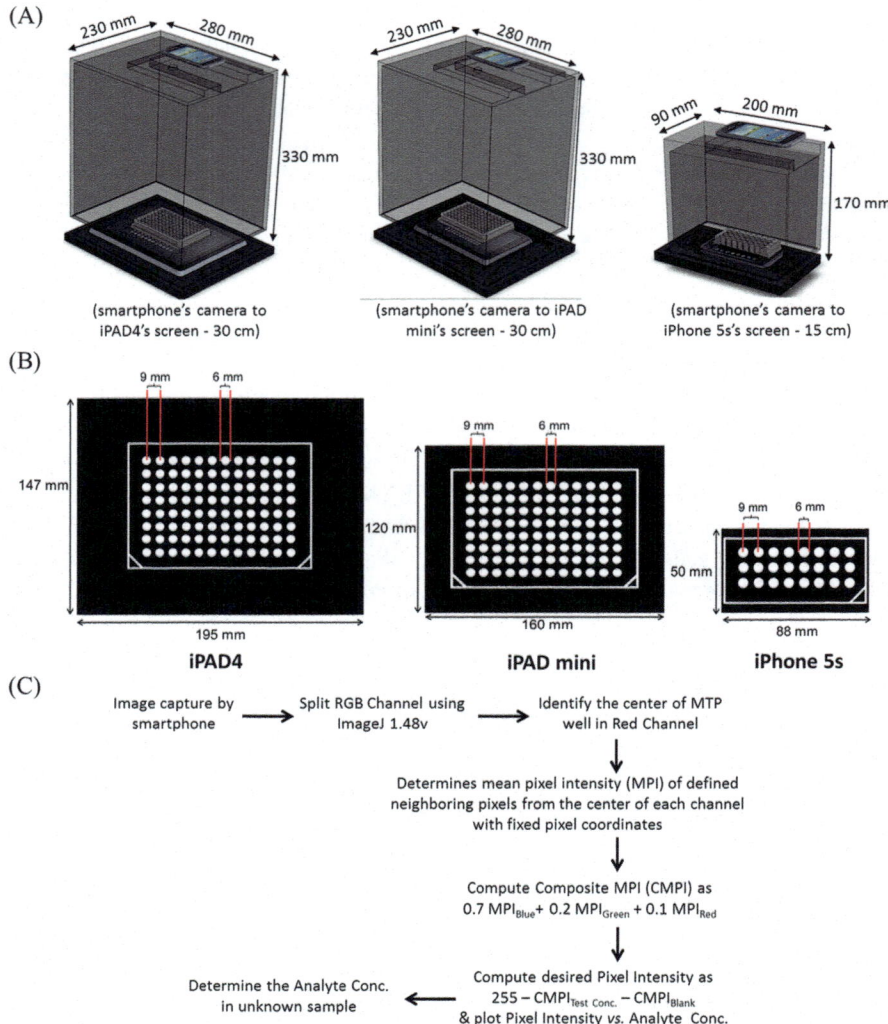

Fig. 2.1 SP-based colorimetric readers (SBCRs) for human CRP sandwich ELISA [35]. (**A**) Schematics of the SBCRs developing using the gadgets' (iPad4, iPad mini, or iPhone 5s) screen-based bottom illumination, Samsung Galaxy SIII mini's back camera (5 MP)-based imaging, and a custom-made polyamide dark hood and polyamide base holder assembly. (**B**) Screensavers used for the screen-based bottom illumination of the 96-well or 24-well microtiter plate (MTP) in gadgets. (**C**) Image processing algorithm employed for the analysis of smartphone-captured colorimetric images. Reproduced with permission from Springer International Publishing AG

A CP-based POC device detects *E.coli* O157: H7 in water and milk with a LOD of ~5–10 CFU/mL by employing a quantum dot (QD)-based sandwich immunoassay that utilizes an anti-*E. coli* O157: H7 antibody-functionalized capillary array [23] (Fig. 2.3). A low-cost, compact (dimensions: ~3.5 cm × 5.5 cm × 2.4 cm), and

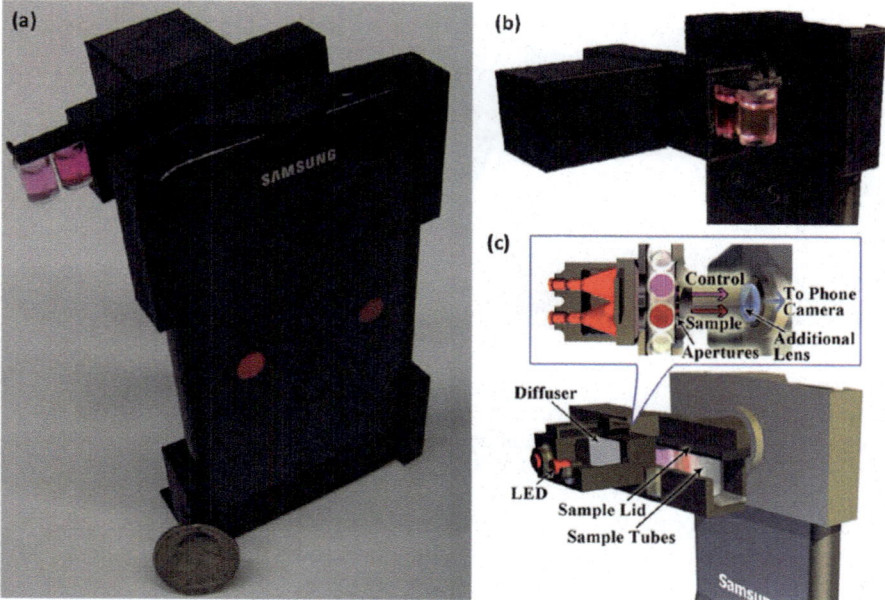

Fig. 2.2 (a) An SP optomechanical attachment, iTube platform, for the SP-based colorimetric readout of food allergen assay. (b) Attachment of the SP attachment at the back of the SP. (c) A schematic diagram of the iTube platform. Reproduced with permission from the Royal Society of Chemistry

lightweight (~28 g) CP optomechanical attachment can monitor ~10 functionalized capillary tubes (length, ~11 mm; inner and outer diameters of ~100 μm and ~170 μm, respectively) with an imaging FOV of 11 mm × 11 mm. The battery-powered ultra-violet LEDs butt-coupled to the capillary array provide the uniform excitation of QD-labeled *E. coli* particles (Fig. 2.3), while an additional lens with a focal length of 15 mm placed between the capillary array and the CP camera enables the emitted fluorescence light to be imaged by the CP. The CP device detects *E.coli* in water and milk samples with a detection limit of ~5–10 CFU/mL.

The SP-based POC device that employs paper microfluidics-based IA and Mie scattering offers the detection of *Salmonella* and *E. coli* [36]. Further, the detection of an HE4 cancer biomarker in urine was demonstrated using a CP-based microchip ELISA [37], with a sensitivity of 89.5% at a specificity of 90%. The analysis on the CP (Sony Ericsson i790, 3.2 MP camera) was done by an automated analysis mobile application. The assay format employed a postage stamp-sized microchip to detect HE4 by a sandwich ELISA, where the urine sample and assay reagents are pipetted manually into the microchannels. The detection of aflatoxin B1 is based on a one-dot LFIA based on a competitive binding format and an SP-based POC reader [38]. Another development is the CP-based imaging of two paper-based analytical

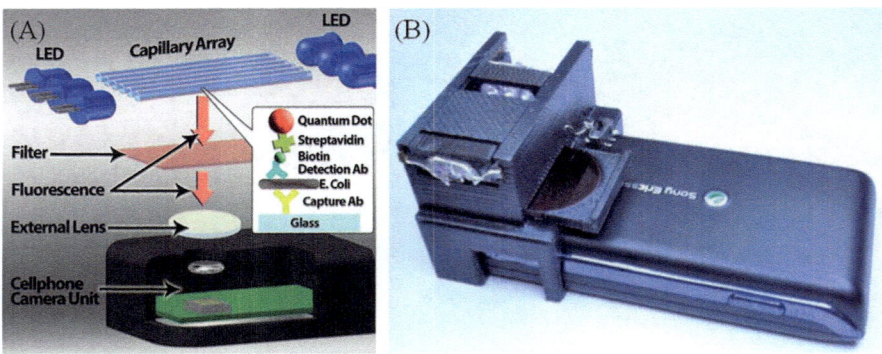

Fig. 2.3 An SP-based optomechanical attachment for fluorescent microscopy-based detection of *E.coli* using the QD-based sandwich immunoassay in glass capillary tubes [23]. Reproduced with permission for the Royal Society of Chemistry

devices (µPADs) for the on-site quantification of organophosphate pesticides based on the inhibition of immobilized acetylcholinesterase by these contaminants [39]. The quantification is based on via an on-site image processing smart application that employs a pixel counting algorithm. The use of test and control µPADs together for the quantification using the smart application reduces the bias resulting from variations in the ambient lighting. The smart application also provides the spatio-temporal tagging of the results and transmits the results in real time to a publically accessible website.

A prospective SP-based handheld POC reader (dimensions: 195 × 98 × 100 mm) (Fig. 2.4) for the colorimetric readout of ELISA in 96-well microplate has been advocated as the readout of various commercial ELISAs for mumps IgG, measles IgG, and herpes simplex virus IgG (HSV-1 and HSV-2) [40]. The reader shows a remarkable accuracy of 99.6%, 98.6%, 99.4%, and 99.4% for mumps, measles, HSV-1, and HSV-2, respectively, in agreement with the clinical spectrophotometric data. The SP reader comprises a Windows-based smartphone (Lumia 1020, Nokia), a 3D-printed optomechanical SP attachment with integrated optical components, a custom smart application, and a Cloud-connected data processing server. The data from the SP is transferred from the SP to the server by a wireless network (cellular data or WiFi) via the smart application. The server (Intel Core i5-760, 2.8 GHz, 16 GB RAM) processes the data using a machine learning algorithm (Fig. 2.5) and sends the results back to the smart application for display in 1 min. The device top part acts as the holder for the SP, the middle part holds the 96-well microplate, and the bottom part houses the fiber-optic array. The middle chamber contains an LED array at the top that illuminates the 96-well microplate. The LED array consists of 24 evenly spaced blue LED with peak wavelength of 464 nm. The device is powered by six AAA batteries and contains a low-noise, low-dropout linear current regulator to provide constant power to all the LEDs. Each LED is located in the center of the

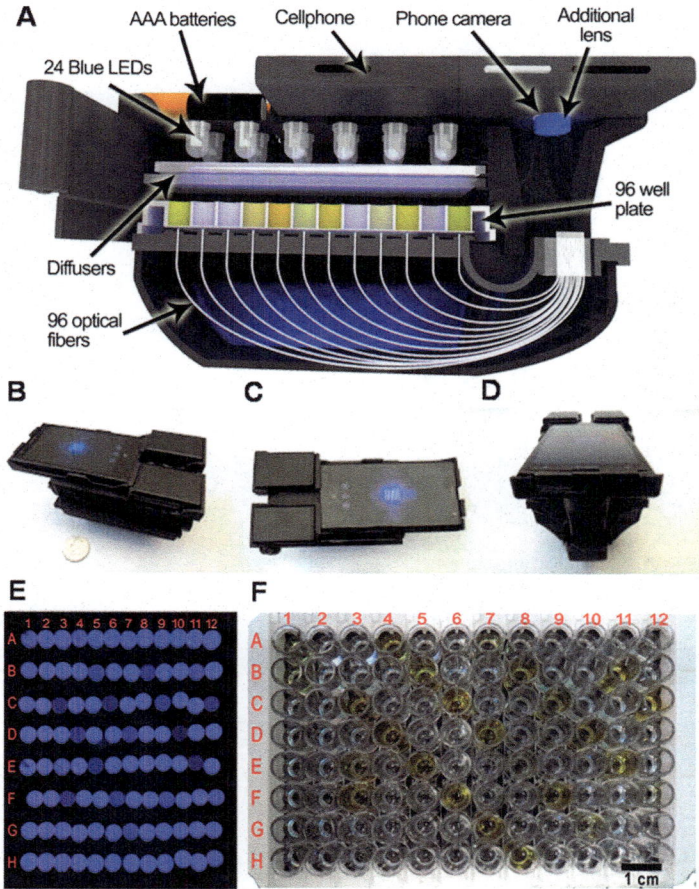

Fig. 2.4 An SP-based POC colorimetric ELISA reader [40]. (**A**) Schematic, (**B–D**) different perspectives. (**E**) Sample image and (**F**) sample 96-well microplate. Reproduced with permission from the American Chemical Society

microplate four wells to illuminate all the wells uniformly. Two layers of plastic diffusers are used between the LED and the microplate to homogenize the illuminated light. The optical fibers located at the base of each well in the microplate collect and guide the transmitted light to the external collection lens (focal length 45 mm), which is placed in front of the SP camera (41 MP, pixel size 1.12 µm). The CP camera captures the colorimetric images in a RAW 10-bit/channel Digital Negative (DNG) image format. The device has a superior design in comparison to other SP-based colorimetric readers. The use of optical fibers transforms the imaging area of 96-well microplate to more than 110-fold smaller imaging area at the end of the fiber bundle, which minimizes the distance between the SP camera and the imaging area.

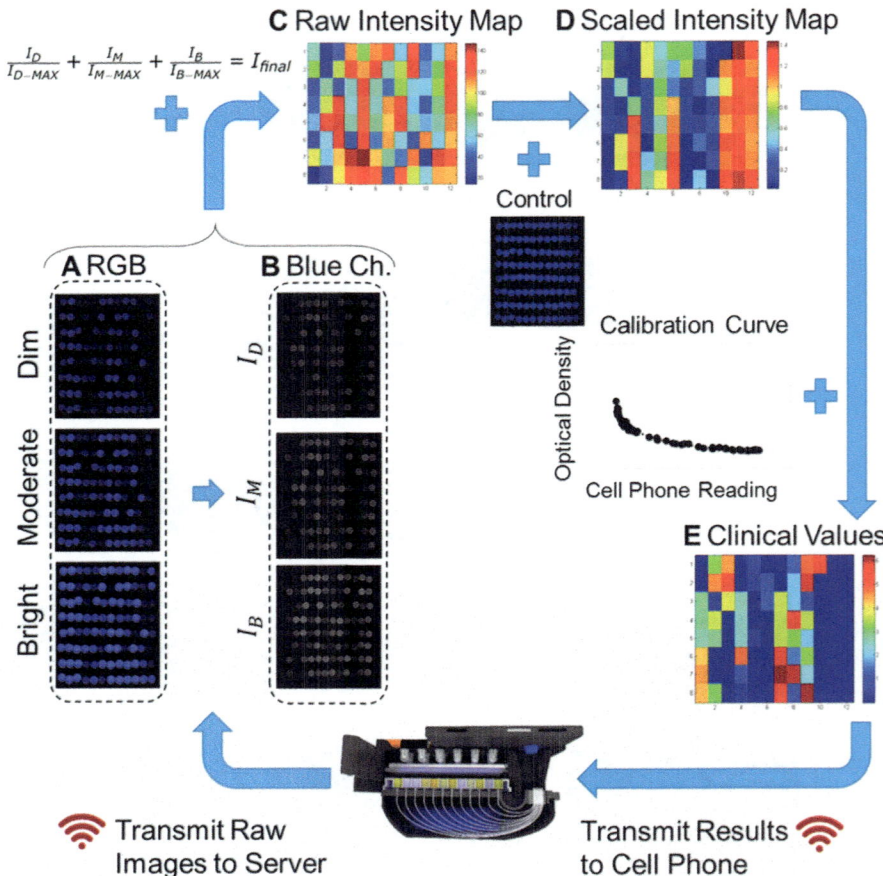

Fig. 2.5 An SP-IVD flowchart showing the data processing steps of the reader. From the raw images (**a**), the blue channel (**b**) is extracted to be used for the rest of the data processing. Dividing the intensities of each well by the intensity of the brightest well, a raw intensity map (**c**) of blue pixel values is generated. Next, by normalizing everything to a control, a scaled intensity map of transmittances (**d**) is formed. Lastly, the transmittances are converted to clinical values (**e**) using a calibration curve

2.2.2 Fluorescence Detection

A wide range of SP-based POC fluorescence readers has been developed for various analytes and multifarious bioanalytical applications, as summarized in Table 2.2. Figure 2.6 shows an SP-based device developed for the POC detection of recombinant bovine somatotropin (rbST) antibodies in milk [94]. It might be used to increase the milk production in cows; however, the administration of rbST to cows is illegal in the EU and a public health concern in the USA. The detection is based on rbST bound covalently to paramagnetic microspheres that bind to anti-rbST Ab in milk,

Table 2.2 SP-based POC fluorescence detection

Analytes detected	Bioanalytical application	Refs.
M. tuberculosis	*M. tuberculosis* bacilli in auramine O-stained sputum smears	[16]
Salmonella typhimurium DNA	An SP-based fluorescent microscope and a paper microfluidic-based assay detected *S. typhimurium* down to 10^3 and 10^4/CFU mL using cellulose and nitrocellulose papers, respectively	[100]
Hepatitis B virus plasmid	An SP-based fluorescent detector was used for the screening Hepatitis B virus plasmid samples by DNA amplification using convective polymerase chain reaction	[101]
rbST Abs	An SP-based fluorescent microscope detected rbST Abs in milk by magnetic polystyrene microsphere-based IA using QD-labeled detection Ab	[94]
Salmonella and *E.coli O157*	An SP-based fluorescent reader detected *Salmonella* and *E. coli O157* via an LFIA with a LOD of 10^5 CFU/mL and a rapid sample-to-answer time of a few minutes. The LFIA employs Ab-bound dye-doped silica NPs	[98]
Salmonella typhimurium and *E.coli K12*	An SP-based fluorescent reader and a droplet-based multiplex IA on Ab-bound polycaprolactone electrospun fiber-coated indium tin oxide glass detects *Salmonella typhimurium* and *E.coli K12* with a LOD of 10^2 CFU/mL	[102]
β-D-galactosidase	An SP-based fluorescence detection device and a paper microfluidic-based IA for detecting β-D-galactosidase in the linear range of 0.7–12 nM with a LOD of 0.7 nM	[103]
Single NPs and viruses	An SP-based fluorescence microscope detected isolated 100 nM fluorescent NPs and fluorescently labeled human cytomegaloviruses	[104]
microRNA	Using the fluorescent molecular beacon assay to detect microRNA with a LOD of 10 pM	[105]
RBCs WBCs Hb	An SP-based imaging cytometry platform detected Hb concentration and the density of RBCs and WBCs using just 10 μL of the whole blood sample. The fluorescently labeled WBCs are detected by fluorescent imaging, unlabeled RBCs are detected by bright-field imaging, and Hb is detected by absorbance	[14]
E. coli	An SP-based fluorescence reader detects *E. coli O157* in fat-free milk by a QD-based sandwich IA in glass capillaries with a LOD of ~5–10 CFU/mL	[23]
WBCs *Giardia lamblia* cysts	An SP-based fluorescent reader detects fluorescently labeled WBCs in the whole blood and waterborne pathogenic *Giardia lamblia* cysts with a resolution of 10 μm and a FOV of 81 mm²	[106]
Trypanosoma cruzi	An SP fluorescence reader detects *T. cruzi* genomic DNA [0.1–100 fg/μL] by PCR reaction	[99]
PSA	An SP-based fluorescence detection system and a miniaturized microcapillary film platform detect PSA via a sandwich IA in the dynamic range of 0.08–60 ng/mL in less than 13 min	[107]

(continued)

Table 2.2 (continued)

Analytes detected	Bioanalytical application	Refs.
pH	An SP-based fluorimeter was developed and used for the determination of pH of environmental water [4–11] using temperature stable 4-aminonaphthalimide fluorophore	[108]
pH	An SP fluorimeter for the detection of pH [4.5–9.77] using temperature stable 4-aminonapthalimide fluorophore	[108]
Basic metabolic panel (Na, K, Cl, Ca, bicarbonate, glucose, urea, and creatinine)	An SP fluorescence reader for the sensing of the metabolites in the basic metabolic panel. Na, K, and pH are detected in the linear ranges of 100–200 mM, 1–20 mM, 6.5–8, respectively. The detection ranges for Ca, Cl, glucose, bicarbonate, urea, and creatinine are 0–5 mM, 25–150 mM, 3–10 mM, 15–25 mM, 1–20 mM, and 10–200 µM, respectively	[109]
Albumin	An SP fluorescence reader detects albumin in urine in about 5 min with a LOD of 10 µg/mL	[95]
Thrombin activity	An SP fluorescence reader and a single-step FRET bioassay, using QDs and an array of paper-in-polydimethylsiloxane (PDMS)-on-glass sample chips, detect the thrombin activity in less than 30 min with a LOD of 18 NIH units/mL using just 12 µL of the whole blood sample	[110]
HIV and hepatitis B	An SP fluorescence reader detects HIV, hepatitis B, hepatitis C, and influenza type A and B viruses down to 1000 viral genetic copies per mL in less than 1 h via a QD barcode-based assay and isothermal amplification	[111]
Collagenase and trypsin	An SP fluorescence detection system detects collagenase and trypsin down to 0.938 µg and 930 pg, respectively	[112]
Avian influenza subtypes, i.e., H5N3, H7N1, and H9N2	A coumarin-derived dendrimer-based fluorescence LFIA detects avian influenza subtypes: H5N3, H7N1, and H9N2 with a sensitivity and specificity of 96.55% and 98.55%, respectively. The lowest detectable virus titers for H5N3, H7N1, and H9N2 are 6.25×10^3, 5.32×10^2, and 5.23×10^1 PFU/mL, respectively	[113]
HSV-2	An SP fluorescent readout-based rapid nucleic acid amplification-based microfluidic LAMP assay detects as few as 100 copies of HSV-2 viral DNA	[97]
Ochratoxin A	An SP fluorescence analyzer detects ochratoxin A in the linear range of 2–20 µg/L with a LOD of 2 µg/L	[114]
Staphylococcus aureus and λ-phage	An SP fluorescence readout-based lab-on-a-drone nucleic acid diagnostic platform for the analysis of the in-flight replication of *Staphylococcus aureus* and λ-phage DNA targets in less than 20 min. The SP fluorescence detector quantitatively analyzes template concentrations down to 1000 copies/µL	[115]
Parasite fecal egg counting	An SP fluorescent imaging system for the automated fluorescently labeled parasite fecal egg counting	[116]

(continued)

Table 2.2 (continued)

Analytes detected	Bioanalytical application	Refs.
GGT	An SP-based fluorescent microscope and an organ-on-a-chip platform enable dual-mode monitoring of drug-induced nephrotoxicity in situ. The presence and release of GGT from the organ-on-a-chip platform are monitored	[117]
Brain-derived exosome biomarkers (GluR2)	An SP fluorescence reader and an optofluidic device for the detection of enzyme amplified exosome biomarkers. The device can isolate and profile brain-derived exosomes in less than an hour	[118]
Human IgM/IgG, IL-6, PSA, AFP, Leptin, TNFα, BNP, HIV p24	An SP fluorescence readout-based POC IA, using inkjet-printed nanoscale polymer brush, for the detection of the mentioned analytes in the sub-picomolar ranges	[119]
KSHV	An SP fluorescence readout-based solar thermal PCR for the analysis of human skin biopsies infected with KSHV in less than 30 min	[120]
17-β-estradiol	An SP fluorescence imaging-based dual-wavelength fluorescence biosensor, employing the binding of target analytes to the split capture and detection aptamer probes, detects 17-β-estradiol [1 pg/mL–100 ng/mL] with a LOD of 1 pg/mL	[121]
Neutrophil and cancer cell chemotaxis	An integrated microfluidic device with SP-based fluorescence readout for the cell migration assay. The device could effectively measure purified neutrophil and cancer cell chemotaxis	[122]
Hg^{2+}	A cysteamine-capped QD-based fluorescence assay, based on the fluorescence quenching by Hg^{2+} and SP fluorescence readout, detects Hg^{2+} in the linear range of 5–200 nM with a LOD of 1 nM	[123]
Chloride in sweat	An SP-based fluorescence readout-based POC assay for chloride in sweat in the linear range of 0.8–200 mM	[96]
Zika virus	An SP fluorescence readout-based diagnostic platform, employing reverse-transcription LAMP and quenching of unincorporated amplification signal reporters (QUASR), detects Zika virus in crude human sample matrices of blood, urine, and saliva	[124]
Separation of prostate, breast, and ovarian cancer cells and differentiation of QTracker 625- and calcein-stained HeyA8 cells	An SP fluorescence imaging device and a POC tool for the density-based cell sorting via magnetic focusing enable the separation of cells	[125]

rbST recombinant bovine somatotropin, *PSA* prostate-specific antigen, *FRET* Förster resonance energy transfer, *HSV-2* herpes simplex virus type 2, *LAMP* loop-mediated isothermal amplification, *GGT* γ-glutamyl transpeptidase, *GluR2* glutamate receptor 2, *AFP* alpha-fetoprotein, *TNFα* tumor necrosis factor alpha, *BNP* B-type natriuretic peptide, *KSHV* Kaposi's sarcoma herpesvirus

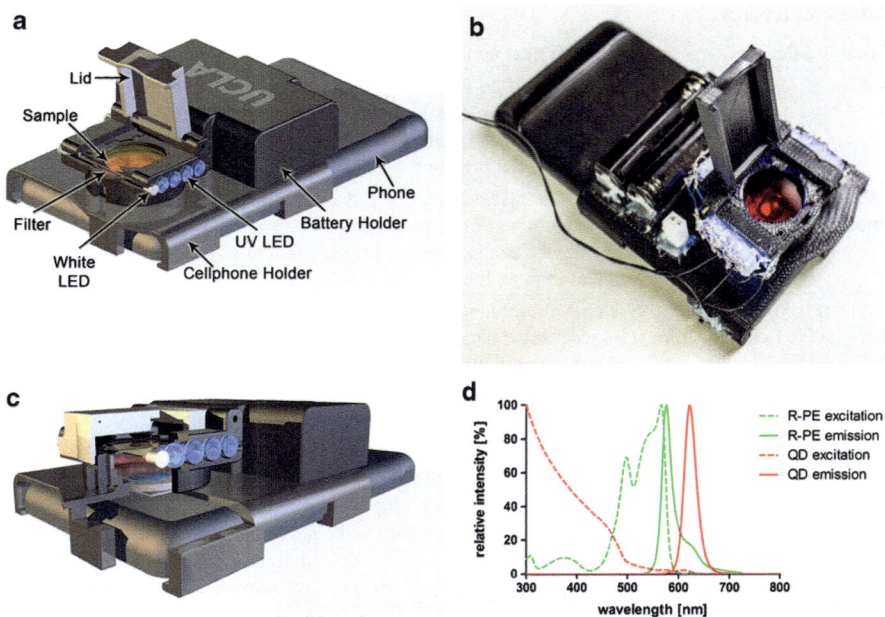

Fig. 2.6 An SP-based POC device for the detection of anti-recombinant somatotropin (rbST) Ab in milk [94]. Schematics (**a**, **c**) and a picture (**b**) of the SP attachment. Excitation (dotted lines) and emission (solid lines) spectra (**d**) of R-phycoerythrin (R-PE, green) and 625-nm emitting quantum dots (QD, red). Reproduced with permission from Springer

followed by the detection of the immune complex by binding to QD-labeled detection Ab (Fig. 2.7). The fluorescence of the bound QD-labeled detection Ab detected by the developed SP attachment has the same bioanalytical performance as the newly developed planar imaging array but with additional features for POC detection: external power supply, wireless connectivity, increased portability, and improved cost-effectiveness. The compact SP attachment (88 × 73 × 31.25 mm) employs a dual-imaging approach for dark-field and fluorescence imaging. It comprises an SP holder that aligns all optical parts with SP camera; 12 ultraviolet LEDs (wavelength 380 nm) for exciting the QDs for fluorescence imaging; 2 white light LEDs for dark-field imaging; an optical filter (long pass 610 nm, 25 mm diameter) for filtering the scattered excitation light from the sample; a sample tray for positioning the sample, i.e., the microsphere suspension sandwiched in between the cover slides; an aspherical lens that increases the FOV by providing ×2 demagnification; a battery compartment; and a mechanical lid to create a dark environment for fluorescence imaging by protecting from the ambient light. The SP imaging is performed by operating it in the "night mode" in order to obtain increased sensitivity.

Another prospective format is SP device for the testing of albumin in urine using a fluorescent assay in disposable test tubes and an SP attachment [95]. The compact and lightweight (148 g) SP attachment is mechanically installed on the existing

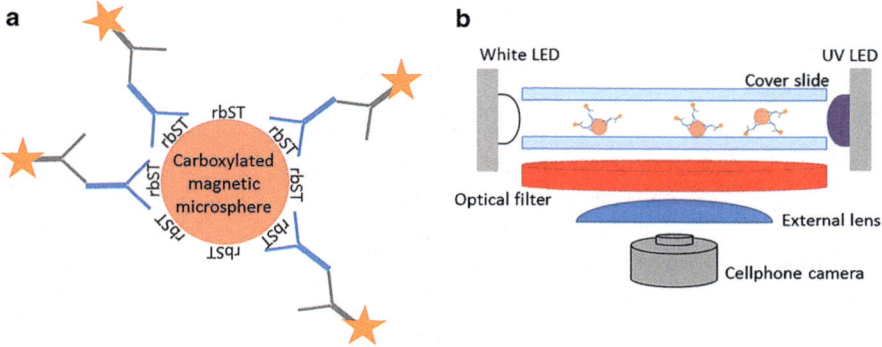

Fig. 2.7 SP-based POC detection of anti-recombinant somatotropin (rbST) Ab in milk [94]. (**a**) Assay principle and (**b**) detection setup for the SP-based platform. Reproduced with permission from Springer

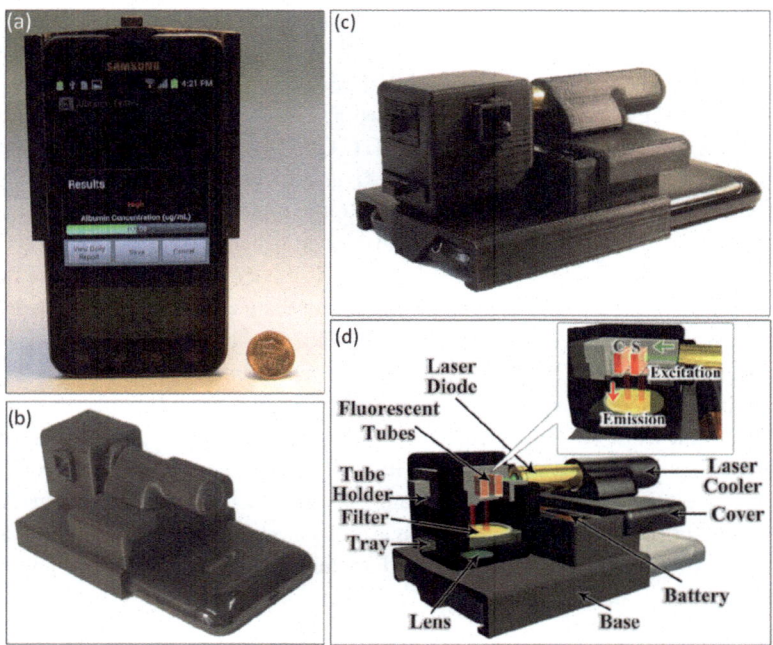

Fig. 2.8 An SP-based device for the testing of albumin in urine [95]. (**a–c**) Different views of the SP attachment. (**d**) Schematic of the SP attachment. Reproduced with permission from the Royal Society of Chemistry

back camera unit of the SP (Fig. 2.8). It involves the insertion of test and control tubes (6 × 2 × 15 mm) from the side followed by their excitation by a battery-powered laser diode (5 mW, 532 nm). The weakly scattered excitation light is rejected by an interference filter. The SP camera captures the images of the fluorescent tubes perpendicular to the direction of excitation using a plano-convex lens (focal length ~28 mm) inserted between the interference filter and the SP back camera. The SP camera collects the fluorescent emission only through the thin side of each tube (2 mm thick) using two rectangular apertures (2 mm × 2 mm). The captured images are processed in 1 s via an Android application running on the SP. The developed albumin assay employs a simple sample preparation and incubation, which takes about 5 min per test and detects albumin in urine with a LOD ~5–10 μg mL^{-1}. A mini-syringe transfers a small volume of the urine sample (25 μL) into the test tube prefilled with all required assay reagents via a PDMS-based injection port.

An SP-based chloridometer for the POC diagnosis of cystic fibrosis using a citrate-derived sensor material that detects chloride in sweat exhibits linearity of 0.8–200 nM chloride [96] (Fig. 2.9). The assay procedure involves the dilution of the chloride sample with citric acid (CA)-cysteine and sulfuric acid in a quartz cuvette. The chloride ions in the sample attenuate the blue fluorescence of CA-cysteine, while the sulfuric acid protonates the sensor's carboxyl groups to maintain reliable performance. The SP device comprises a 3D-printed SP attachment (made from acrylonitrile-butadiene-styrene (ABS) plastic), which houses a UV LED (365 nm, 1 W), powered by a 9 V battery, for the excitation of CA-cysteine. The applied voltage and current to the UV LED are limited to 4.1 V and 700 mA, respectively, using a 7-ohm high power resistor. The blue fluorescent images of the sample in the cuvette are taken by an SP (HTC One M9) by fixing the parameters of the camera to exposure time 10 ms, ISO 100, and focus set at near field. The setup employs a 441.6 nm band-pass filter to obviate the undesired excitation light as the CA-cysteine has maximum fluorescent emission at 441 nm.

An interesting application is the SP-based POC device for the detection of herpes simplex virus type 2 (HSV-2) using a loop-mediated isothermal amplification (LAMP) assay and a microfluidic diagnostic chip (Smart cup) [97] (Fig. 2.10). It could detect as few as 100 copies of HSV-2 viral DNA in POC settings. The excitation of the fluorescent dye (EvaGreen) is feasible using the SP's flashlight via an excitation filter, while the fluorescent emission is measured by the SP's back camera (Samsung Galaxy S3) via an emission filter. The SP images are transferred to a computer, and the average fluorescent intensity of the images is determined by a custom-developed MATLAB-based image analysis software. The SP adapter and the microfluidic chip holder and the cup lid are fabricated by 3D printing. The Smart cup is powered by the water-triggered exothermic chemical reaction based on the generation of heat where water oxidizes the magnesium-iron alloy and induces galvanic corrosion. The device temperature for amplification is regulated using a phase-change material (PCM) at 60–65 °C.

An SP-based fluorescence reader equipped with a monochromatic filter measures the fluorescent signal of a labeled dye [98] such as EvaGreen, a dye used in the polymerase chain reaction (PCR) [99]. Further, an SP-based fluorescent microscope detects *Salmonella typhimurium* DNA using a paper microfluidics-based assay [100].

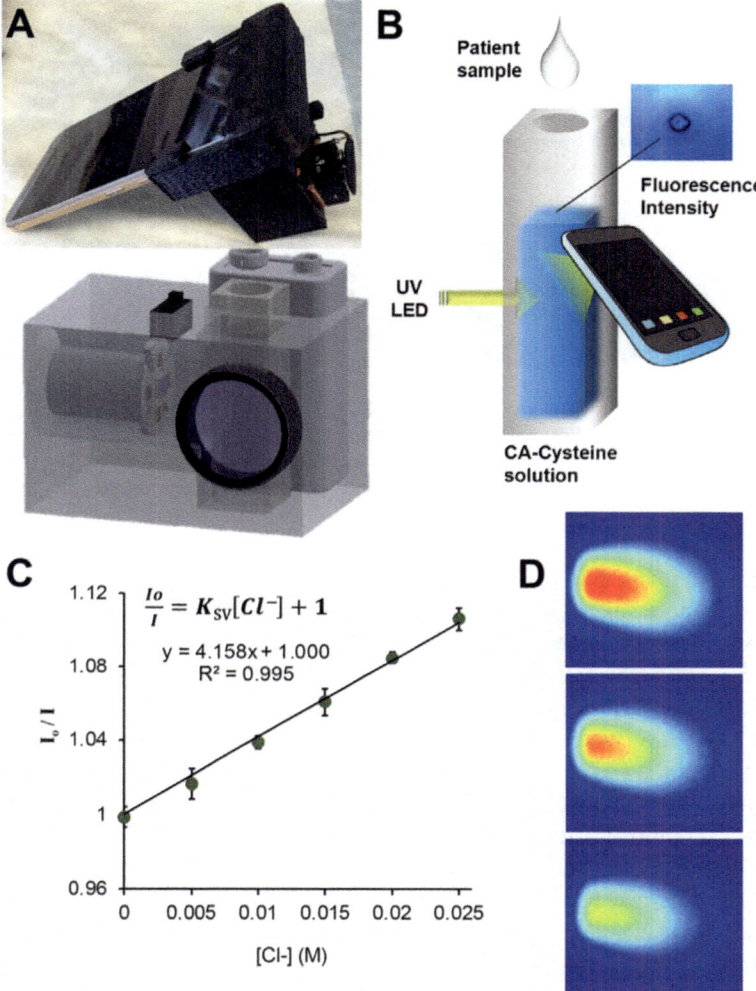

Fig. 2.9 (**a**) (Top) Photograph of the SP-based chloridometer device and (Bottom) a schematic view of SP attachment [96]. (**c**) A calibration curve showing the fluorescence quenching rates (I_0/I) with increasing chloride concentration. (**d**) Raw images of CA-cysteine fluorescence captured by an SP camera in the presence of increasing chloride concentrations. Reproduced with permission from the Elsevier BV

2.2.3 Luminescence Detection

For luminescent detection, the measurement is performed in the dark [126] using a plano-convex lens in front of the SP camera for converging the field of view [127]. Various prospective SP-based POC luminescence detection devices have been developed that enable the determination of many analytes, as summarized in

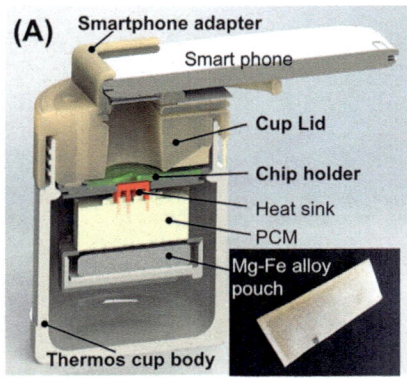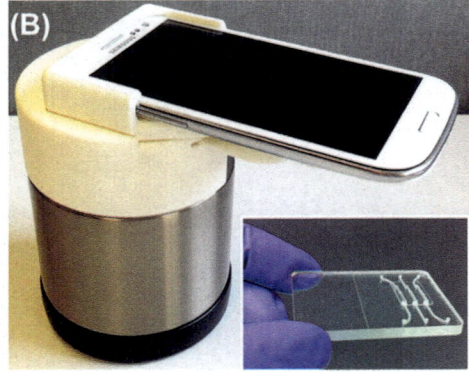

Fig. 2.10 An SP-based POC device (Smart Cup) for the fluorescent detection of HSV-2 [97]. (**A**) Smart Cup. Inset: Mg-Fe alloy pouch used as a heating source. (**B**) A photograph of Smart Cup. Inset: a photograph of an integrated microfluidic chip containing three independent isothermal amplification reactors for nucleic acid extraction and amplification. Reproduced with permission from Elsevier BV

Table 2.3. An interesting approach is an SP-based device developed for the readout of the bioluminescent assay for total bile acids and the chemiluminescence assay for total cholesterol, which are performed in a disposable mini-cartridge within 3 min [127] (Fig. 2.11). It employs low-cost 3D printing for the fabrication of an SP attachment and a compact mini-cartridge (3.5 cm long, 1.2 cm wide, and 5 mm thick), which are made by a thin layer (200 μm) of transparent acrylonitrile-butadiene-styrene (ABS) polymer. The back-illuminated CMOS photodiode integrated into an SP (iPhone 5S, 8 MP back camera) is used as a luminometer. The SP attachment comprises a dark box to shield from ambient light and a lens holder that holds a plano-convex lens (6 mm in diameter). The mini-cartridge comprises a blood separator pad holder with an LF1 glass fiber filter for the one-step serum separation from whole blood. The blood separator pad is connected to a reaction chamber that contains a nitrocellulose disk (4 mm thick) adsorbed with specific enzymes. The reaction chamber is connected to a reservoir that contains the substrate for generating the luminescent assay signal. The mini-cartridge is 3D printed into two pieces that are then glued together. The SP-captured luminescent images are analyzed by the Image J software to quantify the signal over the sample spot area as relative light units (RLUs). The SP-based cholesterol assay exhibits a linear range of 20–386 mg dL^{-1} and a LOD of 20 mg dL^{-1}, while the SP-based 3α-hydroxy bile acid assay has a linear range and a LOD of 0.5–100 μmol L^{-1} and 0.5 μmol L^{-1}, respectively. The developed POC assays detect cholesterol and 3α-hydroxy bile acid in real sample matrices using only minute sample volume, i.e., 15 μL of blood or 50 μL of oral fluid.

Another prospective approach is the SP-based device for the luminescent readout of upconversion paper sensor for pesticide, i.e., thiram [80] (Fig. 2.12). The test paper is fabricated by the fixing of copper ions decorated NaYF$_4$: Yb/Tm upconversion nanoparticles onto a filter paper. Thiram is detected based on the quenching of

Table 2.3 SP-based POC luminescence detection

Analytes detected	Bioanalytical application	Refs.
Bile acid	An LFA mini-cartridge format-based assay determined total bile acid in serum and oral fluid within 3 min with linearity and a LOD of 0.5–100 µM and 0.5 µM, respectively	[127]
Cholesterol	An LFA mini-cartridge format-based assay for total cholesterol in serum within 3 min with linearity and LOD of 20–386 mg/dL^{-1} and 20 mg/dL, respectively	[127]
Salivary cortisol	An LFIA format based on direct competitive IA detects salivary cortisol [0.3–60 ng/mL] with a LOD of 0.3 ng/mL	[129]
Proteolytic activity	Multiplexed homogeneous assays for the proteolytic activity of pM–nM concentration of proteases: trypsin, chymotrypsin, and enterokinase	[42]
ECL	A portable, thermo-powered, high-throughput, electrochemiluminescence visual sensor for the detection of ECL generated by the reaction of DBAE with Ru(bpy)$_3$$^{2+}$-bound ITO surface	[130]
ECL	An SP sensor for the detection of ECL of water-soluble iridium(III) complex	[131]
Thiram	Upconversion paper sensor detects thiram in the linear detection range of 0.1 µM–1 mM with a LOD of 0.1 µM by the luminescence quenching via LRET mechanism	[80]
Photoluminescence of QDs	Demonstrates a model protein binding assay with a LOD of sub-ng/mL and a FRET assay for proteolytic activity	[132]
Toxicity assay	A 3D-printed whole-cell toxicity biosensor with integrated bioluminescent sentinel cells for the toxicity assay within 30 min	[133]
H$_2$O$_2$	A POC assay for H$_2$O$_2$ in human exhaled breath condensates as low as 264 nM	[128]
Antibodies against HIV1-p17, HA, and dengue virus type I	A sensor based on BRET for antibodies against HIV1-p17, HA, and dengue virus type I with a LOD of 10 pM	[134]
C677T SNP of MTHFR gene	A paper-based strip for the genotyping of the C677T SNP of MTHFR gene	[135]
Cocaine	An upconversion nanoparticle-based paper device detects cocaine with a LOD of 50 nM in human saliva using two pieces of aptamer fragments	[136]

Ru(bpy)$_3$$^{2+}$ tris(2,2′-bipyridine)ruthenium(II), *ECL* electrochemiluminescence, *DBAE* 2-(dibutyl-amino)ethanol, *ITO* indium tin oxide, *LRET* luminescence resonance energy transfer, *FRET* Förster resonance energy transfer, *HA* hemagglutinin, *BRET* bioluminescence resonance energy transfer, *SNP* single nucleotide polymorphism, *MTHFR* methylenetetrahydrofolate reductase

the blue luminescence of test paper by thiram via the luminescence resonance energy transfer mechanism. The change in the luminescence signal is monitored by capturing the SP images via the developed SP optomechanical attachment, followed by the determination of blue channel intensities of SP-captured images using the custom-developed Android program installed on the SP. The SP attachment is fabricated by 3D-printed parts that are glued together. It comprises a holder for the mini-laser (180 mW, 980 nm); a dark cavity with an optical filter and a chamber for

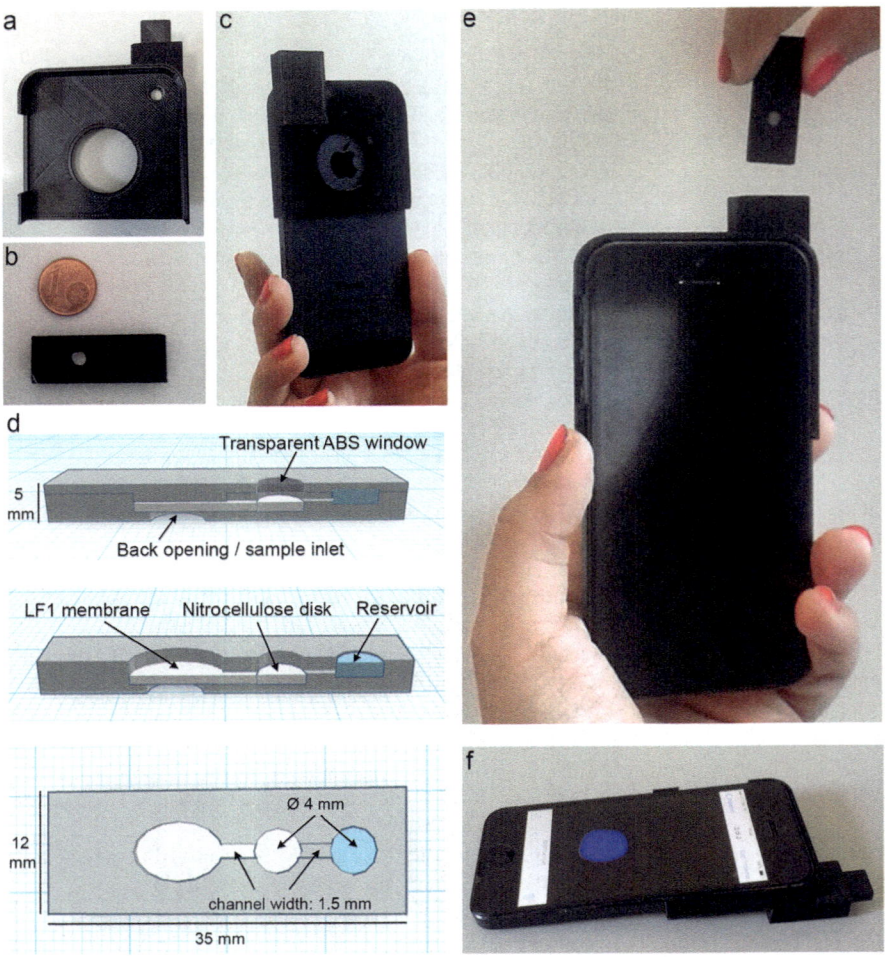

Fig. 2.11 An SP-based device for the detection of luminescence [127]. (**a**) SP attachment. (**b**) Mini-cartridge. (**c**) The SP attachment snapped into the SP. (**d**) Schematic of the mini-cartridge showing the various components, where the transparent ABS window (200 μm thick, 4 mm diameter) allows the imaging of luminescent reaction by the SP back camera. (**e**) Insertion of mini-cartridge into the SP attachment. (**f**) Luminescence signal acquisition by the SP. Reproduced with permission from the American Chemical Society

placing the test paper; and an SP holder with an optical window of 1 cm diameter for SP alignment and imaging. The power to the mini-laser is provided by the USB interface from the SP. The mini-laser is kept an angle of 45 °C from the test paper to prevent the interference from the excitation light, while an optical fiber is placed in front of the SP back camera to avoid the access of excitation light into the SP camera. Thiram is detected with a LOD of 0.1 μM in the linear range of 0.1 μM–1 mM.

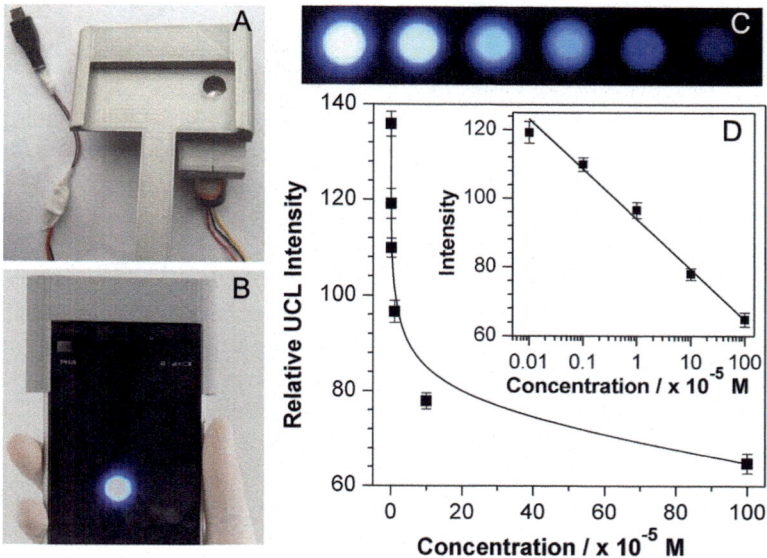

Fig. 2.12 An SP-based device for the detection of thiram by a luminescent assay. (**A**) The SP attachment with a mini-laser, an optical filter, and mini-cavity. (**B**) The SP-based device assembly for luminescence readout. (**C**) The luminescent images of test paper upon additions of different amounts of thiram (left to right: 0.1×10^{-7}, 1×10^{-6}, 1×10^{-5}, 1×10^{-4}, 1×10^{-3}). (**D**) The relative luminescent intensities of SP-captured images determination by the blue channel. The inset figure shows the linearity of mean luminescent intensities with the logarithm of thiram concentrations. Reproduced with permission from Elsevier BV

The SP-based chemiluminescent detection of H_2O_2 in human exhaled breath condensates [128] has a good analytical performance equivalent to the standard Amplex Red assay. It detects H_2O_2 as low as 264 nM in exhaled human breath condensate samples employing specialized photography smart applications (OSnap, VSCO, and stock camera), a custom-made wooden dark box ($5 \times 7.5 \times 5.5$ in.), and an SP (iPhone 6). The walls of the dark box are glued together by epoxy resin, while a plastic SP case is glued to the lid of the dark box such that the aperture for SP back camera is aligned to the 0.5×0.5 in. hole cut in the lid. The SP captures chemiluminescent images that are transferred to a computer and analyzed for pixel intensity using Image J. The mean pixel intensity is evaluated for each image by selecting a circle around the reaction well in Image J.

In photoluminescence-based SP-IVD using QDs and Förster resonance energy transfer, the setup requires a UV lamp (365 nm) for excitation and a long-pass (400 nm cutoff) and a short-pass filter (650 nm cutoff), inserted in front of the SP camera [42]. For multi-sample imaging, a microtiter plate (MTP) with 96 wells is placed on the gadget's screensaver to provide uniform bottom illumination inside a dark hood. The SP is simply placed on top of the hood in containment with an aperture in alignment with the SP back camera [30].

2.2.4 Spectroscopy

Various prospective SP-based POC spectrophotometers have been demonstrated for diversified bioanalytical applications (Table 2.4). A portable SP fluorimeter in the form of a custom-designed cradle could measure the full emission spectrum of any fluorescent light emitter [105]. It employs a transmission diffraction grating in front of the SP back camera (iPhone 4, 5 MP resolution) and an optical setup to collimate the light emitted by a liquid fluorescent sample onto the diffraction grating (Fig. 2.13). The cradle interfaces the SP back camera equipped with a complementary metal-oxide semiconductor (CMOS) image sensor. The mechanical alignment of a diffraction grating (1200 lines/mm), a collimating lens (focal length 75 mm), a cylindrical lens (focal length 40 mm), and a pinhole (aperture 1 mm) are also provided by the cradle. However, a laser excitation source (green laser 532 nm, 300 mW), an optical fiber, a collecting lens (focal length 50 mm), a focusing lens (focal length 40 mm), and a transparent sample cuvette are external to the cradle. The sample is illuminated at an orthogonal angle to the light collection axis to minimize the collection of light from the laser into the optical fiber. The device performs the sensitive molecular beacon Förster resonance energy transfer (FRET) assay for the detection of a specific microRNA sequence with better analytical performance than the conventional laboratory fluorimeter. The FRET assay detects a specific miRNA sequence, which differs from the target sequence by only one base, with a LOD of 10 pM. The fluorescence readout is performed by an advanced image processing algorithm, which involves the transformation of primary RGB colors to an HSV (hue-saturation-value) color map to determine the photon density of each pixel. The SP is used at the maximum exposure time of 1 s to maximize the fluorescent intensity values of the captured image. The device is calibrated using a calibrated fiber-optic spectrophotometer.

The same group also developed an SP-based spectrophotometer for the colorimetric readout of conventional ELISAs [137] (Fig. 2.14). They demonstrated the same analytical sensitivity of IL-6 and Ara h1 (one of the main peanut allergens) ELISAs using the SP device in comparison to the one performed using the standard microplate reader. In fact, the SP-based absorption at 450 nm replicates the microplate reader measurements for the entire range of standard concentrations for IL-6 ELISA. However, the LOD of SP-based readout of Ara h1 ELISA is lower than that of the microplate reader. The optical setup of the developed SP device is similar to that employed for the fluorimeter described above except that it employs a broadband light source (150 W halogen fiber-optic high-intensity illuminator) for the illumination of the sample cuvette. The SP back camera (iPhone 4, Omnivision OV5653 5MP BSI CMOS sensor with f/2.4) detects the wavelengths in the visible range of 400–700 nm. The image analysis procedure involves the SP capture of five consecutive images for each measurement and the use of a MATLAB script for digital image analysis to convert the raw images into absorption spectra. As most ELISAs involve the colorimetric enzyme-substrate reaction using TMB substrate, only the blue channel RGB image is taken into consideration, while red and green channels are omitted.

Table 2.4 SP-based POC spectroscopy detection

Analytes detected	Bioanalytical application	Refs.
Peanut	An SP spectrometer detects 1–25 ppm of peanut within 20 min	[22]
Cisplatin-induced kidney toxicity	An SP spectrometer and a metabolomics platform were used to assess cisplatin-induced kidney toxicity in a rat model	[140]
IL-6 and Ara h1	An SP spectrometer was developed and used for the readout of conventional ELISA for IL-6 biomarker and Ara h1 (a peanut allergen)	[137]
Atmospheric optical depth	An SP sun photometer was developed for the remote sensing of atmospheric optical depth	[141]
microRNA sequences	An SP fluorimeter was developed and used for the detection of specific microRNA-21 sequence and distinguishing a one-point mismatch in target microRNA via a fluorescent molecular beacon FRET assay. It detects specific microRNA sequence with a LOD of 10 pM	[105]
Salmonella typhimurium and *Escherichia coli*	Paper microfluidics-based immunoassays, with readout via a developed SP spectrometer, for the detection of *Salmonella typhimurium* and *Escherichia coli* with a sample-to-answer time of less than 1 min and a LOD of a single cell	[36]
Zn^{2+} in water	A combined dual absorption and fluorescence SP spectrometer for the detection of Zn^{2+} in environmental water [0–50 µM]	[142]
Estimation of banana ripeness	An SP spectrometer determines the banana ripeness by simultaneous analysis of two broad-spectral images of the banana taken under white light and ultraviolet illumination	[143]
Various colored dyes	SP-based evanescent wave coupled spectroscopic sensing for the determination of different colored dyes (safranin orange, methyl orange, methyl violet, sunset yellow, rhodamine 6G, malachite green)	[144]
Analysis of foods and beverages	SP spectroscopy for the analysis of foods and beverages. The addition of three colored additives to a lemon-lime beverage, adulteration of milk with water, changes occurring on a green onion surface over 48 h, and five different cuts from lamb carcasses are assessed	[145]
pH	An SP-based spectrometer for sensing the pH of the ground and river water	[146]
Diffuse tissue and rhodamine 6G dye	An SP-based visible-light spectrometer for the acquisition of a white light transmission spectrum through the diffuse tissue of a human finger and the acquisition of a fluorescence spectrum of rhodamine 6G dye	[15]
Drink powder	An SP spectrometer for determining the absorbance of a cherry-flavored drink powder	[147]
BSA	A G-Fresnel SP spectrometer for the determination of BSA concentration via the Bradford assay	[138]
Creatinine	An SP spectrometer for the determination of creatinine concentration in human urine in the linear range of 160 µM–1.6 mM	[148]

(continued)

Table 2.4 (continued)

Analytes detected	Bioanalytical application	Refs.
Paraoxon	An SP spectrometer for the detection of paraoxon in the range of 5 nM–25 μM with a LOD of 2.9 nM	[149]
Spectral analysis of apple	An optical fiber-based SP endoscopic spectrometer working in the visible-near infrared range for characterizing the changes in the pigment contents within an apple via absorption spectroscopy	[150]
BSA and IL-6	An SP multichannel spectrometer for the measurement of the protein concentration via the Bradford assay and the determination of the IL-6 biomarker concentration via an ELISA	[151]

IL-6, interleukin 6; Ara h1, *Arachis Hypogaea* (Peanut)

Another prospective device is the SP spectrophotometer developed using a G-Fresnel device, with a nanometer resolution in the visible range [138] (Fig. 2.15). The G-Fresnel is a dual-functionality diffractive optical element with low f-number that could simultaneously focus and disperse the incident light. The Fresnel lens side of the G-Fresnel collimates the light coming via the entrance slit, while the grating side of the G-Fresnel disperses the light. The use of the G-Fresnel critically reduces the size of the developed SP spectrophotometer attachment to $1.8 \times 0.8 \times 0.9$ in. The fabrication and working principle of G-Fresnel are described elsewhere [139]. The fabrication of the G-Fresnel involves sandwiching a PDMS prepolymer between the grating and the negative Fresnel lens molds and then curing it. The optical elements are placed in a 3D-printed SP attachment, which has slots to hold the G-Fresnel and the slit at pre-aligned positions. The SP attachment is secured to the SP case and then attached to the SP. The removing and reinstalling of the SP attachment cause only a negligible shift of alignment, thereby providing a compact and stable design. Moreover, the device could use an optical fiber or another light source. The device is used for the Bradford assay for the determination of various concentrations of BSA.

2.2.5 Lateral Flow Assay Readers

Various prospective SP-based lateral flow assay (LFA) readers have been demonstrated for several analytes based on LFA (Table 2.5). An SP-based lateral flow IA (LFIA) format is based on the signal detection at an optimized angle to maximize Mie scattering from a nitrocellulose membrane [18], resulting in maximal Rayleigh scattering from gold nanoparticles (Au NPs) in the LFIA bands. The LFIA is illuminated by the SP embedded flash via an optical fiber and a collimating lens. The quantitative detection of thyroid-stimulating hormone (TSH) by Mie scattering-optimized lateral flow assay (LFA) is demonstrated using an SP-POC device [7]. The developed method detects TSH with a LOD of 0.31 mIU L^{-1}, below the minimum TSH concentration (0.4 mIU L^{-1}) to be measured in case of hyperthyroidism.

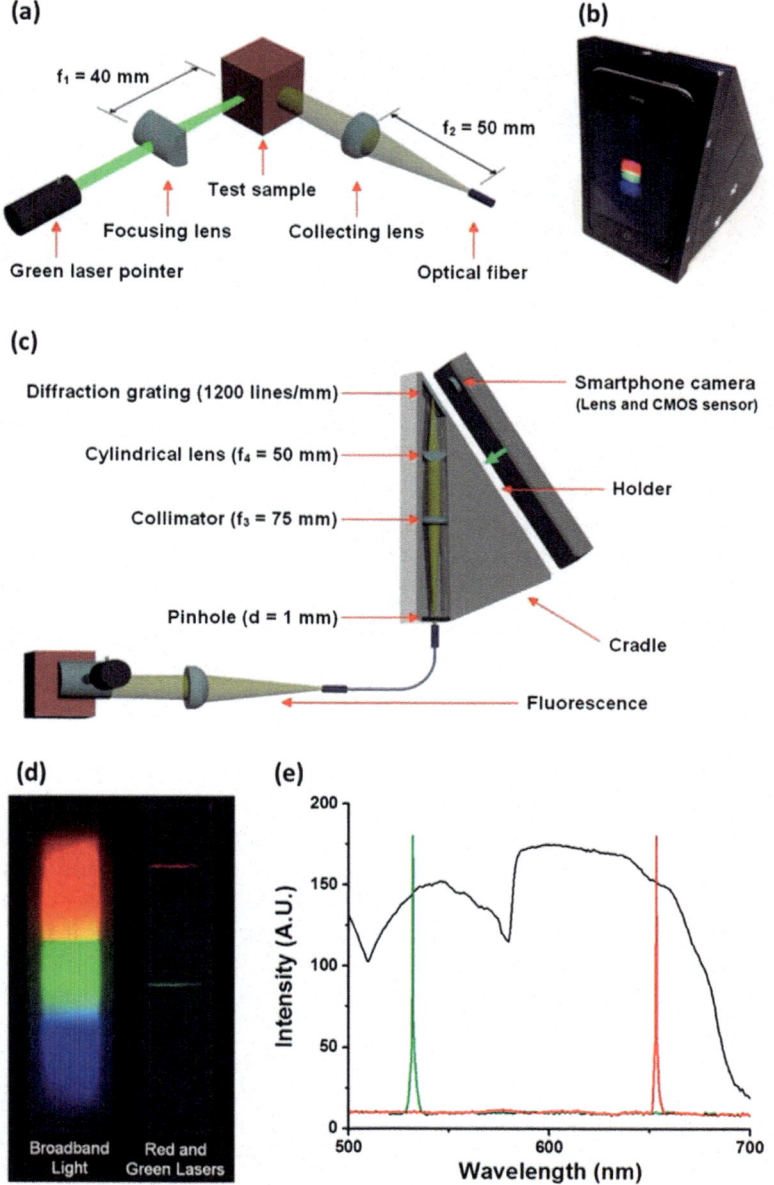

Fig. 2.13 A smartphone fluorimeter [105]. (**a**) The excitation laser (532 nm) illuminates a cuvette containing the probe-target duplexes. Fluorophores linked to one end of the molecular beacon probes are excited to emit fluorescence in all directions. A portion of the emission is gathered by a collecting lens oriented perpendicular to the laser and enters the cradle, where it is further collimated before incidence upon a diffraction grating placed in front of the camera. (**b**) An optical cradle installed on the smartphone. (**c**) The screen of the smartphone shows a spectrum of the transmitted light dispersed by the grating. (**d**) Images of broadband light, red and green laser beams. (**e**) Light intensity distributions of two lasers (solid green line with $\lambda_{green} = 532$ nm and solid red line with $\lambda_{red} = 653$ nm) and a broadband light source (solid black line) measured by the smartphone fluorimeter. Reproduced with permission from the American Chemical Society

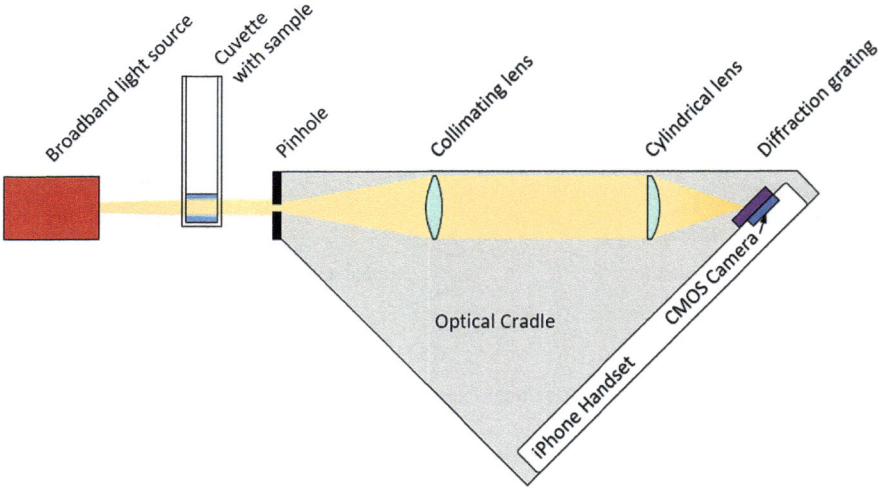

Fig. 2.14 A smartphone-based spectrophotometer for the absorbance readout of colorimetric ELISA [137]. A broadband light source illuminates a cuvette containing the colorimetric solution obtained after ELISA, which absorbs specific wavelengths in the visible range of 400–700 nm. The transmitted light emerging from the cuvette enters the custom-made optical cradle via a 0.1 mm diameter pinhole. It is then collimated, focused into a line, passed through a diffraction grating, and finally collected by the CMOS image sensor of the SP. Reproduced with permission from the OSA Publishing, The Optical Society

It detects TSH in human serum accurately with an error of less than 7% w.r.t. an established TSH clinical immunoassay. The Mie scattering from the nitrocellulose membrane of the LFA is minimized by employing optimized angles of incident light and detection from LFA bands. The minimized Mie scattering results in a high Rayleigh scattering detection from AuNPs embedded in the LFA strip. The integrated flash in the CP is used to illuminate the LFA strip via an optical fiber and a collimating lens. The CP-captured image is digitally processed on a PC using a MATLAB-based image analysis algorithm, which determines the quantified TSH concentration and displays it on the CP.

Cellmic (previously Holomic LLC) has developed various commercial SP-based POC readers for the readout of LFA, i.e., Holomic Rapid Diagnostic Test Reader (HRDR-200) and HRDR-300 [152] (Fig. 2.16). The prototype and working of the device concept used in HRDR-200 are available elsewhere [8]. HRDR-200, registered with FDA as a Class 1 medical device, is a compact, low-cost, and lightweight hand-held SP reader that is compliant with ISO 13485 and could be used either stand-alone or connected to a network. It reads chromatographic and fluorescent assays in various assay formats, i.e., lateral flow, flow-through, and dipstick. Moreover, tests of various sizes or formats, such as strips, cassettes, and multiplexed tests, could be also read. The device comprises an integrated reader housing and an SP, which comes together with a smart application and access to secure Cloud Services and Test Developer. HRDR-200 enables real-time diagnostic data integration with electronic health records

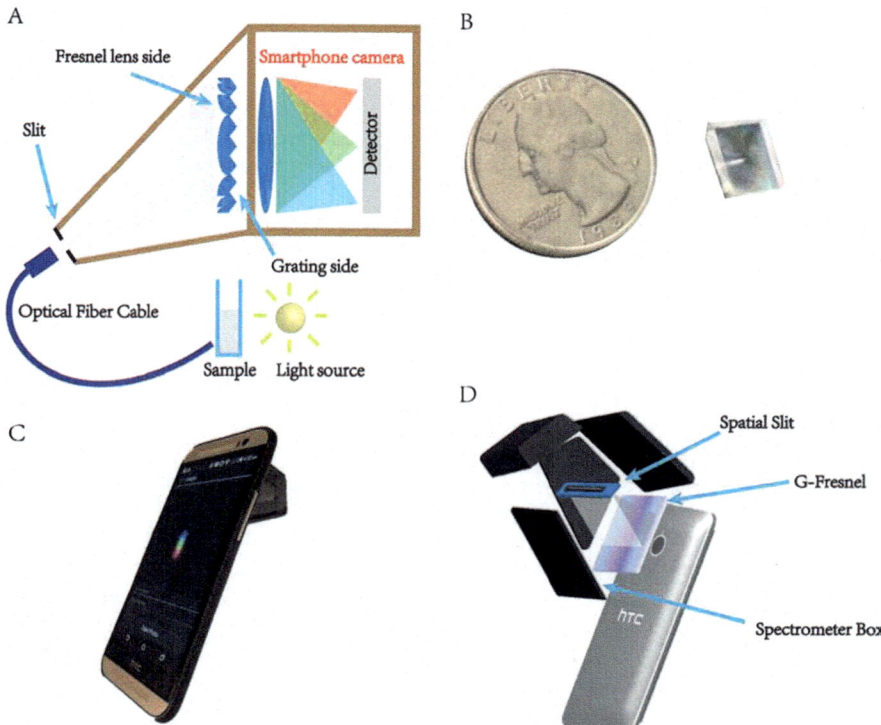

Fig. 2.15 An SP spectrophotometer developed using a G-Fresnel device [138]. (**A**) Schematic. (**B**) A photo of a transmission G-Fresnel device with a US quarter dollar coin. (**C**) Photograph of the device. (**D**) Schematic of the device with the exploded view. Reproduced with permission from the Royal Society of Chemistry

(EHRs), laboratory information system (LIS), and hospital information system (HIS) via a secure Cloud service. The device can be connected to laptops, PCs, printers, routers, and EHRs via wireless, Bluetooth, and USB. The integrated QR code scanner enables the automated identification of the test, lot number, and patient data along with the analysis of the lot expiry. A PC equipped with Test Explorer Software performs the analysis of the data obtained by the SP reader and e-mail, prints or texts the test results.

The company has also developed an SP-based fluorescent reader, i.e., HRDR-300 (Fig. 2.16B), which employs an advanced image processing algorithm for the multicolor imaging readout of the control and test lines of LFA. Cellmic could also customize the device for a particular multiplexed fluorescent assay that would require multiple excitation sources. The users can select the excitation in the range of 350–700 nm and the emission in the range of 300–800 nm. The rest of the device features is similar to that of HRDR-200. It is registered with the FDA as a Class I medical device and ISO 13485 compliant. Cellmic is also working on a new SP reader, namely, HRDR-400, a dual reader that could read chromatographic as well as fluorescent rapid tests in a single device.

Table 2.5 SP-based POC detection of LFA

Analytes detected	Bioanalytical application	Refs.
Salmonella and *E.coli O157*	A fluorescent LFIA detects *Salmonella* and *E. coli O157* with a LOD of 10^5 CFU/mL	[98]
Bile acid	An LFA mini-cartridge format-based luminescent IA detects total bile acid in serum and oral fluid with linearity and a LOD of 0.5–100 µM and 0.5 µM	[127]
Cholesterol	An LFA mini-cartridge format-based luminescent IA detects total cholesterol in serum with linearity and a LOD of 20–386 mg/dL and 20 mg/dL	[127]
Salivary cortisol	A chemiluminescent LFIA based on direct competitive IA format detects salivary cortisol [0.3–60 ng/mL] with an LOD of 0.3 ng/mL	[129]
Salivary cortisol	An LFA detects salivary cortisol [0.01–10 ng/mL] with an LOD of 0.01 ng/mL	[153]
Malaria, TB, HIV	An SP-based rapid diagnostic test reader detects malaria, TB, and HIV by lateral flow immune-chromatographic assays	[8]
TSH	An SP-based Rayleigh/Mie scatter optimized LFA detects TSH with a LOD of 0.31 mIU/L	[7]
AFB1	An LFIA based on a competitive binding format detects AFB1 in the linear range of 5–1000 µg/kg with a LOD of 5 µg/kg	[38]
Antibodies against HCV	A lateral electrophoretic flow assay based on fluorescence readout detects antibodies to HCV in serum in 60 min	[154]
ALP	A disposable lateral flow-through strip detects ALP in milk in the linear detection range of 0.1–150 U/L within 10 min	[155]
NT-proBNP	SP imaging detects NT-proBNP in the range of 60–3000 pg/mL using an LFA strip format in 12 min	[156]
Vitamin B_{12}	A competitive format-based LFA strip detects vitamin B_{12} in 15 min using just 40 µL of the finger prick blood	[157]

TSH thyroid-stimulating hormone, *AFB1* aflatoxin B1, *HCV* hepatitis C virus, *ALP* alkaline phosphatase activity, *NT-proBNP* N-terminal pro-B-type natriuretic peptide

(A)   **(B)**

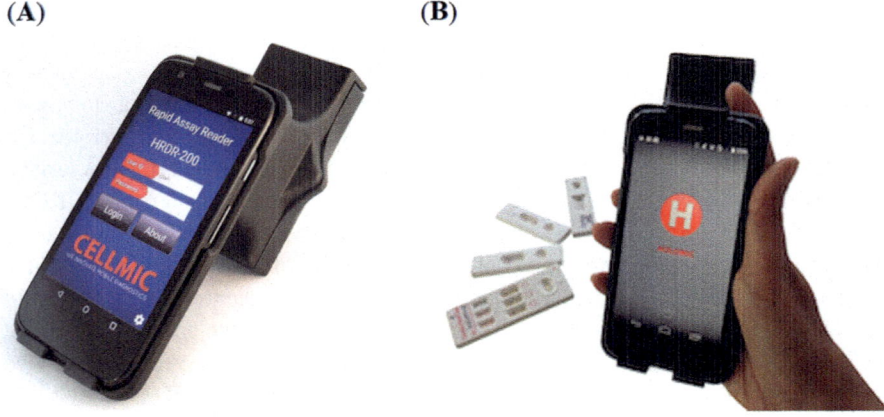

Fig. 2.16 SP-based POC readers for rapid diagnostic tests developed by Cellmic. (**A**) Holomic Rapid Diagnostic Test Reader (HRDR-200). (**B**) HRDR-300. Reproduced with permission from Cellmic

Similarly, a compact and lightweight (~65 g) SP-based universal rapid diagnostic test (RDT) reader [8] can read various LFIAs. The RDT reader has an inexpensive plano-convex lens, three LED arrays (two located underneath the RDT tray for reflection imaging and one at the top for transmission imaging), and a cost-effective microcontroller. The RDT reader is powered by external batteries or the SP battery via a USB connection and analyzes the sample in various types of LFIAs or RDTs in reflection or transmission imaging modes under diffused LED illumination. It provides highly accurate and repeatable digital evaluation of RDTs to differentiate even some minor color signal variation that is difficult to be quantified and assessed by the human eye.

The rapid diagnostic test (RDT) reader prototype [8] used for HRDR-200 is a compact and lightweight (~65 g) device comprising a plano-convex lens, a microcontroller, and three LED arrays. Two LED arrays are positioned underneath the RDT tray for the reflection imaging of RDT, while one LED array is located at the top for the transmission imaging of RDT. The device enables the quantitative determination of an analyte by reflection or transmission imaging modes of RDT under diffused LED illumination. It is powered by external batteries or the SP's internal battery via USB connection. The device exhibits high sensitivity as it detects the minor color signal variation, which could not be visualized. The raw images captured by the SP's camera are processed by a smart application in less than 0.2 s, and the results are shared with a central server that could be assessed by a remote computer using web browsers. A dynamic spatiotemporal map and real-time statistics of various diseases diagnosed by RDTs could also be provided by the smart application, which would be very useful to monitor, track, and analyze the emerging diseases and outbreaks.

Mobile Assay, Inc., developed a cost-effective SP-based LFA reader that employs mobile image ratiometry (MIR) for the quantification of rapid lateral flow test strips in less than 10 min. The appearance of two bands in the test strip occurs when there is no analyte in the sample as the dye would bind to the test as well as the control areas. The relative intensity of test band increases directly with the analyte concentration in the sample. The intensity of the test band is determined by MIR-based image analysis, where MIR subtracts the background noise, selects the test and control signal bands, and provides their pixel density ratio. The sample dispensed at the specified area on the test strip is taken together with the dye-conjugated antibodies, specific for the analyte to be detected, across the test and control areas. The company provides the Data Collection Module for the real-time transfer of data to the Mobile Assay Cloud™, which could be accessed locally and remotely. Moreover, the Tracker Manager™ enables the sending of text alerts to clients. The company demonstrated the use of their SP reader for the detection of drugs (e.g., cocaine and benzoylecgonine), food pathogens (e.g., *Botrytis cinerea*) [11], and aflatoxin. The SP reader and LFA detect cocaine and benzoylecgonine in the concentration range of 0.1–300 ng/mL and 0.003–0.1 ng/mL, respectively. It also detects *Botrytis cinerea*, a fungus causing significant damage to plants and flowers, which might prevent crop losses and lead to increased productivity. Further, it detects food pathogens and tracks the origin and severity of outbreaks, which would be useful to the food producers to take the desired measures to prevent the large-scale distribution of contaminated food products.

A colorimetric detection-based SP-IVD for 25-hydroxyvitamin D is based on an Au NP-based IA [41], the DNA sequences from Kaposi's sarcoma-associated herpes virus (KSHV) using a microfluidic chip and an NP-based colorimetric assay [52], and the total blood cholesterol using the CardioChek test strips [31]. An SP-based reader for one-dot LFIA using a competitive binding format was reported for aflatoxin B1 (AFB1) [38].

Biochemiluminescent detection-based SP-IVD using a lateral flow assay (LFA) mini-cartridge format has been developed for total bile acid [127], total cholesterol [127], and salivary cortisol [126]. A rapid diagnostic test reader (65 g) provides the readout of LFIAs for malaria, tuberculosis (TB), and human immunodeficiency virus (HIV) [8].

2.2.6   Electrochemical Detection

Table 2.6 shows a wide range of SP-based electrochemical detection devices for several bioanalytical applications. A compact SP-POC electrochemical biosensor [17] detects *Plasmodium falciparum* histidine-rich protein 2 (*Pf*HRP2) in human serum in just 15 min with a LOD of 16 ng mL^{-1} and detection in the range of 4–1024 ng mL^{-1}. It has good specificity as it selectively detects the purified *Pf*HRP2 recombinant protein in the presence of five non-specific target proteins that are used at 1 µg mL^{-1}. The procedure employs just two loading steps for sample and reporter (*Pf*HRP2 detection antibodies conjugated to horseradish peroxidase) solutions. It employs a compact embedded circuit for signal processing and data analysis and a disposable SIM card-size microfluidic chip (25 mm × 15 mm) for fluidic handling and sensing. A smart application provides step-by-step instructions on the screen to the user for performing the measurement. The results are displayed on the SP's screen after each measurement and stored in the SP's memory for subsequent data transmission and analysis. A pipette is used to load the sample, which is subsequently driven by a flow capillary. The modified PDMS surface coating of the microfluidic chip facilitates the autonomous capillary-driven flow with a constant flow rate. There are two inlets and one outlet of 1 mm diameter in the microfluidic chip. The appropriate volumes of sample (0.5 µL) and reporter (2 µL) solutions are mixed in a 2 mm chamber before they enter into a zig-zag mixer having serpentine channels with a spacing of 40 µm. The serpentine channels maintain a uniform flow of sample-reporter mixture over the electrochemical sensor, while a secondary serpentine channel (25 cm long, 400 µm wide, and 100 µm high) acts as a capillary pump and a waste reservoir. The sensor chip accommodates the tetramethylbenzidine/hydrogen peroxide (TMB/H$_2$O$_2$) substrate for washing and subsequent enzymatic reaction for amperometric measurement. The anti-*Pf*HRP2 capture antibodies are bound uniformly to the polypyrrole-coated gold electrode surface. If there is no *Pf*HRP2 in the sample, the detection anti-*Pf*HRP2 antibodies cannot bind to the electrode and are thus washed away when the TMB/H$_2$O$_2$substrate is loaded. But the detection antibodies bind to the electrode in the presence of *Pf*HRP2, which results

Table 2.6 SP-based POC technologies for electrochemical detection

Analytes detected	Bioanalytical application	Refs.
*Pf*HRP2	Detects *Pf*HRP2 biomarker for malaria in 15 min with a LOD of 16 ng/mL using a compact embedded circuit, disposable microfluidic chip, and capillary flow	[17]
iHealth Wireless Smart Gluco-Monitoring System	Detects pathophysiological blood glucose concentrations using a miniaturized glucometer interfaced with SP via a smart application	[158]
Nitrate	An audio jack-based electrochemical sensor detects nitrate in water with a LOD of 0.2 ppm and a linear detection range of 1.4–70 ppm within 1 min	[20]
Glucose, *Pf*HRP2, sodium, and trace heavy metals (Pb, Cd, Zn)	A universal SP electrochemical biosensor for glucose in blood (linear range, 50–500 mg/dL); *Pf*HRP2 in clinical sample (linear range, 0–150 ng/mL, LOD 20 ng/mL); sodium in urine; and trace heavy metals (Pb, Cd, Zn) in water (linear range, 4–40 μg/L, LOD = 4 μg/L)	[159]
TNT	An SP-based biosensor using disposable SPE modified with TNT-specific peptides as biosensing element detects TNT as low as 10^{-6} M in 120 s by impedimetric measurement	[160]
E.coli cells	An SP sensor based on electrical impedance spectroscopy employs a microfluidics procedure for the pre-concentration of the bacteria and detects *E.coli* cells in the dynamic range of 10–1000 cells/mL with a LOD of 10 cells/mL	[161]
Potassium ferro-/ferricyanide	A cost-effective SP-based electrochemical biosensor, using a low-power potentiostat that interfaces and harvests power from the audio jack of the SP, is used for cyclic voltammetry experiments using potassium ferro-/ferricyanide	[162]
DBAE and L-Proline	An SP potentiostat using the audio jack of the SP for supplying potential and a low-cost $Ru(bpy)_3^{2+}$-loaded paper-based microfluidic sensor detects DBAE and L-proline. The linear detection range for DBAE is 0.1–5 mM with a LOD of 100 μM, while the linear detection range and a LOD for L-proline are 0.1–10 mM and 100 μM, respectively	[163]
BSA and thrombin	An SP electrochemical biosensor using antibodies and peptides immobilized printed carbon electrodes for the detection of BSA and thrombin as low as 1.78 μg/mL and 2.97 μg/mL, respectively	[164]
SLPI	An efficient power harvesting SP-based electrochemical biosensor, consuming only 6.9 MW peak power and measuring <1 nA bidirectional current, detects SLPI with a LOD of 1 nM using disposable SPEs coated with antihuman SLPI and a sandwich IA	[165]
HCV	An SP-based electrochemical biosensor, using genetically engineered yeast cell lines with displayed HCV core antigen linked to GBP, detects anti-HCV core antibody by immunefluorescent and electrochemical assays The dynamic range and LOD of the immunefluorescent assay are 30 pM–3 nM and 12.3 pM, respectively. The electrochemical assay has a dynamic range of 4–250 nM and a LOD of 2 nM	[166]

(continued)

Table 2.6 (continued)

Analytes detected	Bioanalytical application	Refs.
Honey	An SP-based electrochemical platform, using a custom-made potentiostat and an Android smart application for multivariate data processing, is applicable for the fingerprinting of Brazilian honey samples according to their botanical and geographical origins	[167]
Glucose	An SP-based cyclic voltammetry, using reduced graphene oxide modified SPEs and APBA, detects glucose with a LOD of 0.026 mM	[168]
ERα	A fully disposable microfluidic electrochemical array device, with the working electrodes modified with DNA sequences specific for the binding of ERα, and paramagnetic particles bound to anti-ERα antibody and HRP, detects ERα with a LOD of 10 fg/mL. It detects ERα in calf serum in the range of 16.6–513.3 fg/mL and showed good recoveries for the determination of ERα in MCF-7 cell lysate	[169]

*Pf*HRP2, *Plasmodium falciparum* histidine-rich protein 2; TNT, 2,4,6-trinitrotoluene; DBAE, 2-(dibutylamino)ethanol; SLPI, secretory leukocyte protease inhibitor; SPEs, screen-printed electrodes; HCV, hepatitis C core antibody; GBP, gold-binding peptide; APBA, 3-amino phenylboronic acid; ERα, estrogen receptor alpha

in an electrochemical current that is proportional to the *Pf*HRP2 concentration when the electrode is poised at a fixed potential.

Similarly, iHealth Lab [158] has developed two prominent blood glucose meters for the electrochemical detection of glucose: Wireless Smart Gluco-Monitoring System and iHealth Align, which are Food and Drug Administration (FDA) approved, Conformité Européenne (CE) compliant, and meet the ISO 15197:2003 in vitro blood glucose monitoring requirements. The iHealth Gluco, a free smart application for iOS and Android stores, is required for the operation of these devices. The smart application is personalized as it requires the users to log in to their iHealth account using their specific details.

The iHealth Align is the world's smallest blood glucose meter that plugs directly into the headphone jack of the SP and is connected to the SP by Bluetooth. It detects the entire pathophysiological range of blood glucose in diabetics, i.e., 1.1–33.3 M in just 5 s using a conventional amperometric detection method based on glucose oxidase. The procedure involves the finger pricking so that 0.7 µL of fresh capillary whole blood is loaded onto the test strip plugged into the iHealth Align. The blood glucose measurements are shown on the SP screen and stored securely inside the iHealth Gluco-Smart application, which allows users to view the trend and statistics of their blood glucose measurements for up to 90 days. Moreover, the smart app automatically determines the remaining test strips in the vial along with their expiry date to issue alerts to the users for buying a new vial. The app allows users to add notes to their stored readings, record pre- and post-meal glucose, and set up reminders for medication and insulin dosages. Moreover, it allows the users to share their measurements with their friends, family members, caregivers, and doctors.

The Wireless Smart Gluco-Monitoring System [158] is a stand-alone next-generation glucose monitoring device for diabetic monitoring and management, which is powered by a built-in, rechargeable battery, and has a light-emitting diode (LED) display. The device is interfaced with the smartphone via the Bluetooth and

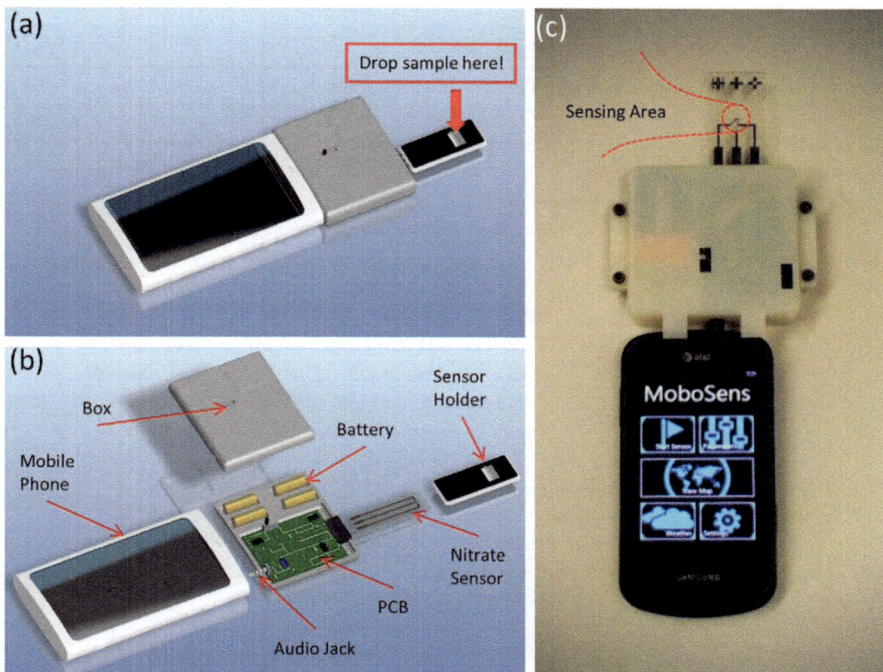

Fig. 2.17 (**a**) An assembly view of an audio jack-based electrochemical sensor, MoboSens, for the detection of nitrate concentration in water. (**b**) Detailed components of MoboSens. (**c**) Actual photograph of the complete MoboSens system. Reproduced with permission from Elsevier BV

the smart app. It could store up to 500 blood glucose test results, track the progress of the results, and set up medication alerts. Moreover, it also automatically warns the user in case of the test strip expiry, to prevent potential false evaluation.

An audio jack-based miniaturized SP electrochemical sensing platform (~65 g) has also been demonstrated for analysis of nitrate in field water samples [20] (Fig. 2.17). It comprises a microfabricated three-electrode sensor, a smart application, and a circuit board to drive with the sensor.

2.2.7 Microscopy

Various prospective SP-based lateral flow assay (LFA) readers have been demonstrated for the detection of several analytes based on LFA (Table 2.7). A low-cost CP-mounted light microscope, using LED-based excitation, was developed and used for the bright-field imaging of *P. falciparum*-infected and sickle red blood cells (RBC) and the fluorescence imaging of *M. tuberculosis*-infected sputum samples [16]. Of interest is the development of CP-based optical microscope and visible-light spectrophotometer [15]. The CP microscope enables transmission and

Table 2.7 SP-based POC microscopes

Analytes detected	Bioanalytical application	Refs.
M. tuberculosis	An SP-based fluorescent microscope detects *M. tuberculosis* bacilli in auramine O-stained sputum smears	[16]
Salmonella typhimurium DNA	An SP-based fluorescent microscope and a paper microfluidics-based assay for detecting *S. typhimurium* down to 10^4 CFU/mL	[100]
Single NPs and viruses	An SP-based fluorescent microscope for the detection of isolated 100 nM fluorescent NPs and human cytomegaloviruses	[104]
Single DNA strands	An SP-based microscope enabled the imaging and determination of length of DNA strands over a FOV of ~2 mm^2	[173]
WBCs *Giardia lamblia* cysts	An SP-based fluorescent microscope for the imaging of labeled WBCs in whole blood and waterborne pathogenic *Giardia lamblia* cysts with a resolution of ~10 μm and FOV of ~81 mm^2	[106]
Giardia lamblia cysts	An SP-based fluorescent microscope with machine learning detects and quantifies *Giardia lamblia* cysts with a LOD of 12 cysts per 10 mL	[172]
Blood smears and diffuse tissue	An SP-based microscope for the imaging of stained and unstained blood smears and an SP-based spectrometer for the transmission and fluorescence spectroscopy of diffuse tissue	[15]
Blood smears containing granulocytes and RBCs	An SP-based microscope for the imaging of Wright-stained blood smear containing granulocytes and RBCs	[174]
Colonic mucosa and lymphoma	Various commercial SP-based adapters for microscopy for the imaging of colonic mucosa and lymphoma	[175]
RBCs and WBCs	An SP-based microscope employing glass-based tapered fiber-optic array for the multi-frame contact imaging of RBCs and WBCs in transmission mode	[171]
Microparticles, skin tissue, and a resolution test target	An SP-based lens-free dual-mode holographic microscope, which can image specimens in transmission and reflection modes, is useful for the imaging of microparticles, a histopathology slide of skin tissue, and a US Air Force resolution test target	[176]
P. falciparum-infected and sickle RBCs	A smartphone-based microscope for the bright-field imaging of *P. falciparum*-infected and sickle RBCs in blood smears	[16]
In situ, dual-mode monitoring of OOC	An SP-based fluorescence microscope for the monitoring of fluorescence NP IA into an OOC enabled monitoring of drug-induced nephrotoxicity in situ	[117]
Semen analysis	An automated SP-based diagnostic assay using an innovative microfluidic device for the POC semen analysis in unwashed, unprocessed liquefied semen sample in less than 5 s with an accuracy of ~98%	[177]

OOC organ-on-a-chip

polarized microscopy with a resolution of ~1.5 μm over an imaging FOV of ~150 μm × 150 μm, while the CP spectrophotometer has a bandwidth of 300 nm with a spectral resolution of ~5 nm.

Prof. Ozcan's group at UCLA developed various low-cost, compact, and lightweight CP microscopes using partially coherent lens-free digital in-line holography.

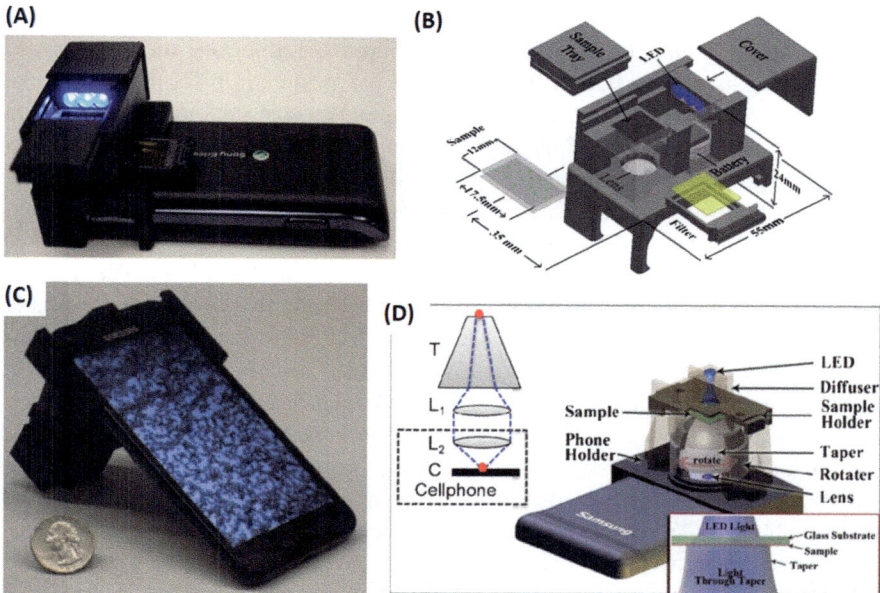

Fig. 2.18 (**A**) An SP-based POC device for wide-field fluorescent and dark-field imaging and (**B**) its schematic [106]. Reproduced with permission from The Royal Society of Chemistry. (**C**) SP-based contact microscopy platform and (**D**) its schematic [171]. Reproduced with permission from The Royal Society of Chemistry

Initially, the group developed a USB-powered stand-alone portable microscope that weighed just ~46 g [12]. This prototype involved the illumination of the sample, loaded on a sample tray on the side of the microscope, using a single LED and a large pinhole of ~100 μm in front of it. A CP-based fluorescent and dark-field microscope was demonstrated using a compact (~28 g) and low-cost optomechanical attachment for a CP that employs battery-powered butt-coupled LEDs to illuminate the loaded target sample in a cuvette [106] (Fig. 2.18a, b). The sample in the cuvette acts as an optofluidic waveguide that enables uniform sample excitation. The fluorescent imaging is done by the CP via an additional lens, i.e., a plastic color filter in front of the CP's camera, which filters the specific fluorescent emission of the target sample. However, the plastic color filter is not used for dark-field microscopy. The CP microscope imaged the waterborne parasites in drinking water and the labeled white blood cells (WBCs) in whole blood samples. Further, an inexpensive CP microscope was developed using a simple and lightweight (~38 g) optomechanical attachment that is installed at the back of the CP's camera [170]. The sample is illuminated using a battery-powered LED via a large pinhole, while the CMOS imager chip in the CP's camera is used to capture the lens-free holographic images of the samples. The procedure involves the interaction of spatially filtered LED light with the sample, which creates holographic signatures of individual particles/cells that are captured by a complementary metal-oxide semiconductor (CMOS) imager chip in the CP's camera. The lens-free holograms, formed by the interference between the unscattered background light and the scattered object fields, are processed instantaneously using custom holographic reconstruction algorithms that provide amplitude and phase images of the samples. The CP microscope was used for the imaging of white blood cells (WBCs), red blood cells (RBCs), platelets, waterborne parasites, and microparticles. The lens-free holographic on-chip microscopy has much wider FOV that could easily reach >20–30 mm^2 as the entire active imaging area of the imaging sensor could be used as the object FOV. The microscopy approach was improved further by the same group by developing a portable lens-free pixel super-resolution microscope, which demonstrated submicron resolution over the same imaging FOV, i.e., ~24 mm^2 [13].

In another approach, a contact microscopic platform (76 g) was developed employing a glass-based tapered fiber array illuminated by a LED (Fig. 2.18c, d) [171]. It was used for the imaging of highly dense samples in the transmission mode with 3× magnification in each direction, which is followed by the projection of the image on the CMOS sensor of the SP using two lenses. The resolution of the captured image is improved, and spatial artifacts are obviated by employing a "shift and add" algorithm for the digital fusion of multi-frame images.

An SP-based POC device for fluorescence microscopy employing a portable (~186 g) optomechanical attachment was developed and used for the imaging of 100 nm fluorescent polystyrene beads and individual human cytomegaloviruses [104] (Fig. 2.19). It comprises a high-power compact laser diode (450 nm, 75 mW); a long-pass thin-film interference filter (blocking wavelength of 500 nm and sharp transmission slope) to reject the scattered excitation light; an external lens with a low numerical aperture to have 2× optical magnification lens; and a coarse mechanical translation stage for focus adjustment. The compact laser diode creates oblique excitation on the sample plane with a high incidence angle of ~75°. The excitation laser beam has a small spot size of ~1.8 mm in diameter. The use of a high-power laser diode as the excitation source enhanced the fluorescence emission, while the use of a thin-film interference filter and a high illumination angle suppressed the background noise, thereby providing critically improved signal-to-noise ratio.

Two SP attachments were developed to transform an SP into a 350× microscope and a visible-light spectrophotometer [15]. Of notice is a 78 g smartphone-based contact microscopy platform using a glass-based tapered fiber-optic array and multi-frame imaging [171] for RBCs and WBCs (Fig. 2.4e, f). Another development is an SP-based high-resolution microscope for bright-field imaging of *P. falciparum*-infected and sickle RBCs in blood smears [16].

A compact and lightweight (~205 g) SP-based fluorescent microscope with FOV of ~0.8 cm^2 was attempted for the detection of *Giardia lamblia* cysts [172]. It employs an optomechanical attachment coupled to an SP, which detects *Giardia lamblia* cysts in disposable water sample cassettes, comprising absorbent pads and mechanical filter membranes, with LOD of ~12 cysts per 10 mL. Similarly, the detection of *M. tuberculosis* bacilli in auramine O-stained sputum smears [16] by an

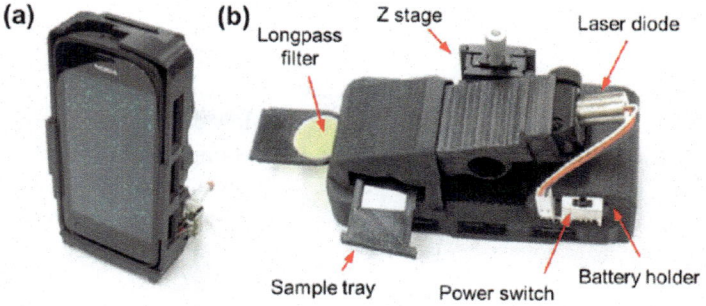

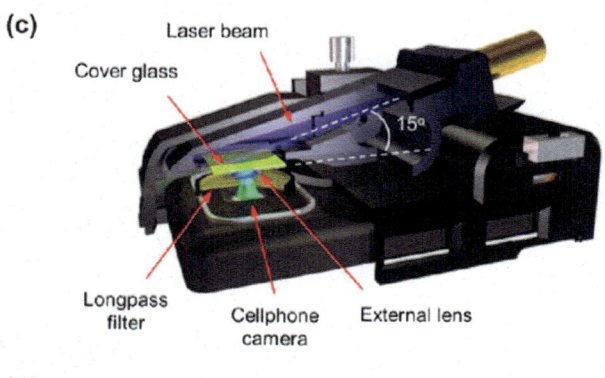

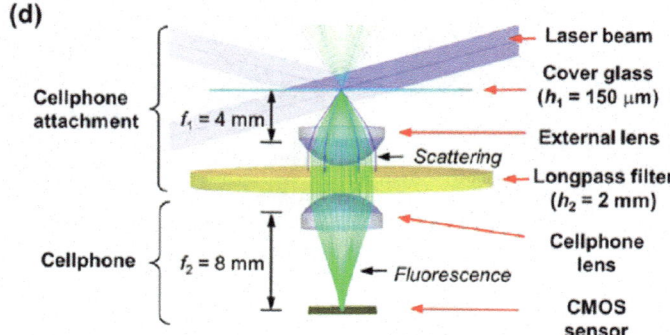

Fig. 2.19 An SP-based fluorescent microscope [104]. Photographs (**a**) Front view and (**b**) back view. The SP screen in (**a**) shows the fluorescent image of 1 μm diameter green fluorescent beads. (**c**) Schematic view. (**d**) Ray-tracing diagram. The excitation and scattered beams are shown as solid blue rays, while the fluorescent emission is indicated with solid green rays. Reproduced with permission from the American Chemical Society

SP-based POC fluorescent microscope has also been demonstrated. Further, a compact and lightweight SP-based fluorescent microscope was developed and used for imaging and sizing of single DNA molecules of λ and T7 bacteriophages [173] with sizing accuracy of <1 kb-pairs over a FOV of ~2 mm^2.

2.2.8   Cytometry

Table 2.8 shows various prospective SP-based lateral flow assay (LFA) readers for several analytes based on LFA. An SP-based POC flow cytometer employs optofluidic fluorescent imaging for the analysis of large sample volumes of more than 0.1 mL [13]. The device comprises a compact, lightweight (~18 g), and low-cost optomechanical SP attachment, which employs very low-cost components: an inexpensive lens, a plastic color filter (~0.1 USD), two LEDs (~0.6 USD), and coin cell batteries (cost ~0.5 USD). A syringe pump facilitates the continuous delivery of the sample to the imaging volume via a disposable microfluidic channel that acts as a multilayered optofluidic waveguide (Fig. 2.20). The plastic absorption filter creates

Table 2.8 SP-based POC cytometers

Analytes detected	Bioanalytical application	Refs.
Optofluidic fluorescent imaging-based flow cytometer	A compact, lightweight, and cost-effective SP-based flow cytometer with a fluorescent resolution of ~2 μm and capability to analyze samples >0.1 mL	[27]
RBCs, WBCs, and Hb	Determines the density of RBCs, WBCs, and Hb in blood using just 10 μL sample	[14]

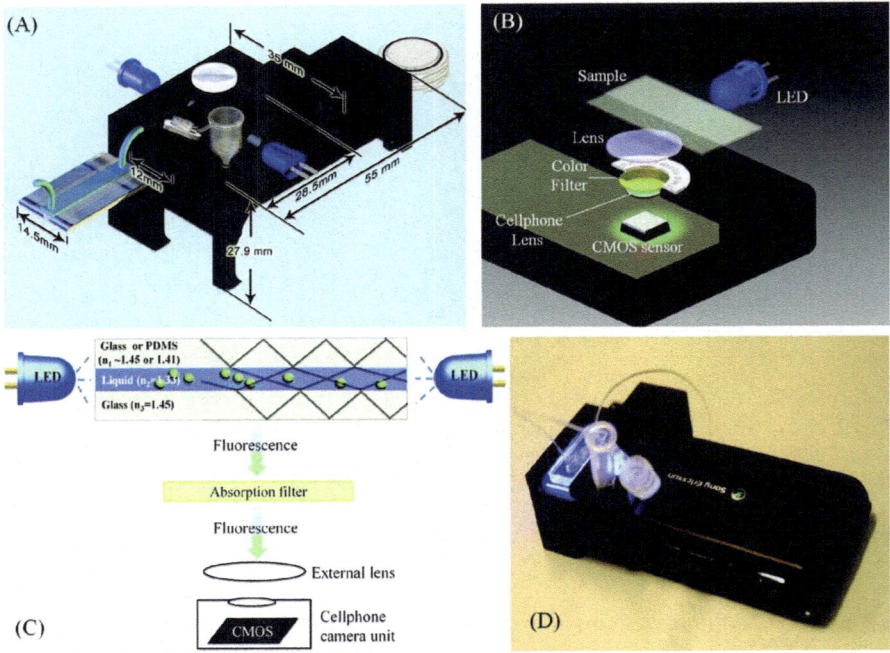

Fig. 2.20 A CP-based POC flow cytometer [27]. (**A–C**) Schematics of the optical attachment for optofluidic fluorescent imaging cytometry on a CP, which can be repeatedly attached or detached to the CP body without the need for fine alignment. (**D**) Actual CP-based optofluidic fluorescent imaging cytometer. Reproduced with permission from the American Chemical Society

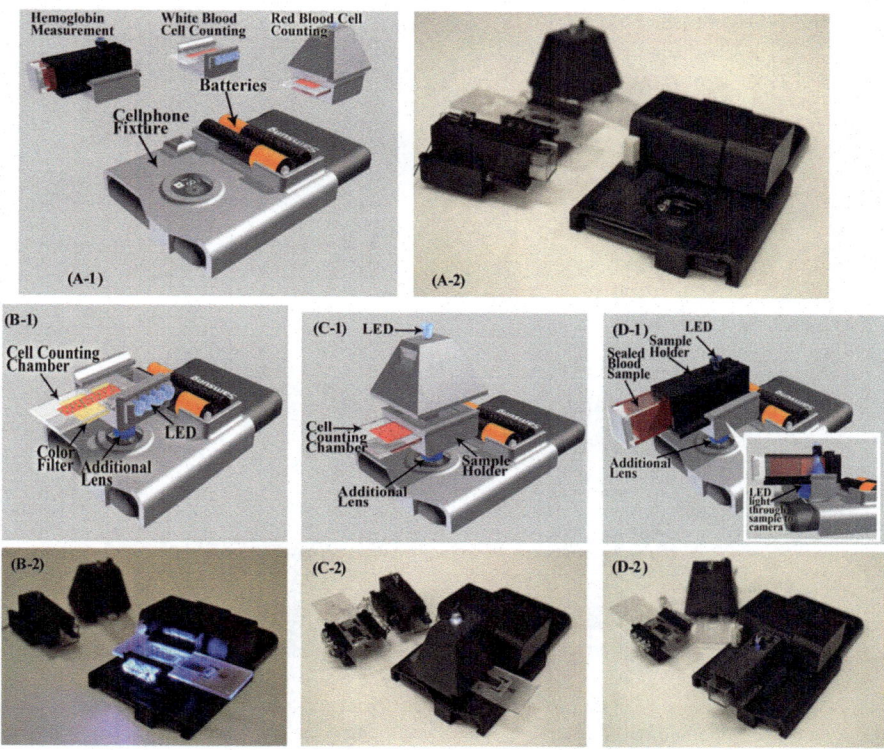

Fig. 2.21 An SP-based POC cytometry platform [14]. (**A**-1) and (**A**-2) Illustration and picture of SP-based blood analysis platform comprising of a base attachment with two AA batteries and a universal port for adopting three different add-on components for WBC counting, RBC counting, and hemoglobin (Hb) measurements. (**B**-1) and (**B**-2) Illustration and picture of the WBC counting device. (**C**-1) and (**C**-2) Illustration and picture of the RBC counting device. (**D**-1) and (**D**-2) Illustration and picture of Hb measurement device. Reproduced with permission from the Royal Society of Chemistry

the dark-field background because the guided excitation light propagates perpendicular to the detection path. The cell count and density are determined by recording and processing the cell movement through the microfluidic channel. The device has a fluorescence resolution of ~2 μm, which is appropriate for whole blood analysis and screening of waterborne parasites.

A further miniaturized and low-cost SP imaging-based cytometry device and a smart application were developed by the same group for rapid blood analysis using only ~10 μL of the sample [106] (Fig. 2.21). It determines the density of RBCs and WBCs by imaging them in bright-field and fluorescent modes apart from simultaneously determining the hemoglobin (Hb) concentration in human blood samples. The universal base of the device is attached to the CP's camera unit and three "add-on" components for WBC/RBC counting and hemoglobin (Hb) density measurement. The desired "add-on" components can be clicked into the same port on the base

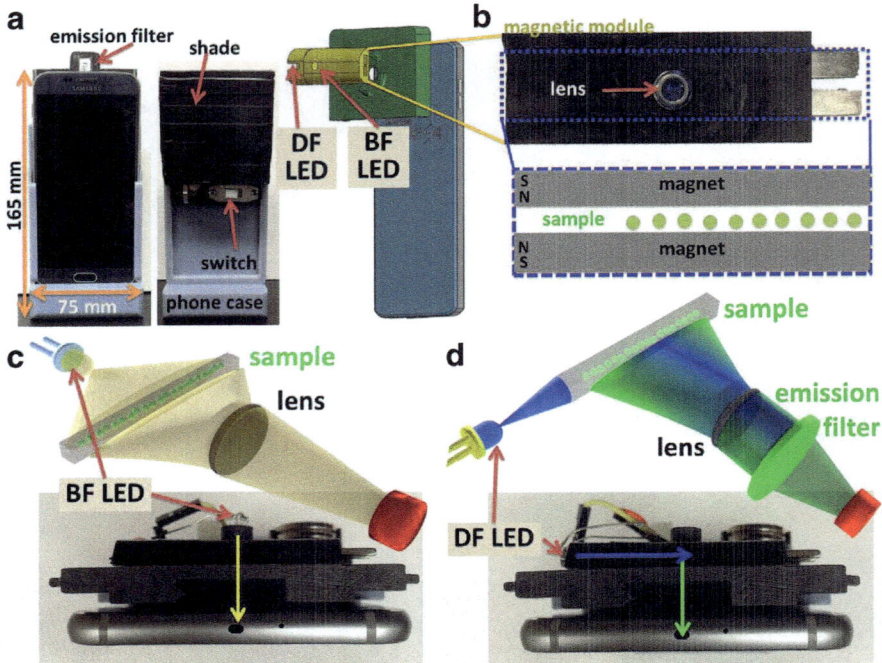

Fig. 2.22 An SP-based device for cytometry [125]. (**a**) Front and back views of the SP-based fluorescence microscope without the shade to show components such as an emission filter, a phone case, and an optical component. The optical component pictured in the back view includes LED locations for both bright-field (BF) and dark-field (DF) configurations, magnets, a switch, and batteries. At the right is a back view of the SP-based fluorescence microscope with the shade on, depicting the dark-field configuration. The inlay shows the magnetic focusing piece of the optical component including lens, magnets, and sample. (**b**) Schematic (top) of light path in bright-field imaging configuration, with a top view of the microscope (bottom) to show the simplified light path in the setup. (**c**) Schematic (top) of light path in dark-field imaging configuration for a sample excited by blue light and emitting green light. A top view of the microscope (bottom) shows a simplified light path in the setup. (**d**) Reproduced with permission from the Royal Society of Chemistry

attachment to perform the measurements via the smart application running on the CP. The analytical performance of the SP device was comparable to that of a standard benchtop Sysmex KN21 hematology analyzer.

Figure 2.22 shows a prospective SP-based device for cytometry for density-based cell separation using two permanent magnets and employs fluorescence microscopic imaging for multiplex detection [125]. Being low-cost (~100 USD), compact, and portable, it could be employed for cell sorting and imaging of cells in dark-field, bright-field, or fluorescent modes. The combination of magnetic focusing and fluorescence microscopy in a single device would lead to prospective POC applications. The SP attachment, comprising an SP case, emission filter folders, a two-piece optical component and a shade, is fabricated by 3D printing. The device employs SP back camera (Samsung Galaxy S6) for high-resolution imaging and the dark-field configuration for desired reproducible imaging by avoiding the need for expensive components such as a dichroic mirror. The excitation of the sample is done by low-cost LEDs (powered by two 3 V batteries), while an emission filter takes out the undesired light. The magnetic focusing using two permanent magnets focuses microparticles into the focal plane of the SP camera for density-based cell separation. The SP-captured images via Camera FV-5 application are analyzed by Image J to determine the fluorescent pixel intensity. As the SP attachment has modular components that could be easily exchanged, the LEDs, emission filters, and other components are easily exchanged as desired for a particular application. Each use of the device requires a microcapillary tube and sample preparation in paramagnetic solution. The device is applicable for the imaging of microspheres of different sizes (5.35–79 μm) using both transmitted light for bright-field imaging and reflected light for dark-field imaging. The fluorescence is studied using red-, green-, and blue-colored fluorescent microspheres, where each type of microsphere is imaged with no, red, green, and blue emission filters. The device is also used for the fluorescent imaging of breast cancer cells stained with calcein, a green cytoplasmic stain, using blue LED for excitation and green emission filters. The fluorescent imaging of prostate cancer cells stained with QTracker 625, a red cytoplasmic stain, was also demonstrated using blue LED for excitation and red emission filters. The limits of cell counting and cell detection are determined using ovarian cancer cells stained with calcein. Moreover, the device was also employed to analyze the differences in two cell populations, i.e., QTracker 625-stained HeyA8 cells and calcein-stained HeyA8 cells. It was also used to evaluate the use of acridine orange for the identification of cells as cancer cells fluorescence redder than other cells due to high replication rate. Acridine red stains single-stranded RNA fluorescence red and double-stranded DNA fluorescence green.

2.2.9 Surface Plasmon Resonance Detection

Various prospective SP-based lateral flow assay (LFA) readers have been demonstrated for the detection of several analytes based on LFA (Table 2.9). An angle-resolved SPR-based SP device [25] was demonstrated based on the gentle attachment of a disposable SPR coupler to the SP screen and the optical detection of the SPR signal by the SP's front camera. A red triangle displayed on the SP screen acts as a light source, while a white frame guides the placement of the SPR coupler on the screen. The controlled illumination provided by the CP's display provides the wide-angle illumination for angle-resolved SPR. The Au-coated glass on top of the SPR coupler serves as the sensing surface. The SPR coupler is made up of polydimethylsiloxane (PDMS) prism and epoxy and has a refractive index of 1.5 same as that of glass. The PDMS plano-cylindrical element collects the illumination from the red triangle and directs it to the Au interface to reflect the light containing the angle-resolved SPR signal. The reflected light is steered by total internal reflection inside a PDMS prism to the SP's front camera. The custom-made SPR chip has three

Table 2.9 SP-based POC SPR detection

Analytes detected	Bioanalytical application	Refs.
β2M	An angle-resolved SPR detection system based on a single disposable device detects β2M with a LOD of 0.1 µg/mL	[25]
Glycerol	A fiber-optic SPR sensor detected various volume concentrations of glycerol, i.e., 0–20% with a sensitivity of 1.83×10^{-3} RIU/pixel	[178]
Bovine IgG	A fiber-optic SPR biosensor detected various concentrations of bovine IgG with a LOD of 47.4 nM	[179]
Imidacloprid	An SPR biosensor detects imidacloprid pesticide with a LOD of 1 ppb by an indirect competitive IA	[180]
BSA and trypsin	An LSPR platform-based biosensor detects BSA and trypsin with a LOD of 19.2 µg/mL and 25.7 µg/mL, respectively	[181]
CEA and ATP	An LSPR platform-based sensor detects CEA and ATP by IA and aptamer-based assay, respectively. It detects CEA in the range of 16–512 pg/mL with a LOD of 6.1 pg/mL, while it determines ATP in the linear detection range of 20–320 µM with a LOD of 11 µM	[182]
Mouse IgG	An SPRi platform using low-cost disposable SPR substrates detects mouse IgG antibodies in the range of 1.33–830 nM with a LOD in nM level	[183]
Liposaccharides	An SP-based grating-coupled SPR biosensor detects lipopolysaccharides in routine clinical injectable fluids in the range of 50 ng/mL–1 µg/mL with a LOD of 32.5 ng/mL	[184]

β2M β_2 microglobulin, *LSPR* localized surface plasmon resonance, *CEA* carcinoembryonic antigen, *ATP* adenosine triphosphate

channels: two calibration channels for high and low concentrations and the test channel. An iOS-based smart application controls the camera exposure, i.e., exposure time and ISO number (sensitivity), which provides reproducible image acquisition under identical conditions. The device detects β_2 microglobulin (β_2M), a biomarker for cancer, kidney disease, and inflammatory disorders, in the desired pathophysiological range with a LOD of 0.1 µg/mL [25]. The SPR-based detection of β_2M was demonstrated using a commercial Biacore sensor chip CM5 and a custom-made chip that was bound to monoclonal mouse-antihuman β_2M.

2.3 Conclusions

SP-based POC technologies, based on different detection schemes, have been advocated for numerous bioanalytical applications. These devices with advanced features are paving the way for the next generation of POC devices to be deployed at home, office, remote locations, physician office lab, and decentralized settings. The trend inclines to the fabrication of low-cost and compact SP-based devices as mobile healthcare tools to speed up the outreach of healthcare in the developing countries with scarce resources. The analytical performance of most updated SP-based POC devices is comparable to that of costly and bulky lab-based instruments. Doubtlessly, the continuously improving features of the SP (camera, processor, storage, security, and other technology features), Cloud computing, smart applications, and data storage and security, would further enhance the performance and capabilities of SP-based POC devices in the near future. The advancement in complementary technologies, such as lab-on-a-chip-based integrated microfluidic platforms, simple assay procedures, novel biosensor concepts, and prolonged reagent storage strategies, would further lead to highly innovative bioanalytical applications based on the SP-based POC signal detection.

References

1. Measuring the information Society Report. 2017. https://www.itu.int/en/ITU-D/Statistics/Pages/publications/mis2017.aspx.
2. Vashist SK, Mudanyali O, Schneider EM, Zengerle R, Ozcan A. Cellphone-based devices for bioanalytical sciences. Anal Bioanal Chem. 2014;406(14):3263–77.
3. Vashist SK, Luppa PB, Yeo LY, Ozcan A, Luong JHT. Emerging technologies for next-generation point-of-care testing. Trends Biotechnol. 2015;33(11):692–705.
4. Vashist SK, Luong JHT. Smartphone-based immunoassays. Handbook of immunoassay technologies. Elsevier; 2018. p. 433–53. ISBN: 9780128117620.
5. Ozcan A. Mobile phones democratize and cultivate next-generation imaging, diagnostics and measurement tools. Lab Chip. 2014;14(17):3187–94.
6. Erickson D, O'Dell D, Jiang L, Oncescu V, Gumus A, Lee S, et al. Smartphone technology can be transformative to the deployment of lab-on-chip diagnostics. Lab Chip. 2014;14(17):3159–64.
7. You DJ, Park TS, Yoon JY. Cell-phone-based measurement of TSH using Mie scatter optimized lateral flow assays. Biosens Bioelectron. 2013;40(1):180–5.
8. Mudanyali O, Dimitrov S, Sikora U, Padmanabhan S, Navruz I, Ozcan A. Integrated rapid-diagnostic-test reader platform on a cellphone. Lab Chip. 2012;12(15):2678–86.
9. Cooper DC, Callahan B, Callahan P, Burnett L. Mobile image ratiometry: a new method for instantaneous analysis of rapid test strips. Nat Preced. 2012; https://doi.org/10.1038/npre201268271.
10. Cadle BA, Rasmus KC, Varela JA, Leverich LS, O'Neill CE, Bachtell RK, et al. Cellular phone-based image acquisition and quantitative ratiometric method for detecting cocaine and benzoylecgonine for biological and forensic applications. Subst Abus. 2010;4:21–33.
11. Cooper DC. Mobile image ratiometry for the detection of Botrytis cinerea (Gray Mold). Nat Preced. 2012; https://doi.org/10.1038/npre201269891.
12. Mudanyali O, Tseng D, Oh C, Isikman SO, Sencan I, Bishara W, et al. Compact, light-weight and cost-effective microscope based on lensless incoherent holography for telemedicine applications. Lab Chip. 2010;10(11):1417–28.
13. Bishara W, Sikora U, Mudanyali O, Su TW, Yaglidere O, Luckhart S, et al. Holographic pixel super-resolution in portable lensless on-chip microscopy using a fiber-optic array. Lab Chip. 2011;11(7):1276–9.
14. Zhu H, Sencan I, Wong J, Dimitrov S, Tseng D, Nagashima K, et al. Cost-effective and rapid blood analysis on a cell-phone. Lab Chip. 2013;13(7):1282–8.
15. Smith ZJ, Chu K, Espenson AR, Rahimzadeh M, Gryshuk A, Molinaro M, et al. Cell-phone-based platform for biomedical device development and education applications. PLoS One. 2011;6(3):e17150.
16. Breslauer DN, Maamari RN, Switz NA, Lam WA, Fletcher DA. Mobile phone based clinical microscopy for global health applications. PLoS One. 2009;4(7):e6320.

17. Lillehoj PB, Huang MC, Truong N, Ho CM. Rapid electrochemical detection on a mobile phone. Lab Chip. 2013;13(15):2950–5.
18. Oberding JW, Geiger GE, White KD, Ward RN. Blood glucose meter/modem interface arrangement. U.S. Patent Application No. 7,181,350.B2.2007.
19. Peeters JP. Diagnostic radio frequency identification sensors and applications thereof. U.S. Patent No. 8,077,042.
20. Wang X, Gartia MR, Jiang J, Chang T-W, Qian J, Liu Y, et al. Audio jack based miniaturized mobile phone electrochemical sensing platform. Sensors Actuators B Chem. 2014;209:677–85.
21. Lu Y, Shi W, Qin J, Lin B. Low cost, portable detection of gold nanoparticle-labeled microfluidic immunoassay with camera cell phone. Electrophoresis. 2009;30(4):579–82.
22. Coskun AF, Wong J, Khodadadi D, Nagi R, Tey A, Ozcan A. A personalized food allergen testing platform on a cellphone. Lab Chip. 2013;13(4):636–40.
23. Zhu H, Sikora U, Ozcan A. Quantum dot enabled detection of *Escherichia coli* using a cellphone. Analyst. 2012;137(11):2541–4.
24. McGeough CM, O'Driscoll S. Camera phone-based quantitative analysis of C-reactive protein ELISA. IEEE Trans Biomed Circuits Syst. 2013;7(5):655–9.
25. Preechaburana P, Gonzalez MC, Suska A, Filippini D. Surface plasmon resonance chemical sensing on cell phones. Angew Chem. 2012;51(46):11585–8.
26. Coskun AF, Cetin AE, Galarreta BC, Alvarez DA, Altug H, Ozcan A. Lensfree optofluidic plasmonic sensor for real-time and label-free monitoring of molecular binding events over a wide field-of-view. Sci Rep. 2014;4:6789.
27. Zhu H, Mavandadi S, Coskun AF, Yaglidere O, Ozcan A. Optofluidic fluorescent imaging cytometry on a cell phone. Anal Chem. 2011;83(17):6641–7.
28. Shen L, Hagen JA, Papautsky I. Point-of-care colorimetric detection with a smartphone. Lab Chip. 2012;12(21):4240–3.
29. Vashist SK, Marion Schneider E, Zengerle R, von Stetten F, Luong JHT. Graphene-based rapid and highly-sensitive immunoassay for C-reactive protein using a smartphone-based colorimetric reader. Biosens Bioelectron. 2015;66:169–76.
30. Vashist SK, van Oordt T, Schneider EM, Zengerle R, von Stetten F, Luong JHT. A smartphone-based colorimetric reader for bioanalytical applications using the screen-based bottom illumination provided by gadgets. Biosens Bioelectron. 2015;67:248–55.
31. Oncescu V, Mancuso M, Erickson D. Cholesterol testing on a smartphone. Lab Chip. 2014;14(4):759–63.
32. Vashist SK, Schneider EM, Luong JHT. Commercial smartphone-based devices and smart applications for personalized healthcare monitoring and management. Diagnostics. 2014;4(3):104–28.
33. Vashist SK, Luong JHT. Trends in in vitro diagnostics and mobile healthcare. Biotechnol Adv. 2016;34(3):137–8.
34. Wei Q, Nagi R, Sadeghi K, Feng S, Yan E, Ki SJ, et al. Detection and spatial mapping of mercury contamination in water samples using a smart-phone. ACS Nano. 2014;8(2):1121–9.
35. Venkatesh AG, van Oordt T, Schneider EM, Zengerle R, von Stetten F, Luong JHT, et al. A smartphone-based colorimetric reader for human C-reactive protein immunoassay. Methods Mol Biol. 2017;1571:343–56.
36. Park TS, Li W, McCracken KE, Yoon JY. Smartphone quantifies *Salmonella* from paper microfluidics. Lab Chip. 2013;13(24):4832–40.
37. Wang S, Zhao X, Khimji I, Akbas R, Qiu W, Edwards D, et al. Integration of cell phone imaging with microchip ELISA to detect ovarian cancer HE4 biomarker in urine at the point-of-care. Lab Chip. 2011;11(20):3411–8.
38. Lee S, Kim G, Moon J. Performance improvement of the one-dot lateral flow immunoassay for aflatoxin B1 by using a smartphone-based reading system. Sensors. 2013;13(4):5109–16.

39. Sicard C, Glen C, Aubie B, Wallace D, Jahanshahi-Anbuhi S, Pennings K, et al. Tools for water quality monitoring and mapping using paper-based sensors and cell phones. Water Res. 2015;70:360–9.
40. Berg B, Cortazar B, Tseng D, Ozkan H, Feng S, Wei Q, et al. Cellphone-based hand-held microplate reader for point-of-care testing of enzyme-linked immunosorbent assays. ACS Nano. 2015;9(8):7857–66.
41. Lee S, Oncescu V, Mancuso M, Mehta S, Erickson D. A smartphone platform for the quantification of vitamin D levels. Lab Chip. 2014;14(8):1437–42.
42. Petryayeva E, Algar WR. Multiplexed homogeneous assays of proteolytic activity using a smartphone and quantum dots. Anal Chem. 2014;86(6):3195–202.
43. Smith JE, Griffin DK, Leny JK, Hagen JA, Chavez JL, Kelley-Loughnane N. Colorimetric detection with aptamer-gold nanoparticle conjugates coupled to an android-based color analysis application for use in the field. Talanta. 2014;121:247–55.
44. El Kaoutit H, Estévez P, García FC, Serna F, García JM. Sub-ppm quantification of Hg(II) in aqueous media using both the naked eye and digital information from pictures of a colorimetric sensory polymer membrane taken with the digital camera of a conventional mobile phone. Anal Methods. 2013;5(1):54–8.
45. Xiao W, Xiao M, Fu Q, Yu S, Shen H, Bian H, et al. A portable smart-phone readout device for the detection of mercury contamination based on an aptamer-assay nanosensor. Sensors. 2016;16(11):1871.
46. Sumriddetchkajorn S, Chaitavon K, Intaravanne Y. Mobile-platform based colorimeter for monitoring chlorine concentration in water. Sensors Actuators B Chem. 2014;191:561–6.
47. Sumriddetchkajorn S, Chaitavon K, Intaravanne Y. Mobile device-based self-referencing colorimeter for monitoring chlorine concentration in water. Sensors Actuators B Chem. 2013;182:592–7.
48. Chen A, Wang R, Bever CR, Xing S, Hammock BD, Pan T. Smartphone-interfaced lab-on-a-chip devices for field-deployable enzyme-linked immunosorbent assay. Biomicrofluidics. 2014;8(6):064101.
49. Salles MO, Meloni GN, de Araujo WR, Paixão TRLC. Explosive colorimetric discrimination using a smartphone, paper device and chemometrical approach. Anal Methods. 2014;6(7):2047–52.
50. Oncescu V, O'Dell D, Erickson D. Smartphone based health accessory for colorimetric detection of biomarkers in sweat and saliva. Lab Chip. 2013;13(16):3232–8.
51. Hong JI, Chang BY. Development of the smartphone-based colorimetry for multi-analyte sensing arrays. Lab Chip. 2014;14(10):1725–32.
52. Mancuso M, Cesarman E, Erickson D. Detection of Kaposi's sarcoma associated herpesvirus nucleic acids using a smartphone accessory. Lab Chip. 2014;14(19):3809–16.
53. Mancuso M, Jiang L, Cesarman E, Erickson D. Multiplexed colorimetric detection of Kaposi's sarcoma associated herpesvirus and Bartonella DNA using gold and silver nanoparticles. Nanoscale. 2013;5(4):1678–86.
54. García A, Erenas M, Marinetto ED, Abad CA, de Orbe-Paya I, Palma AJ, et al. Mobile phone platform as portable chemical analyzer. Sensors Actuators B: Chemical. 2011;156(1):350–9.
55. Chen W, Cao F, Zheng W, Tian Y, Xianyu Y, Xu P, et al. Detection of the nanomolar level of total Cr[(III) and (VI)] by functionalized gold nanoparticles and a smartphone with the assistance of theoretical calculation models. Nanoscale. 2015;7(5):2042–9.
56. Koesdjojo MT, Pengpumkiat S, Wu Y, Boonloed A, Huynh D, Remcho TP, et al. Cost effective paper-based colorimetric microfluidic devices and mobile phone camera readers for the classroom. J Chem Educ. 2015;92(4):737–41.
57. Su K, Zou Q, Zhou J, Zou L, Li H, Wang T, et al. High-sensitive and high-efficient biochemical analysis method using a bionic electronic eye in combination with a smartphone-based colorimetric reader system. Sensors Actuators B: Chemical. 2015;216:134–40.
58. Masawat P, Harfield A, Namwong A. An iPhone-based digital image colorimeter for detecting tetracycline in milk. Food Chem. 2015;184:23–9.

59. Nie H, Wang W, Li W, Nie Z, Yao S. A colorimetric and smartphone readable method for uracil-DNA glycosylase detection based on the target-triggered formation of G-quadruplex. Analyst. 2015;140(8):2771–7.
60. Martinez AW, Phillips ST, Carrilho E, Thomas SW III, Sindi H, Whitesides GM. Simple telemedicine for developing regions: camera phones and paper-based microfluidic devices for real-time, off-site diagnosis. Anal Chem. 2008;80(10):3699–707.
61. Wang S, Tasoglu S, Chen PZ, Chen M, Akbas R, Wach S, et al. Micro-a-fluidics ELISA for rapid CD4 cell count at the point-of-care. Sci Rep. 2014;4:3796.
62. Wang H, Li YJ, Wei JF, Xu JR, Wang YH, Zheng GX. Paper-based three-dimensional micro-fluidic device for monitoring of heavy metals with a camera cell phone. Anal Bioanal Chem. 2014;406(12):2799–807.
63. Yetisen AK, Martinez-Hurtado JL, Garcia-Melendrez A, da Cruz Vasconcellos F, Lowe CR. A smartphone algorithm with inter-phone repeatability for the analysis of colorimetric tests. Sensors Actuators B Chem. 2014;196:156–60.
64. Laksanasopin T, Guo TW, Nayak S, Sridhara AA, Xie S, Olowookere OO, et al. A smart-phone dongle for diagnosis of infectious diseases at the point of care. Sci Transl Med. 2015;7(273):273re1-re1.
65. Gómez-Robledo L, López-Ruiz N, Melgosa M, Palma AJ, Capitán-Vallvey LF, Sánchez-Marañón M. Using the mobile phone as Munsell soil-colour sensor: an experiment under controlled illumination conditions. Comput Electron Agric. 2013;99:200–8.
66. Moonrungsee N, Pencharee S, Jakmunee J. Colorimetric analyzer based on mobile phone camera for determination of available phosphorus in soil. Talanta. 2015;136:204–9.
67. Vesali F, Omid M, Kaleita A, Mobli H. Development of an android app to estimate chlorophyll content of corn leaves based on contact imaging. Comput Electron Agric. 2015;116:211–20.
68. Intaravanne Y, Sumriddetchkajorn S. Android-based rice leaf color analyzer for estimating the needed amount of nitrogen fertilizer. Comput Electron Agric. 2015;116:228–33.
69. Pohanka M. Photography by cameras integrated in smartphones as a tool for analytical chem-istry represented by an butyrylcholinesterase activity assay. Sensors. 2015;15(6):13752–62.
70. Wu Y, Boonloed A, Sleszynski N, Koesdjojo M, Armstrong C, Bracha S, et al. Clinical chem-istry measurements with commercially available test slides on a smartphone platform: colo-rimetric determination of glucose and urea. Clin Chim Acta. 2015;448:133–8.
71. Thiha A, Ibrahim F. A colorimetric enzyme-linked immunosorbent assay (ELISA) detec-tion platform for a point-of-care dengue detection system on a lab-on-compact-disc. Sensors. 2015;15(5):11431–41.
72. Moonrungsee N, Pencharee S, Peamaroon N. Determination of iron in zeolite catalysts by a smartphone camera-based colorimetric analyzer. Instrum Sci Technol. 2016;44(4):401–9.
73. Levin S, Krishnan S, Rajkumar S, Halery N, Balkunde P. Monitoring of fluoride in water samples using a smartphone. Sci Total Environ. 2016;551–552:101–7.
74. Wang L, Li B, Xu F, Shi X, Feng D, Wei D, et al. High-yield synthesis of strong photolumi-nescent N-doped carbon nanodots derived from hydrosoluble chitosan for mercury ion sens-ing via smartphone APP. Biosens Bioelectron. 2016;79:1–8.
75. Im SH, Kim KR, Park YM, Yoon JH, Hong JW, Yoon HC. An animal cell culture monitoring system using a smartphone-mountable paper-based analytical device. Sensors Actuators B: Chemical. 2016;229:166–73.
76. http://wp.moca-tech.net/news/global-mobile-statistics-2016.html.
77. Su K, Qiu X, Fang J, Zou Q, Wang P. An improved efficient biochemical detection method to marine toxins with a smartphone-based portable system—Bionic e-Eye. Sensors Actuators B: Chemical. 2017;238:1165–72.
78. Abderrahim M, MA S, Condezo-Hoyos L. A novel high-throughput image based rapid Folin-Ciocalteau assay for assessment of reducing capacity in foods. Talanta. 2016;152:82–9.
79. Yang X, Wang Y, Liu W, Zhang Y, Zheng F, Wang S, et al. A portable system for on-site quan-tification of formaldehyde in air based on G-quadruplex halves coupled with a smartphone reader. Biosens Bioelectron. 2016;75:48–54.

80. Mei Q, Jing H, Li Y, Yisibashaer W, Chen J, Nan Li B, et al. Smartphone based visual and quantitative assays on upconversional paper sensor. Biosens Bioelectron. 2016;75:427–32.
81. Wang Y, Liu X, Chen P, Tran NT, Zhang J, Chia WS, et al. Smartphone spectrometer for colorimetric biosensing. Analyst. 2016;141(11):3233–8.
82. Oliveira KA, Damasceno D, de Oliveira CR, da Silveira LA, de Oliveira AE, Coltro WK. Dengue diagnosis on laser printed microzones using smartphone-based detection and multivariate image analysis. Anal Methods. 2016;8(35):6506–11.
83. Yang J-S, Shin J, Choi S, Jung H-I. Smartphone Diagnostics Unit (SDU) for the assessment of human stress and inflammation level assisted by biomarker ink, fountain pen, and origami holder for strip biosensor. Sensors Actuators B: Chemical. 2017;241:80–4.
84. Kim SW, Cho IH, Lim GS, Park GN, Paek SH. Biochemical-immunological hybrid biosensor based on two-dimensional chromatography for on-site sepsis diagnosis. Biosens Bioelectron. 2017;98:7–14.
85. Kostelnik A, Cegan A, Pohanka M. Acetylcholinesterase inhibitors assay using colorimetric pH sensitive strips and image analysis by a smartphone. Int J Anal Chem. 2017;2017:3712384.
86. Shin J, Choi S, Yang J-S, Song J, Choi J-S, Jung H-I. Smart Forensic Phone: colorimetric analysis of a bloodstain for age estimation using a smartphone. Sensors Actuators B: Chemical. 2017;243:221–5.
87. Li L, Liu Z, Zhang H, Yue W, Li C-W, Yi C. A point-of-need enzyme linked aptamer assay for *Mycobacterium tuberculosis* detection using a smartphone. Sensors Actuators B: Chemical. 2017;254:337–46.
88. Kim SC, Jalal UM, Im SB, Ko S, Shim JS. A smartphone-based optical platform for colorimetric analysis of microfluidic device. Sensors Actuators B Chem. 2017;239:52–9.
89. Calabria D, Caliceti C, Zangheri M, Mirasoli M, Simoni P, Roda A. Smartphone–based enzymatic biosensor for oral fluid L-lactate detection in one minute using confined multilayer paper reflectometry. Biosens Bioelectron. 2017;94:124–30.
90. Amirjani A, Fatmehsari DH. Colorimetric detection of ammonia using smartphones based on localized surface plasmon resonance of silver nanoparticles. Talanta. 2017;176:242–6.
91. Machado JMD, Soares RRG, Chu V, Conde JP. Multiplexed capillary microfluidic immunoassay with smartphone data acquisition for parallel mycotoxin detection. Biosens Bioelectron. 2018;99:40–6.
92. Su K, Pan Y, Wan Z, Zhong L, Fang J, Zou Q, et al. Smartphone-based portable biosensing system using cell viability biosensor for okadaic acid detection. Sensors Actuators B: Chemical. 2017;251:134–43.
93. Liu Z, Zhang Y, Xu S, Zhang H, Tan Y, Ma C, et al. A 3D printed smartphone optosensing platform for point-of-need food safety inspection. Anal Chim Acta. 2017;966:81–9.
94. Ludwig SK, Zhu H, Phillips S, Shiledar A, Feng S, Tseng D, et al. Cellphone-based detection platform for rbST biomarker analysis in milk extracts using a microsphere fluorescence immunoassay. Anal Bioanal Chem. 2014;406(27):6857–66.
95. Coskun AF, Nagi R, Sadeghi K, Phillips S, Ozcan A. Albumin testing in urine using a smartphone. Lab Chip. 2013;13(21):4231–8.
96. Zhang C, Kim JP, Creer M, Yang J, Liu Z. A smartphone-based chloridometer for point-of-care diagnostics of cystic fibrosis. Biosens Bioelectron. 2017;97:164–8.
97. Liao SC, Peng J, Mauk MG, Awasthi S, Song J, Friedman H, et al. Smart Cup: a minimally-instrumented, smartphone-based point-of-care molecular diagnostic device. Sensors Actuators B: Chemical. 2016;229:232–8.
98. Rajendran VK, Bakthavathsalam P, Jaffar Ali BM. Smartphone based bacterial detection using biofunctionalized fluorescent nanoparticles. Microchim Acta. 2014;181(15–16):1815–21.
99. Walker FM, Ahmad KM, Eisenstein M, Soh HT. Transformation of personal computers and mobile phones into genetic diagnostic systems. Anal Chem. 2014;86(18):9236–41.
100. Fronczek CF, Park TS, Harshman DK, Nicolini AM, Yoon J-Y. Paper microfluidic extraction and direct smartphone-based identification of pathogenic nucleic acids from field and clinical samples. RSC Adv. 2014;4(22):11103.

101. Lee D, Chou WP, Yeh SH, Chen PJ, Chen PH. DNA detection using commercial mobile phones. Biosens Bioelectron. 2011;26(11):4349–54.
102. Nicolini AM, Fronczek CF, Yoon JY. Droplet-based immunoassay on a 'sticky' nanofibrous surface for multiplexed and dual detection of bacteria using smartphones. Biosens Bioelectron. 2015;67:560–9.
103. Thom NK, Lewis GG, Yeung K, Phillips ST. Quantitative fluorescence assays using a self-powered paper-based microfluidic device and a camera-equipped cellular phone. RSC Adv. 2014;4(3):1334–40.
104. Wei Q, Qi H, Luo W, Tseng D, Ki SJ, Wan Z, et al. Fluorescent imaging of single nanoparticles and viruses on a smart phone. ACS Nano. 2013;7(10):9147–55.
105. Yu H, Tan Y, Cunningham BT. Smartphone fluorescence spectroscopy. Anal Chem. 2014;86(17):8805–13.
106. Zhu H, Yaglidere O, Su TW, Tseng D, Ozcan A. Cost-effective and compact wide-field fluorescent imaging on a cell-phone. Lab Chip. 2011;11(2):315–22.
107. Barbosa AI, Gehlot P, Sidapra K, Edwards AD, Reis NM. Portable smartphone quantitation of prostate specific antigen (PSA) in a fluoropolymer microfluidic device. Biosens Bioelectron. 2015;70:5–14.
108. Hossain A, Canning J, Ast S, Rutledge PJ, Teh Li Y, Jamalipour A. Lab-in-a-Phone: smartphone-based portable fluorometer for pH measurements of environmental water. IEEE Sensors J. 2015;15(9):5095–102.
109. Awqatty B, Samaddar S, Cash KJ, Clark HA, Dubach JM. Fluorescent sensors for the basic metabolic panel enable measurement with a smart phone device over the physiological range. Analyst. 2014;139(20):5230–8.
110. Petryayeva E, Algar WR. Single-step bioassays in serum and whole blood with a smartphone, quantum dots and paper-in-PDMS chips. Analyst. 2015;140(12):4037–45.
111. Ming K, Kim J, Biondi MJ, Syed A, Chen K, Lam A, et al. Integrated quantum dot barcode smartphone optical device for wireless multiplexed diagnosis of infected patients. ACS Nano. 2015;9(3):3060–74.
112. Wargocki P, Deng W, Anwer AG, Goldys EM. Medically relevant assays with a simple smartphone and tablet based fluorescence detection system. Sensors. 2015;15(5):11653–64.
113. Yeo SJ, Choi K, Cuc BT, Hong NN, Bao DT, Ngoc NM, et al. Smartphone-based fluorescent diagnostic system for highly pathogenic H5N1 viruses. Theranostics. 2016;6(2):231–42.
114. Bueno D, Muñoz R, Marty JL. Fluorescence analyzer based on smartphone camera and wireless for detection of Ochratoxin A. Sensors Actuators B: Chemical. 2016;232:462–8.
115. Priye A, Wong S, Bi Y, Carpio M, Chang J, Coen M, et al. Lab-on-a-Drone: toward pinpoint deployment of smartphone-enabled nucleic acid-based diagnostics for mobile health care. Anal Chem. 2016;88(9):4651–60.
116. Slusarewicz P, Pagano S, Mills C, Popa G, Chow KM, Mendenhall M, et al. Automated parasite faecal egg counting using fluorescence labelling, smartphone image capture and computational image analysis. Int J Parasitol. 2016;46(8):485–93.
117. Cho S, Islas-Robles A, Nicolini AM, Monks TJ, Yoon JY. In situ, dual-mode monitoring of organ-on-a-chip with smartphone-based fluorescence microscope. Biosens Bioelectron. 2016;86:697–705.
118. Ko J, Hemphill MA, Gabrieli D, Wu L, Yelleswarapu V, Lawrence G, et al. Smartphone-enabled optofluidic exosome diagnostic for concussion recovery. Sci Rep. 2016;6:31215.
119. Joh DY, Hucknall AM, Wei Q, Mason KA, Lund ML, Fontes CM, et al. Inkjet-printed point-of-care immunoassay on a nanoscale polymer brush enables subpicomolar detection of analytes in blood. Proc Natl Acad Sci U S A. 2017;114(34):E7054–E62.
120. Jiang L, Mancuso M, Lu Z, Akar G, Cesarman E, Erickson D. Solar thermal polymerase chain reaction for smartphone-assisted molecular diagnostics. Sci Rep. 2014;4:4137.
121. Lee WI, Shrivastava S, Duy LT, Yeong Kim B, Son YM, Lee NE. A smartphone imaging-based label-free and dual-wavelength fluorescent biosensor with high sensitivity and accuracy. Biosens Bioelectron. 2017;94:643–50.

122. Yang K, Wu J, Peretz-Soroka H, Zhu L, Li Z, Sang Y, et al. M kit: a cell migration assay based on microfluidic device and smartphone. Biosens Bioelectron. 2017;99:259–67.
123. Chen B, Ma J, Yang T, Chen L, Gao PF, Huang CZ. A portable RGB sensing gadget for sensitive detection of Hg^{2+} using cysteamine-capped QDs as fluorescence probe. Biosens Bioelectron. 2017;98:36–40.
124. Priye A, Bird SW, Light YK, Ball CS, Negrete OA, Meagher RJ. A smartphone-based diagnostic platform for rapid detection of Zika, chikungunya, and dengue viruses. Sci Rep. 2017;7:44778.
125. Knowlton S, Joshi A, Syrrist P, Coskun AF, Tasoglu S. 3D-printed smartphone-based point of care tool for fluorescence- and magnetophoresis-based cytometry. Lab Chip. 2017;17(16):2839–51.
126. Zangheri M, Cevenini L, Anfossi L, Baggiani C, Simoni P, Di Nardo F, et al. A simple and compact smartphone accessory for quantitative chemiluminescence-based lateral flow immunoassay for salivary cortisol detection. Biosens Bioelectron. 2015;64:63–8.
127. Roda A, Michelini E, Cevenini L, Calabria D, Calabretta MM, Simoni P. Integrating bio-chemiluminescence detection on smartphones: mobile chemistry platform for point-of-need analysis. Anal Chem. 2014;86(15):7299–304.
128. Quimbar ME, Krenek KM, Lippert AR. A chemiluminescent platform for smartphone monitoring of H_2O_2 in human exhaled breath condensates. Methods. 2016;109:123–30.
129. Zangheri M, Cevenini L, Anfossi L, Baggiani C, Simoni P, Di Nardo F, et al. A simple and compact smartphone accessory for quantitative chemiluminescence-based lateral flow immunoassay for salivary cortisol detection. Biosens Bioelectron. 2014;64:63–8.
130. Hao N, Xiong M, Zhang JD, Xu JJ, Chen HY. Portable thermo-powered high-throughput visual electrochemiluminescence sensor. Anal Chem. 2013;85(24):11715–9.
131. Doeven EH, Barbante GJ, Harsant AJ, Donnelly PS, Connell TU, Hogan CF, et al. Mobile phone-based electrochemiluminescence sensing exploiting the 'USB on–the-go' protocol. Sensors Actuators B: Chemical. 2015;216:608–13.
132. Petryayeva E, Algar WR. A job for quantum dots: use of a smartphone and 3D-printed accessory for all-in-one excitation and imaging of photoluminescence. Anal Bioanal Chem. 2016;408(11):2913–25.
133. Cevenini L, Calabretta MM, Tarantino G, Michelini E, Roda A. Smartphone-interfaced 3D printed toxicity biosensor integrating bioluminescent "sentinel cells". Sensors Actuators B: Chemical. 2016;225:249–57.
134. Arts R, Den Hartog I, Zijlema SE, Thijssen V, van der Beelen SH, Merkx M. Detection of antibodies in blood plasma using bioluminescent sensor proteins and a smartphone. Anal Chem. 2016;88(8):4525–32.
135. Spyrou EM, Kalogianni DP, Tragoulias SS, Ioannou PC, Christopoulos TK. Digital camera and smartphone as detectors in paper-based chemiluminometric genotyping of single nucleotide polymorphisms. Anal Bioanal Chem. 2016;408:7393–402.
136. He M, Li Z, Ge Y, Liu Z. Portable upconversion nanoparticles-based paper device for field testing of drug abuse. Anal Chem. 2016;88(3):1530–4.
137. Long KD, Yu H, Cunningham BT. Smartphone instrument for portable enzyme-linked immunosorbent assays. Biomed Opt Express. 2014;5(11):3792–806.
138. Zhang C, Cheng G, Edwards P, Zhou MD, Zheng S, Liu Z. G-Fresnel smartphone spectrometer. Lab Chip. 2016;16(2):246–50.
139. Yang C, Shi K, Edwards P, Liu Z. Demonstration of a PDMS based hybrid grating and Fresnel lens (G-Fresnel) device. Opt Express. 2010;18(23):23529–34.
140. Kwon H, Park J, An Y, Sim J, Park S. A smartphone metabolomics platform and its application to the assessment of cisplatin-induced kidney toxicity. Anal Chim Acta. 2014;845:15–22.
141. Cao T, Thompson JE. Remote sensing of atmospheric optical depth using a smartphone sun photometer. PLoS One. 2014;9(1):e84119.
142. Arafat Hossain M, Canning J, Ast S, Cook K, Rutledge PJ, Jamalipour A. Combined "dual" absorption and fluorescence smartphone spectrometers. Opt Lett. 2015;40(8):1737–40.

143. Intaravanne Y, Sumriddetchkajorn S, Nukeaw J. Cell phone-based two-dimensional spectral analysis for banana ripeness estimation. Sensors Actuators B: Chemical. 2012;168:390–4.
144. Dutta S, Choudhury A, Nath P. Evanescent wave coupled spectroscopic sensing using smartphone. IEEE Photon Technol Lett. 2014;26(6):568–70.
145. Iqbal Z, Bjorklund RB. Assessment of a mobile phone for use as a spectroscopic analytical tool for foods and beverages. Int J Food Sci Technol. 2011;46(11):2428–36.
146. Dutta S, Sarma D, Nath P. Ground and river water quality monitoring using a smartphone-based pH sensor. AIP Adv. 2015;5(5):057151.
147. Grasse EK, Torcasio MH, Smith AW. Teaching UV–Vis spectroscopy with a 3D-printable smartphone spectrophotometer. J Chem Educ. 2015;93(1):146–51.
148. Debus B, Kirsanov D, Yaroshenko I, Sidorova A, Piven A, Legin A. Two low-cost digital camera-based platforms for quantitative creatinine analysis in urine. Anal Chim Acta. 2015;895:71–9.
149. Wang L-J, Chang Y-C, Ge X, Osmanson AT, Du D, Lin Y, et al. Smartphone optosensing platform using a DVD grating to detect neurotoxins. ACS Sensors. 2016;1(4):366–73.
150. Hossain MA, Canning J, Cook K, Jamalipour A. Optical fiber smartphone spectrometer. Opt Lett. 2016;41(10):2237–40.
151. Wang LJ, Chang YC, Sun R, Li L. A multichannel smartphone optical biosensor for high-throughput point-of-care diagnostics. Biosens Bioelectron. 2017;87:686–92.
152. http://www.cellmic.com/.
153. Choi S, Kim S, Yang J-S, Lee J-H, Joo C, Jung H-I. Real-time measurement of human salivary cortisol for the assessment of psychological stress using a smartphone. Sens Bio-Sens Res. 2014;2:8–11.
154. Lin R, Skandarajah A, Gerver RE, Neira HD, Fletcher DA, Herr AE. A lateral electrophoretic flow diagnostic assay. Lab Chip. 2015;15(6):1488–96.
155. Yu L, Shi Z, Fang C, Zhang Y, Liu Y, Li C. Disposable lateral flow-through strip for smartphone-camera to quantitatively detect alkaline phosphatase activity in milk. Biosens Bioelectron. 2015;69:307–15.
156. Preechaburana P, Macken S, Suska A, Filippini D. HDR imaging evaluation of a NT-proBNP test with a mobile phone. Biosens Bioelectron. 2011;26(5):2107–13.
157. Lee S, O'Dell D, Hohenstein J, Colt S, Mehta S, Erickson D. NutriPhone: a mobile platform for low-cost point-of-care quantification of vitamin B12 concentrations. Sci Rep. 2016;6:28237.
158. Wireless Smart Gluco-Monitoring System. http://www.ihealthlabs.com/glucometer/wireless-smart-gluco-monitoring-system/.
159. Nemiroski A, Christodouleas DC, Hennek JW, Kumar AA, Maxwell EJ, Fernández-Abedul MT, et al. Universal mobile electrochemical detector designed for use in resource-limited applications. Proc Natl Acad Sci U S A. 2014;111(33):11984–9.
160. Zhang D, Jiang J, Chen J, Zhang Q, Lu Y, Yao Y, et al. Smartphone-based portable biosensing system using impedance measurement with printed electrodes for 2, 4, 6-trinitrotoluene (TNT) detection. Biosens Bioelectron. 2015;70:81–8.
161. Jiang J, Wang X, Chao R, Ren Y, Hu C, Xu Z, et al. Smartphone based portable bacteria pre-concentrating microfluidic sensor and impedance sensing system. Sensors Actuators B: Chemical. 2014;193:653–9.
162. Sun A, Wambach T, Venkatesh A, Hall DA, editors. A low-cost smartphone-based electrochemical biosensor for point-of-care diagnostics. Biomedical Circuits and Systems Conference (BioCAS), IEEE; 2014. p. 312–5.
163. Delaney JL, Doeven EH, Harsant AJ, Hogan CF. Use of a mobile phone for potentiostatic control with low cost paper-based microfluidic sensors. Anal Chim Acta. 2013;790:56–60.
164. Zhang D, Lu Y, Zhang Q, Liu L, Li S, Yao Y, et al. Protein detecting with smartphone-controlled electrochemical impedance spectroscopy for point-of-care applications. Sensors Actuators B: Chemical. 2016;222:994–1002.

165. Sun AC, Yao C, Venkatesh AG, Hall DA. An efficient power harvesting mobile phone-based electrochemical biosensor for point-of-care health monitoring. Sensors Actuators B: Chemical. 2016;235:126–35.

166. Aronoff-Spencer E, Venkatesh AG, Sun A, Brickner H, Looney D, Hall DA. Detection of Hepatitis C core antibody by dual-affinity yeast chimera and smartphone-based electrochemical sensing. Biosens Bioelectron. 2016;86:690–6.

167. Giordano GF, Vicentini MB, Murer RC, Augusto F, Ferrão MF, Helfer GA, et al. Point-of-use electroanalytical platform based on homemade potentiostat and smartphone for multivariate data processing. Electrochim Acta. 2016;219:170–7.

168. Ji D, Liu L, Li S, Chen C, Lu Y, Wu J, et al. Smartphone-based cyclic voltammetry system with graphene modified screen printed electrodes for glucose detection. Biosens Bioelectron. 2017;98:449–56.

169. Uliana CV, Peverari CR, Afonso AS, Cominetti MR, Faria RC. Fully disposable microfluidic electrochemical device for detection of estrogen receptor alpha breast cancer biomarker. Biosens Bioelectron. 2018;99:156–62.

170. Tseng D, Mudanyali O, Oztoprak C, Isikman SO, Sencan I, Yaglidere O, et al. Lensfree microscopy on a cellphone. Lab Chip. 2010;10(14):1787–92.

171. Navruz I, Coskun AF, Wong J, Mohammad S, Tseng D, Nagi R, et al. Smart-phone based computational microscopy using multi-frame contact imaging on a fiber-optic array. Lab Chip. 2013;13(20):4015–23.

172. Koydemir HC, Gorocs Z, Tseng D, Cortazar B, Feng S, Chan RYL, et al. Rapid imaging, detection and quantification of Giardia lamblia cysts using mobile-phone based fluorescent microscopy and machine learning. Lab Chip. 2014;15(5):1284–93.

173. Wei Q, Luo W, Chiang S, Kappel T, Mejia C, Tseng D, et al. Imaging and sizing of single DNA molecules on a mobile phone. ACS Nano. 2014;8(12):12725–33.

174. Skandarajah A, Reber CD, Switz NA, Fletcher DA. Quantitative imaging with a mobile phone microscope. PLoS One. 2014;9(5):e96906.

175. Roy S, Pantanowitz L, Amin M, Seethala RR, Ishtiaque A, Yousem SA, et al. Smartphone adapters for digital photomicrography. J Pathol. 2014;1:24.

176. Lee M, Yaglidere O, Ozcan A. Field-portable reflection and transmission microscopy based on lensless holography. Biomed Optics Exp. 2011;2(9):2721–30.

177. Kanakasabapathy MK, Sadasivam M, Singh A, Preston C, Thirumalaraju P, Venkataraman M, et al. An automated smartphone-based diagnostic assay for point-of-care semen analysis. Sci Transl Med. 2017;9(382):eaai7863.

178. Bremer K, Roth B. Fibre optic surface plasmon resonance sensor system designed for smartphones. Opt Express. 2015;23(13):17179–84.

179. Liu Y, Liu Q, Chen S, Cheng F, Wang H, Peng W. Surface plasmon resonance biosensor based on smart phone platforms. Sci Rep. 2015;5:12864.

180. Lee KL, You ML, Tsai CH, Lin EH, Hsieh SY, Ho MH, et al. Nanoplasmonic biochips for rapid label-free detection of imidacloprid pesticides with a smartphone. Biosens Bioelectron. 2016;75:88–95.

181. Dutta S, Saikia K, Nath P. Smartphone based LSPR sensing platform for bio-conjugation detection and quantification. RSC Adv. 2016;6(26):21871–80.

182. Fu Q, Wu Z, Xu F, Li X, Yao C, Xu M, et al. A portable smart phone-based plasmonic nanosensor readout platform that measures transmitted light intensities of nanosubstrates using an ambient light sensor. Lab Chip. 2016;16(10):1927–33.

183. Guner H, Ozgur E, Kokturk G, Celik M, Esen E, Topal AE, et al. A smartphone based surface plasmon resonance imaging (SPRi) platform for on-site biodetection. Sensors Actuators B: Chemical. 2017;239:571–7.

184. Zhang J, Khan I, Zhang Q, Liu X, Dostalek J, Liedberg B, et al. Lipopolysaccharides detection on a grating-coupled surface plasmon resonance smartphone biosensor. Biosens Bioelectron. 2018;99:312–7.

Chapter 3
Commercially Available Smartphone-Based Personalized Mobile Healthcare Technologies

Sandeep Kumar Vashist and John H. T. Luong

Contents

3.1 Introduction

SPMHDs have emerged as a prospective technology solution for cost-effective personalized healthcare monitoring at any place and time without the need for skilled healthcare professionals and healthcare facilities. Commercially available SPMHDs are highly cost-effective and affordable, which renders them ideal for delivering mH to remote, resource-deficient, decentralized, and personalized settings. The current generation of smartphones is equipped with sophisticated features, data processing capabilities, and various sensors including light detectors, proximity sensors, fingerprinting, and high-resolution cameras. They collect the real-time spatiotemporal tagged data and have excellent connectivity to the personal Cloud and secure central

© Springer Nature Switzerland AG 2019
S. K. Vashist, J. H. T. Luong, *Point-of-Care Technologies Enabling
Next-Generation Healthcare Monitoring and Management*,
https://doi.org/10.1007/978-3-030-11416-9_3

server. Therefore, they have extensive telemedicine applications as the personalized data can be assessed by certified healthcare professionals from remote locations, which would be useful for tackling epidemics and emergency cases [1]. Cell phones are ubiquitous as they are available for over 95% of the world population. Among 7 billion cell phone subscribers worldwide, 3 billion have the Internet on their cellphones [2], and the cell phone subscribers would reach 8.5 billion by the end of 2016 [3]. The continuously increasing capabilities of smartphones and evolving technological features with additional functionalities provide an impetus for the development of truly powerful SPMHDs.

About 70% of the smartphone users are actually from the developing countries, where there is an enormous need for cost-effective mH. Therefore, SPMHDs would play a critical role in healthcare and establish a new trend in healthcare delivery. Apart from significantly cutting down the healthcare costs with better health outcomes, SPMHDs will create new businesses and opportunities. They will lead to health conscious and better-informed society as the patients become active decisionmakers in their healthcare monitoring and management.

Smartphone-based devices for a broad range of bioanalytical applications [4] have been discussed in the previous chapter. These applications include lateral flow assays [5–10], microscopy [11–15], electrochemical sensing [16–19], colorimetric detection [20], immunoassays [21–25], surface plasmon resonance-based biosensing [26], and flow cytometry [27, 28]. Thus, this chapter provides a comprehensive review of commercially available SPMHDs (Table 3.1) taking into account their technology features, applications, and prospects. Only the main commercial SPMHDs capturing the significant share of the consumer mH market are mentioned here. Most of the mentioned SPMHDs in this chapter are based on our ongoing research efforts and business operations in the field of personalized mH. SPMHDs from GENTAG, Inc., Mobile Assay, Inc., Samsung, Garmin, Nuband, Nonin Medical, Inc., and Circlet were searched from the respective company's websites. The product specifications and features of the SPMHDs were taken from the product manuals and the published literature, while the prices of most of the SBDAs were taken directly from the websites. The price of the SPMHD from Nonin Medical, Inc. was taken from the contact person in the company.

The personalized healthcare monitoring is useful in managing chronic health conditions such as diabetes, obesity, and psychological stress [1, 29–47]. Therefore, SPMHDs will play a critical role in the real time and frequent monitoring of such basic physiological parameters to provide improved personalized mH [48–50]. The centralized mH by SPMHDs would increase the healthcare outreach by connecting isolated remote laboratories [50, 51]. It also improves the adherence of end users to checkups, treatment, and medication [24, 52–56]. Further, mH would enable the effective management of chronic diseases [57, 58], improved communication between healthcare professionals [59, 60], and the prevention of infectious and sexually transmitted diseases [61, 62]. Some important mH applications include delivering education [63, 64], large-scale screening of community for a particular disease [65], and improved adherence of the parents to the immunization schedules [66] of their children. It also facilitates the spatiotemporal mapping of disease incidence [67] and improved general healthcare management [68].

Table 3.1 Commercially available smartphone-based personalized mobile healthcare devices (SPMHDs)

Company	Commercial SPMHDs	Type of mobile platform	Clearance/ marking	Price (in US$)	Refs.
iHealth Lab, Inc.	• iHealth Core	iOS, Android	FDA, CE	129.95	[69]
	• Wireless body analysis scale	iOS, Android	FDA, CE	99.95	
	• iHealth Lite wireless scale	iOS, Android	FDA, CE	79.95	
	• Wireless blood pressure (BP) Monitor	iOS, Android	FDA, CE, ESH, EC Medical	99.95	
	• Wireless BP Wrist Monitor	iOS, Android	FDA, CE, ESH, EC Medical	79.95	
	• BP Dock	iOS, Android	FDA, CE, ESH, EC Medical	39.99	
	• iHealth View Wireless Ease BP Monitor	iOS, Android	FDA, CE, ESH, EC Medical	99.99	
	• iHealth Wireless Ease BP Monitor	iOS, Android	FDA, CE, ESH, EC Medical	39.99	
	• iHealth Track	iOS, Android	FDA, CE, ESH, EC Medical	39.95 €	
	• iHealth Wireless Smart Gluco-Monitoring System	iOS, Android	FDA, CE, ISO 15197:2013	29.95	
	• iHealth Align	iOS, Android	FDA, CE	16.95	
	• iHealth Blood Glucose Test Strips (1 pack of 50 strips)	iOS, Android	FDA, CE	12.50	
	• Wireless Pulse Oximeter	iOS, Android	FDA, CE	69.95	
	• iHealth Edge	iOS, Android	CE	69.95	
	• iHealth Wave	iOS, Android	CE	79.95	
	• iHealth Rhythm	iOS, Android	CE	150.00	
	• CardioLab	iOS, Android	FDA, CE	599.00 €	
Cellmic	• Smartphone-based Holomic Integrated rapid diagnostic test reader (HRDR-200)	iOS, Android	FDA Class I device, ISO13485	N.M.[a]	[70]
	• HRDR-300	iOS, Android	FDA Class I device, ISO13485	N.M.[a]	
	• Holomic Substance Test Assistant	iOS, Android	FDA Class I device, ISO13485	N.M.[a]	

(continued)

Table 3.1 (continued)

Company	Commercial SPMHDs	Type of mobile platform	Clearance/ marking	Price (in US$)	Refs.
AliveCor, Inc.	• Kardia Mobile	iOS, Android	FDA, CE	99	[71]
GENTAG, Inc.	• Near Field Communications (NFC) SensorLinkers • NFC tags • NFC diagnostic skin patches • NFC sensors • NFC-radio frequency identification device (RFID) sensors • NFC immunoassays • NFC-Bluetooth weight management kit • Radar responsive (RR) tags • Cellphone-based home monitoring solutions • Transdermal glucose sensing and monitoring system • Customizable spectroscopic radiation detection cellphone	N.M.[a]	N.M.[a]	N.M.[a]	[72]
Apple	• Apple Watch	iOS	CE	549–1099	[73]
Samsung	• Gear S2	Android	CE	299.99–449.99	[74]
	• Gear Fit2	Android	CE	179.99	[75]
	• Simband	Android	CE	N.M.[a]	[76]
Runtastic GmbH	• Runtastic Heart Rate Combo Monitor	iOS, Android, Windows	FDA, CE	69.99	[77]
	• Runtastic Activity Tracker and Heart Rate Monitor	Windows PC or Mac (require Runtastic Connect Software)	FDA, CE	149.99	
	• Runtastic Orbit	iOS, Android, Windows	FDA, CE	99.99	
	• Runtastic Libra	iOS, Android	FDA, CE	121.31	
	• Runtastic Speed and Cadence Sensor	iOS, Android	FDA, CE	58.62	

(continued)

Table 3.1 (continued)

Company	Commercial SPMHDs	Type of mobile platform	Clearance/ marking	Price (in US$)	Refs.
Bühlmann Labs	• IB*Doc*® Calprotectin Home Testing system	iOS, Android	CE	N.M.[a]	[78]
Mobile Assay, Inc.	• Mobile diagnostic reader (mReader™)	iOS, Android, Windows	N.M.[a]	N.M.[a]	[79]
CellScope	• "CellScope Oto" digital Otoscope	iOS	FDA Class I device	N.M.[a]	[80]
	• "CellScope Derm" Dermascope				
Nonin	• Onyx® II 9560 Wireless Finger Pulse Oximeter	iOS, Android	FCC Class B digital device, ISO 10993-1, IEC 60601-1-2, SSP, HDP with security mode 2, IEEE11073, Continua	666	[81]
Cicret	• Cicret Bracelet	iOS, Android	CE	250	[82]
Fitbit	• Fitbit Alta™	iOS, Android	CE	129.95	[83]
	• Fitbit Blaze™	iOS, Android	CE	229.95	
	• Fitbit Surge™	iOS, Android	CE	129.95	
	• Aria® Wi-Fi smart scale	iOS, Android	CE	129.95	
Garmin	• Vivoactive®	iOS, Android	CE	156.59	[84]
	• Vivoactive® HR	iOS, Android	CE	249.99	
	• Vivofit® 3	iOS, Android	CE	99.99	
	• Vivosmart® HR	iOS, Android	CE	149.99	
	• Vivosmart® HR+	iOS, Android	CE	219.99	
Nuband	• Nuband	iOS, Android	CE	87.23	[85]
	• Nuband Activ+	iOS, Android	CE	49.99	[86]

Prices were taken directly from the respective websites on June 18, 2016
[a]N.M.—not mentioned

3.2 Commercial Smartphone-Based Personalized Mobile Healthcare Devices

3.2.1 iHealth Labs, Inc.

A wide range of SPMHDs has been developed by iHealth Lab, Inc. [69] for the monitoring of basic physiological parameters as shown in Fig. 3.1. The physiological data from all SPMHDs is integrated into the smartphone via a single smart application called iHealth MyVitals. This smart app is free to download on all iOS and Android smartphones and provides a dashboard view of all physiological parameters, including the trend in data and the actual data. The only exception is the blood glucose measurements, which are stored separately in a dedicated smart application called iHealth Gluco-Smart. The company has also developed highly sophisticated and specialized smart applications for physicians to facilitate patient management, i.e., iHealth Pro. The user is asked to create a unique iHealth ID for the use of the smart applications to access free and secure iHealth Cloud services. All SPMHDs can be used by multiple users on iOS and Android devices.

3.2.1.1 Body Composition

The wireless body composition scale, i.e., iHealth Core, is a Food and Drug Administration (FDA)- and Conformité Européenne (CE)-approved SPMHD, which measures the body analysis parameters using four electronic sensors and advanced data processing algorithms for measuring body compositions. The SPMHD measures the body analysis parameters of weight, basal metabolic index (BMI), body fat, lean mass, muscle mass, bone mass, body water, daily calorie intake (DCI), and visceral fat rating of individuals. The user is required to switch on the iHealth MyVitals app after switching on the Bluetooth, which interfaces it to the scale and then takes the measurement and synchronizes the data to get the information on the mobile. The scale requires four 1.5 V AAA batteries and weighs about 2.5 kg. The measurement ranges for body weight, body fat, body water, and visceral fat are 5–180 kg, 5–65%, 20–85%, and 1–59, respectively. The wireless body analysis scale is currently being sold in the United States for US$129.95. The company also sells the comparatively lesser advanced previous models, i.e., the wireless body analysis scale at US$99.95 and iHealth Lite weighing scale for US$79.95.

3.2.1.2 Blood Pressure

iHealth offers various FDA-cleared and ESH- and EC Medical-certified BP monitors. The users simply turn on the Bluetooth on the phone, start the iHealth MyVitals app, interface it to the BP monitor, and perform the BP measurement. The smartphone's screen shows whether the hand posture is perfect or must be modified for

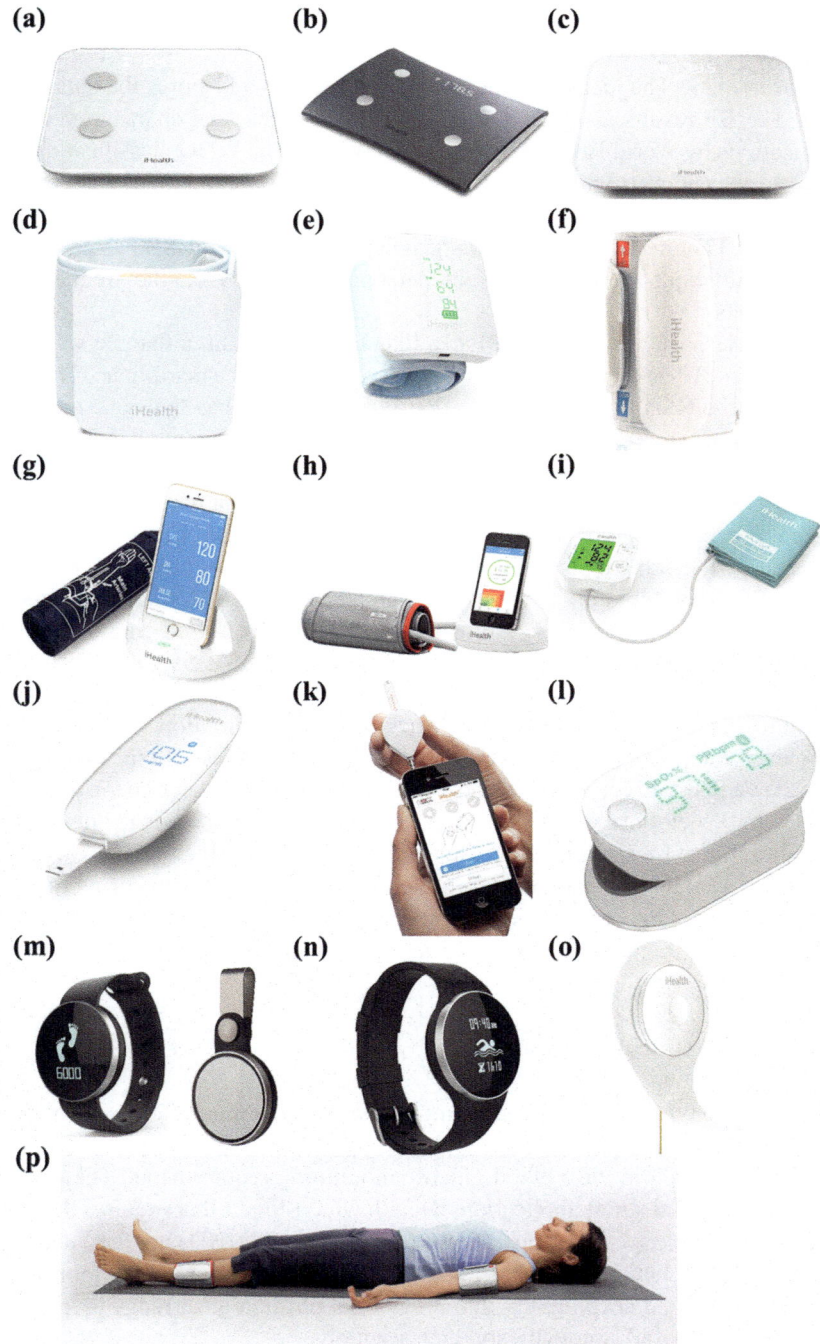

Fig. 3.1 Smartphone-based devices (SBD) developed by iHealth Lab Inc. (**a**) iHealth Core. (**b**) Wireless body analysis scale. (**c**) iHealth Lite. (**d**) Wireless Blood Pressure (BP) Wrist Monitor. (**e**) iHealth View Wireless BP Wrist Monitor. (**f**) Wireless BP Monitor. (**g**) iHealth Wireless Ease BP Monitor. (**h**) iHealth BP dock. (**i**) iHealth Track. (**j**) iHealth Wireless Smart Gluco-Monitoring System. (**k**) iHealth Align. (**l**) Wireless Pulse Oximeter. (**m**) iHealth Edge. (**n**) iHealth Wave. Reproduced with permission from iHealth Lab Inc.

the measurement. The measurement takes a few seconds and stores the data on the phone. The BP results are presented in the form of the visual chart based on the classifications by World Health Organization (WHO). The WHO classification provides a very easy chart with the analysis to indicate the normal, moderate, or high BP range as well as the trend in the BP readings. The BP monitors have integrated rechargeable batteries that can be recharged using the provided USB cable. A single charge is sufficient for many days of personal use based on the frequency of measurements.

The Wireless BP Wrist Monitor looks like a watch with an inflatable wristband to monitor the BP on the wrist and display the reading on the smartphone. The newest version, the iHealth View Wireless BP Wrist Monitor, has the same operation and function but shows the reading on the device itself. Further, another SPMHD is the Wireless BP Monitor, which is quite similar to the conventional clinical BP monitor, as it takes the BP measurement from the upper arm using the same measurement procedure via the smartphone. The previous versions of the BP monitors being sold by iHealth are the iHealth Wireless Ease BP Monitor and BP Dock. The Wireless BP Wrist Monitor, iHealth View Wireless BP Wrist Monitor, Wireless BP Monitor, iHealth Wireless Ease BP Monitor, and BP Dock are being sold in the United States for US$79.95, US$99.99, US$99.95, US$39.99, and US$39.99, respectively.

A more recent version is the iHealth Track, a smart BP monitor, which is easy to use by everyone, with and without a smartphone. It is a Class IIa medical device with an awarded CE certification and can store up to 60 measurements before it needs to be synchronized with the smartphone. The data is sent to the iHealth MyVitals app just by a single click. The device is only available in EU for 39.95 €, and it is not available for sale on the US website. The frequent monitoring of BP is an essential part of hypertension management and treatment, enabling the users and their doctors or caregivers to predict the cardiovascular risks.

3.2.1.3 Blood Glucose

iHealth has two types of blood glucose monitors: Wireless Smart Gluco-Monitoring System and iHealth Align. They are approved by FDA and CE compliant and meet the ISO 15197:2003 in vitro blood glucose monitoring requirements. They can be used via a dedicated smart application, iHealth Gluco-Smart that requires the users to log in using their specific registration details. These SPMHDs are very useful as they enable the diabetics to effective manage their diabetes via frequent monitoring of blood glucose and keeping it within the normal physiological range by physical activity and diet-based simple lifestyle interventions.

iHealth Align is the smallest commercial glucose meter available, which plugs directly into the headphone jack of the smartphone. It is connected to the smartphone by Bluetooth technology. Once the users perform the blood glucose measurement by pricking their finger and uploading the sample onto the test strip plugged into the iHealth Align, the results are displayed in a few seconds on the smartphone's screen and logged securely inside the smart app. The glucose measurement is performed by the standard amperometric detection of blood glucose using glucose oxidase. The glucose meter requires only 0.7 µL of fresh capillary whole blood and detects glucose within the entire diabetic pathophysiological range, 1.1–33.3 mM in just 5 s. This SPMHD can be purchased online for US$ 16.95, but it can use only iHealth test strips. The smart app enables the users to view the trends and statistics of their blood glucose readings for up to 90 days. It automatically determines the remaining test strips in the vial and their expiry based on which it alerts the users to buy a new vial and prevents the error of false evaluation. Further, it empowers the users with the potential technology, which enables them to share the results with family members, friends, caregivers, and doctors. The smart app acts as an automatic logbook to facilitate the addition of notes to the stored readings and setting up of reminders for medication and insulin dosages and recording of pre- and post-meals glucose. The single pack of iHealth Blood Glucose Test Strips costs only US$12.50 and works with both iHealth meters.

The Wireless Smart Gluco-Monitoring System is standalone and sleek (90 mm × 34.5 mm × 19 mm) blood glucose meter, which is interfaced wirelessly with the smartphone via the Bluetooth technology and the smart app. It is powered by a built-in, rechargeable battery and comes with an easy-to-read light-emitting diode (LED) display. This SPMHD has a unique advantage that once the meter is synced with the smartphone, it can be used for glucose measurements without the smartphone. Up to 500 readings are stored in the device in this offline mode, which can then be transferred to the smartphone. The meter can be purchased online for US$29.95. All other features are the same as in iHealth Align.

The monitoring of blood glucose is an essential part of diabetes management as keeping the blood glucose level within the normal physiological range. Consequently, diabetics can live a healthy lifestyle and avoid the costly and painful diabetic complications. Hence, the developed SPMHDs provides the most effective technology solution for the much better management of diabetes.

3.2.1.4 Blood Oxygen Saturation

The Wireless Pulse Oximeter is a sleek (62 × 33 × 28 mm) and lightweight SPMHD developed by iHealth for the noninvasive spot-check determination of blood oxygen saturation (SpO_2) and the pulse rate at the fingertip by shining two light beams into the small blood vessels or finger capillaries. It is an FDA-cleared and CE-marked device, with a tagged online price of US$69.95. The device runs on an integrated rechargeable battery (3.7 V Li-ion, 300 mAh) that can be recharged using the provided USB cable. A single charge is adequate for many days of personal use, depending upon the frequency of measurements. It is useful for athletes or users to understand how their bodies work during recreation activities and high-intensity sports or exercises. Further, it is beneficial for patients with breathing difficulties (pulmonary dysfunction), COPD (chronic obstructive pulmonary disease), coronary heart diseases, and other vascular conditions. The device is interfaced and connected to the smartphone by the Bluetooth technology and iHealth MyVitals app. The current measurements are displayed on the oximeter's screen and recorded into the device's memory. The smart app offers to view the trends in measurements and share the information with other family members, friends, doctors, or caregivers. The SpO_2 level, indicating the amount of oxygen in the blood as a percentage of the maximum carrying amount, is between 96% and 99% for a healthy individual. However, it is affected by many factors including high altitudes. The device measure SpO_2 in the range of 70–99% with the accuracy of ±2%. The normal resting pulse rate in humans is between 60 and 100 beats per minute (bpm), but it is also dependent on the fitness level, body weight, emotional state, medication, body position, and the involvement in physical activities. The optimum reading guidelines provided in the product insert must be followed as several factors can affect the reading and lead to inaccuracy in results. The most common factors are cold hands, fingernail polish, acrylic nails, hand movements, and weak pulse.

3.2.1.5 Activity and Sleep

The iHealth Edge is the wireless activity and sleep tracker, which can be worn on the wrist like a watch or is put in the pants' pocket on the hip in the form of a clip's attachment. The SPMHD can be purchased online for US$69.95. The watch-shaped lightweight device tracks the daily activity and sleep. It consists of a three-axis accelerometer that detects the 3D-motion patterns and counts the number of steps taken, the distance traveled, and the burnt calories. It automatically provides a snapshot of the data at the end of the activity. The data stored continuously within the device's internal memory is transferred to the iHealth MyVitals app on iOS or Android-equipped smartphone during syncing via the Bluetooth technology. The device has advanced power-saving algorithms that enable a single recharge to last for many days. Further, the device continuously observes the sleep efficiency score and the sleep duration by automatically switching modes. The device is sweat, rain, and splash proof and made of hypoallergenic and skin-friendly TPU rubber, i.e., latex- and PVC-free. The smart app provides an option to data sharing with family members, friends, doctors, or caregivers. The internal rechargeable lithium-polymer battery is charged using the supplied USB charging cable with the magnetic contactor, which contains contact pads that align and attach to the charge pins provided at the device base. One charge of the device is good for 5 days of continuous operations.

The company has recently launched a new version of the device, iHealth Wave, which has the same functions but with the added functionality to track swimming with respect to the type of swim stroke (breaststroke, crawl, and backstroke), a number of movements, movements per minute, and burnt calories. The waterproof device weighs just 35 g and operates via an internal rechargeable 3.7 V Li-ion battery 100 mAh with a battery life of 3 years. A single recharge works for about 7 days. The price in Europe is 79.95 €, but this device is not available on the US website. The device is of immense utility as it facilitates the general healthcare management. Swimming is one of the complete recreation and sports activities that are highly useful for the cardiovascular system. It helps in the development of muscles and is especially recommended for obese persons. It soothes and relaxes the body apart from relieving the stress in the joints.

3.2.1.6 Electrocardiogram

iHealth Rhythm is a recently launched CE-marked smart one lead ECG, which is provided only by the doctor. It is a small (10 cm) and lightweight (20 g) device consisting of a single ultra-flat recorder that clips onto a consumable three-electrode patch. Being light, wearable, and invisible under the clothes, the device monitors the cardiac activity of the patient for up to 72 h, when it is positioned on the patient sternum. It can detect four types of arrhythmia as well as atrial fibrillation and has an "event recorder" button that marks the time whenever the symptoms of abnormal heart activity appear. The patients can press the "event recorder" button on the device when they are experiencing abnormal chest pain. This will enable the device to precisely indicate the anomaly on the ECG report. It synchronizes the ECGs taken by iHealth Rhythm via Bluetooth connection on the free iHealth PRO app for iPad. The app enables the healthcare professionals to visualize, store, and organize ECG results, which simplifies the patient monitoring. The reports can be edited in PDF format and shared with colleagues. iHealth Rhythm can be purchased online at a price of US$150. It is a Class IIa regulated medical device that carries CE0197 mark while the FDA approval is still pending. The device would not interfere with the normal patient activities as the subject can wear it even when taking a shower.

3.2.1.7 Cardiovascular Health

iHealth has recently launched the iHealth CardioLab, which enables the general practitioners (GP) to obtain a detailed cardiovascular assessment of their patients in less than 2 min. It results in better and sustainable cardiovascular healthcare for the patients as it provides the physicians a quick and detailed cardiovascular evaluation, which allows them to anticipate many health problems such as the early detection of peripheral arterial disease (PAD). It provides a simple, accurate, and efficient way of calculating the risk of PAD, strokes, and infarcts. The device will enable the general practitioner to refer the patient to a cardiologist based on the detection of early-stage abnormalities in the evaluation. CardioLab is CE-marked and FDA-approved device, which can be purchased online at a price of 599 € in Europe. Further, it is a Class IIa regulated medical device that carries CE0197 mark. The device employs two measurement cuffs for the upper arm and lower leg, each weighing 135 g and using a universal cuff of circumference 22–42 cm. The measurements are done using an oscillometric method that involves automatic inflation and deflation. It enables the measurement of various cardiovascular health parameters such as BP, heart rate, mean arterial pressure (MAP), ankle-brachial index (ABI), pulse pressure (PP), stroke volume (SV), and cardiac output (CO). These parameters are calculated from the measurement of BP using the algorithms validated and used by cardiologists. The ABI is one of the most effective indicators for the diagnosis, screening, and prevention of PAD. It is calculated by the ratio of systolic pressure at the ankle to the systolic BP of the arm. The results are transmitted in real time by Bluetooth connection to the iHealth PRO app on the iPad, which measures and calculates all these parameters. The rechargeable battery (DC: 5 V, 1 A, 1 × 3.7 V, Li-ion 400 mAh) is charged by a USB cable. The measurement ranges of iHealth Rhythm for systolic pressure, diastolic pressure, and pulse rate are 60–260 mm Hg, 40–199 mm Hg, and 40–180 bpm, respectively.

3.2.2 Cellmic

Cellmic, formerly Holomic LLC, was established in 2011 to commercialize the SBDs developed at Prof. Ozcan's laboratory at UCLA, USA. It has two main product lines: rapid assay readers and mobile microscopy and sensing.

The primary product launched initially was the smartphone-based Holomic Rapid Diagnostic Test Reader (HRDR-200) [87] (Fig. 3.2a), which enables the readout of lateral flow assays (LFA) with high sensitivity and precision. HRDR-200 is equipped with a smartphone, an integrated reader housing, smart application, and access to secure Cloud Services (HIPAA compliant and compatible with HL7 standards) and Test Developer. It is lightweight, handheld, economical, compliant with ISO13485, registered with FDA as a Class I medical device, and CE marked. It is available globally but only allowed for research use in the United States. The reader enables real-time diagnostic data integration via a secure Cloud service and integration with electronics health records (EHRs), laboratory information system (LIS),

(a)   **(b)**

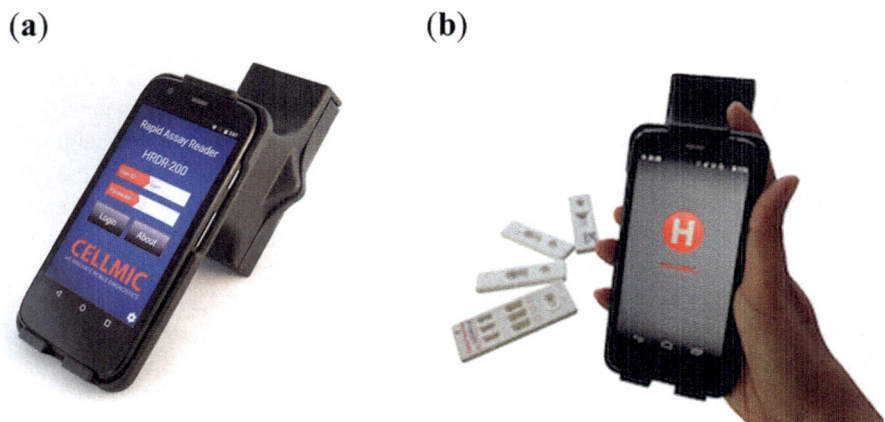

Fig. 3.2 SPMHDs developed by Cellmic. (**a**) Holomic Rapid Diagnostic Test Reader (HRDR-200). (**b**) HRDR-300. Reproduced with permission from Cellmic

and hospital information system (HIS). HRDR-200 is a universal reader that can read chromatographic and fluorescent assays in lateral flow, flow-through, and dipstick test formats with high precision. It can also read tests of various sizes or formats, including strips, cassettes, and multiplexed tests. It can be used standalone or connected to a network. The device can identify the test, lot number, and patient data. Moreover, it is equipped with QR code for automatic entry of test and patient data and issues the lot expiration warning. It is connected to laptops, PCs, printers, routers, and EHRs via wireless, Bluetooth, and USB. The data analysis is performed on a PC with Test Explorer Software, while the test results can be printed, e-mailed, or texted. The lot calibration and distribution can be done with the Test Developer Software. The Cellmic's secure Cloud services are hosted by HIPAA compliant TrueVault in compliance with HL7 standards. The device prototype and its operation have been demonstrated in a pioneering publication by Prof. Ozcan's group [6].

HRDR-300 (Fig. 3.2b) is the recently developed fluorescent reader that enables the multicolor imaging-based readout of the control and test lines of LFA with high accuracy using an advanced image processing algorithm. The users can select the excitation and emission in the regions between 350–700 nm and 300–800 nm, respectively. The device can also be customized according to the needs of the multiplexed fluorescent assay, such as the requirement of multiple excitation sources. All other features are the same as those of chromatographic HRDR-200. The device is also ISO 13485 compliant and registered with the FDA as a Class I medical device. The company is working on the development of HRDR-400, a dual reader for chromatographic and fluorescent rapid tests in a single device.

Holomic Substance Test Assistant (HSTA) is a handheld, economical, and high-performance tool, which acts as a single chromatographic and fluorescent viewer for alcohol and substance abuse tests of different sizes or formats, including saliva tests. All the device features are similar to that of HRDR-200. The company has also developed a desktop application called Test Developer for the LFA test manufacturers, which enables the quality control of the test during development and the calibration of the HRDR-200 reader.

Cellmic provides the services for the development of customized readers for their clients based on their specific requirements. An example is the development of a benchtop model of the smartphone-based HRDR-200 with a smartphone and a portable printer built into the instrument. Further, Cellmic is also developing a broad range of mobile microscopy and sensing technologies.

The development and working of the rapid diagnostic test (RDT) reader prototype [6] that was used for arriving at HRDR-200 are briefly illustrated here. The RDT reader has a plano-convex lens, a microcontroller, and three LED arrays (two located underneath the RDT tray for reflection imaging and one at the top for transmission imaging). It analyzes various types of lateral flow immunoassays and RDTs in reflection or transmission imaging modes under diffused LED illumination and provides a quantitative determination of analytes (Fig. 3.3). The device can run on external batteries or the smartphone battery via USB connection. The highly sensitive RDT reader can detect even the minor color signal variation that cannot be observed by visualization. A smart application, which can be installed on the

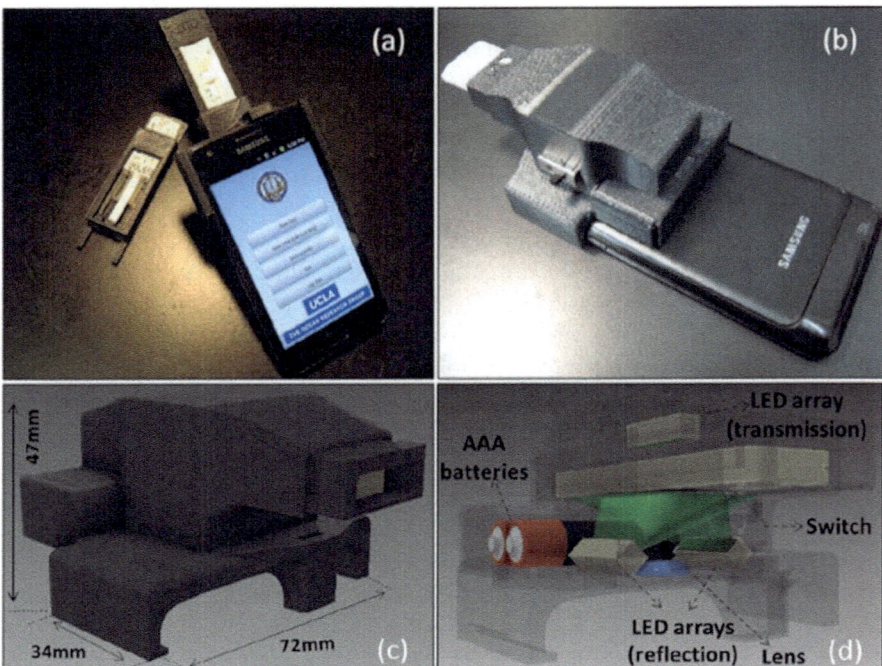

Fig. 3.3 (**a**) and (**b**) Different views of the smartphone-based integrated rapid diagnostic test reader. (**c**) and (**d**) Schematic diagrams of the optical RDT reader attachment. Reproduced with permission from the Royal Society of Chemistry [6]

Android- and iOS-based smartphones, processes the raw images taken by the smartphone's camera within <0.2 s and shares the results with a central server apart from storing the information on the smartphone. The results can also be assessed by a remote computer using web browsers. The software application provides a dynamic spatiotemporal map and real-time statistics for various diseases that can be diagnosed by RDTs, thereby enabling healthcare professionals and policymakers to monitor, track, and analyze emerging diseases and outbreaks.

3.2.3   AliveCor, Inc.

Dr. David Albert founded the AliveCor, Inc. [71] based on his unique concept of iPhone-based electrocardiogram (ECG). Kardia (Fig. 3.4) is the first FDA-cleared and CE-marked device for smartphone- and smartwatch-based ECG that has been cleared for sale in most countries including the United States. It is the clinically validated mobile ECG that allows users to capture medical-grade ECG in just 30 s and interpret it immediately via instant ECG analysis (employing FDA-cleared machine learning algorithms) and consultation with board-certified cardiologists.

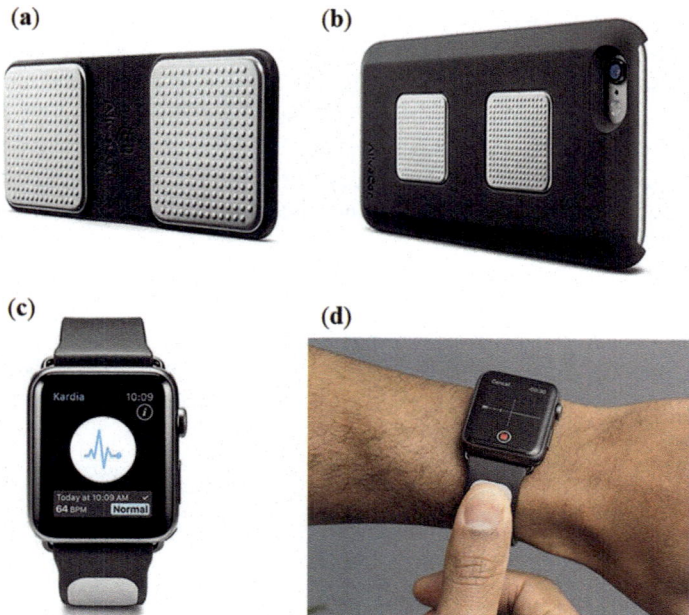

Fig. 3.4 SPMHDs developed by AliveCor, Inc. (**a**) Kardia Mobile. (**b**) Kardia Mobile in iPhone 6 cover accessory. (**c**) Kardia Band. (**d**) Kardia Band's operational procedure. Reproduced with permission from AliveCor, Inc. Images provided are courtesy of AliveCor, Inc.

The device can record, display, store, and evaluate single-channel ECG rhythms and heart rates. The company markets three types of products: Kardia Mobile, Kardia accessories, and Kardia Band. Kardia Mobile is a miniaturized credit card-sized (8.2 cm × 3.2 cm × 0.35 cm) and lightweight (18 g) ECG device with two stainless steel electrodes (2.3 cm × 3 cm), which is sold for US$99. Kardia accessories include the smartphone cases for iPhone 5/5s and iPhone 6/6s that are sold for US$10 and US$15, respectively. These cases have dedicated slots in which the Kardia Mobile can be inserted to have a smartphone cover equipped with ECG. The Kardia Band is the wrist band for Apple Watch that contains the mobile ECG. But it is not yet approved for sale in the United States as it is pending 510k clearance. All the devices run via a dedicated smart app, Kardia App, which can be free downloaded from the App Store and Google Play but requires an initial account setup to make it personalized. The devices are compatible with many models of iOS- and Android-equipped smartphones and gadgets. The ECG data and information are stored via Cloud on a secure server that can be remotely accessed.

Kardia Mobile runs on a 3 V CR2016 coin cell battery with 200 h of operation and can last for 1 year. The single lead ECG is generated by resting the electrodes on the fingers from each hand. The device can take ECG of 30 s to 5 min duration with 300 samples per second sampling rate, 16-bit resolution, and 10 mV peak-to-peak input dynamic range. The measurement involves putting the fingers from the left and right hands on the left and right electrodes, respectively, of Kardia Mobile.

The Kardia App initiates the ECG recording after establishing electrode-finger contact. The Kardia Mobile employs a proprietary technology, which converts the electrical impulses into the ultrasound signals. The ultrasound signals are transmitted to the smartphone's microphone using an enhanced filtering technology that minimizes artifacts and provides medical-grade Lead I ECG. Several clinical trials have already demonstrated the clinical accuracy of the device. It is highly cost-effective for monitoring the patient's heart rate and rhythm, a useful device for the users to take care of their heart. Moreover, it does not add any extra cost to the users as the device is paid in the United States by Medicare and other private insurance companies.

The company has also started Kardiac Premium services at the monthly fees of US$10 to provide detailed ECG reports and visualizations over time and provides personalized reports supplemented with analysis and actionable advice to maintain a healthy heart.

3.2.4   GENTAG, Inc.

GENTAG [72] offers a broad range of mH technologies. Once such technology is a near-field communication (NFC)-based low-cost disposable wireless sensors, the data from which can be read together with spatiotemporal tagging by NFC-capable smartphones (Fig. 3.5a), tablets, or personal computers. This low-cost alternative compared to Bluetooth® facilitates the reading of NFC-based sensors or other customized sensors within the range of 15 miles. The company has developed wireless NFC SensorLinkers, which are portable, lightweight (74 g), and battery-powered devices for home medical monitoring applications, smart homes, and machine-to-machine applications (Fig. 3.5b). The devices comply with ISO13485, MDDS Class-1 FDA clearance, and Continua certification. The NFC SensorLinker has the NFC NXP PN544 Reader integrated circuit (IC) with a proprietary long-range antenna, 2.4 GHz Wi-Fi, Bluetooth 4 Dual Mode, USB port, and a lithium-ion rechargeable battery. It comes with a rechargeable cradle and a USB charger. The SensorLinker runs on any SIM-based GPRS or 3G WCDMA cellular network. It can be paired with existing Bluetooth devices or bundled with custom-made NFC sensors. Its primary applications are the wireless monitoring of elderly people and children, increasing the compliance with treatment, monitoring of medication, and use in wireless hospital discharge kits and hybrid Wi-Fi/Bluetooth/NFC sensor applications. The technology also offers the direct reading and monitoring of implantable NFC sensors and devices such as pacemakers but with an ultralow power requirement. The NFC SensorLinker technology can also be integrated with FDA-approved general healthcare devices such as those for measuring BP, weight, glucose, oxygen, activity, etc., which employ the interface with the Bluetooth technology at the moment.

The company has used their NFC expertise to develop several lines of products, including disposable wireless skin patches, personal drug delivery systems, and smartphone-based sensors. The wireless skin patches are waterproof, showerproof,

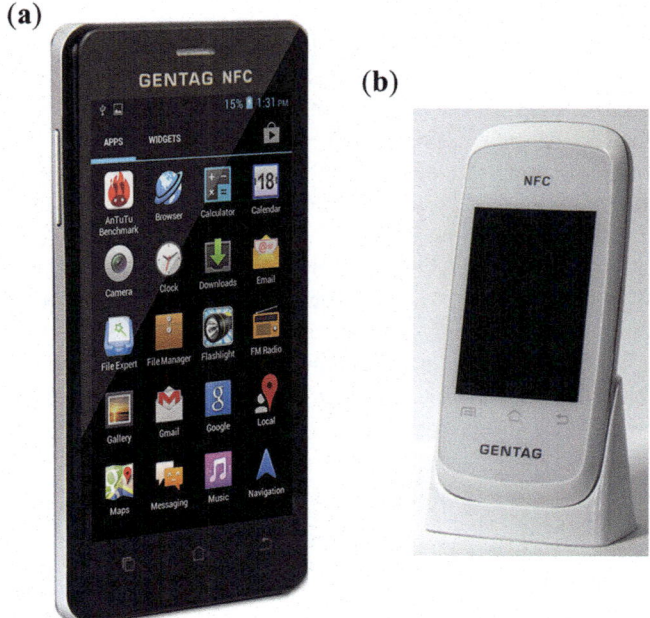

Fig. 3.5 SPMHDs by GENTAG, Inc. (**a**) NFC Smart Cell Phone and (**b**) NFC Sensorlinker. Images provided by Dr. John P. Peeters, GENTAG, Inc. Reproduced with permission from MDPI [92]

and non-allergic, based on low-cost passive technology (battery-less). The FDA-cleared adhesive lasts up to 2 weeks, and the used frequency of 13.56 MHz is the global standard in healthcare. Further, the patches have a unique ID and a radar-responsive (RR) tag, enabling a precise wide area non-GPS wireless geolocation and geofencing over a radius of several miles. The technology can be used for several prospective applications for the monitoring and the location of patients with Alzheimer's dementia. GENTAG has further developed several products and applications such as (1) a NFC-radio frequency identification device (RFID) sensor; (2) NFC immunoassay for prostate cancer; (3) a NFC tag to prevent counterfeit drugs or products; (4) NFC sensors to monitor temperature, radiation, chemicals, and pressure; (5) smartphone-based devices for home monitoring, such as NFC thermometer, NFC-Bluetooth® weight management kit, NFC custom blister packs and medication sensors, and remote wireless monitoring of elderly or at-risk patients directly in their homes by taking BP, fever, and medication data; (6) RR tags; and (7) NFC diagnostic skin patches for fever monitoring, drug delivery, glucose monitoring, post-orthopedics surgery/post-hospital discharge monitoring, and the prevention of hospital errors (due to mismatches from patient-surgery, patient-drug delivery/medication, mother-baby, etc.).

GENTAG has developed low-cost disposable skin patches with wireless sensors for the smartphone-based transdermal glucose sensing and monitoring [19]. These patches are painless as they obviate finger pricking and are more cost-effective than the existing glucose monitoring devices [88–90]. They offer annual savings of US$3000 and US$300 for Type 1 and Type 2 diabetics per patient, respectively. The smartphone can be used for the geolocation of patients in emergency and can also be programmed for the delivery of insulin.

The company has also developed in collaboration with MacroArray Technologies, LLC, a smartphone-based disposable noninvasive immunoassay for the early-stage diagnosis of prostate cancer by detecting a proprietary PCADM-1 biomarker in urine. Considering the cost-effective and more frequent analysis of prostate cancer by this assay, it might replace the existing prostate-specific antigen (PSA)-based blood test being used in hospitals, which is highly affected by various physiological factors [91]. Its second product is a customizable spectroscopic radiation detection cell phone, based on the sensor technology from eV Products, Inc. to discriminate hazardous γ-rays from normal γ-rays.

3.2.5   Apple

Apple Watch [73] (Fig. 3.6) is the latest SPMHD that has captured much attention for general healthcare. With trendy outlooks and designs, the device can be customized further by choosing the specific accessories. This wearable gadget is available online from Apple Store at a price range of US$549–1099, depending on the customized accessories and specifications. The watch outlook on the screen is customized by

Fig. 3.6 Apple Watch. Reproduced with permission from Apple

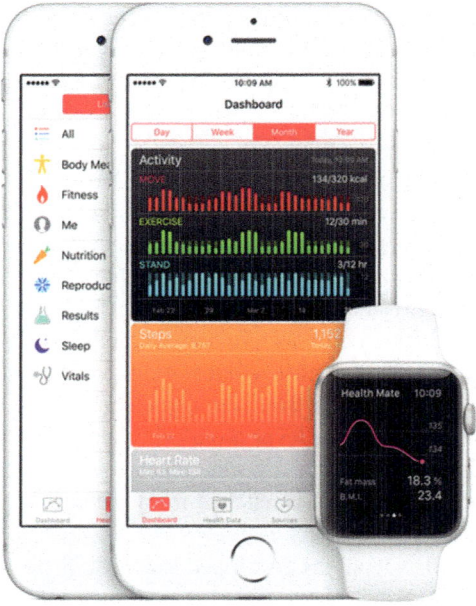

pressing the watch face. The watch monitors the physical activity, heart rate, sleep, and calories burnt throughout the day via the Health app. The Watch has robust and highly sensitive sensors: heart rate monitor, accelerometer, gyroscope, barometer, ambient light sensor, and microphone apart from solid data analysis and power-saving algorithms. It provides an easy-to-read dashboard of the health and fitness data of the user on the screen. The user can enjoy many of the advanced features including notifications and message alerts on the Watch's screen, which ensure much better compliance. It facilitates navigation by tapping on the wrist whether the user has to take a right or left turn. Moreover, it has Siri as the virtual assistant for various things. The Workout app also provides a personalized list of exercises along with the last and best results for each activity. The users can also create their emergency card, providing information on their blood type, allergies, and disease conditions, which is available even on the lock screen of the Watch. Moreover, the users have complete control over their data and decide which data they want to share with the individual health and fitness applications. The Health app data can also be backed up in the iCloud account of the user. The company has implemented stringent guidelines for data security and privacy and complied with the regulatory requirements.

The Watch also enables the user to make a phone call via the Watch, when it is interfaced and connected by Wi-Fi to the smartphone. The watch also has a pay without delay feature that aids easy payments via Apply Pay. Moreover, it controls the Apple TV with the Remote app and finds the misplaced iPhone by playing an audible alert. Further, it plays music and operates interfaced HomeKit devices without iPhone. Apple provides HealthKit to developers so that they can make health and fitness applications. The company also provides the ResearchKit and CareKit, which are open-source software frameworks for medical researchers, doctors, and users. The developers can use ResearchKit to create the applications that will enable medical researchers to gather the desired data for their studies. Similarly, the developers can make applications for users, who want to take more active role in their own well-being. The company is pursuing intensive research in human health via dedicated highly specialized labs for sports and health. This will enable Apple to implement robust health monitoring technologies and sophisticated algorithms in their Watch and iPhone after fine-tuning the sensors, radios, and other components.

Most of the users are looking forward to more healthcare capabilities, such as a pulse oximeter and a glucose sensor, in the Apple Watch2. Apparently, most of the noninvasive technologies should not be a problem to integrate, but the company might require the FDA approval if invasive testing is added.

The company has just announced the Breathe app for Apple Watch 2, which is scheduled to be launched by the end of 2016. The app guides the users through breathing exercises that will enable the users to calm down in stressful situations and would result in a feeling of complete relaxation within a minute. After hitting the start of the Breathe app, the users would see the visualizations of blue-green petals on the Watch's screen when they inhale, which will shrink as they breathe out. Apple has also unveiled the watchOS 3, which is expected to launch the watch apps seven times faster. Moreover, it has a macOS-style dock and a new Control Center, which make the navigation much quicker and simpler. The Activity app has new sharing features and allows the users to compete against their loved ones. The most important is the SOS app, which gets activated by holding the side button. It will send the user's location and a message to a registered contact and emergency services.

3.2.6   Samsung

Samsung also launched the smartwatch, Gear S2 [74] (Fig. 3.7a), which has quite similar functions to Apple Watch. It has a circular face and a rotating bezel that make it easy to navigate through notifications, applications, and widgets. The users can select their customized watch faces on the screen. Once it is interfaced and connected to the smartphone, the user can receive calendar notifications, texts, and new updates on the Gear 2. The charging is simply done by putting the watch onto the wireless charging dock. The Gear 2 has integrated accelerometer, gyroscope, heart rate sensor, ambient light sensor, and barometer. There is a dedicated smart app called S Health app, which allows the users to track their steps and heart rate and get

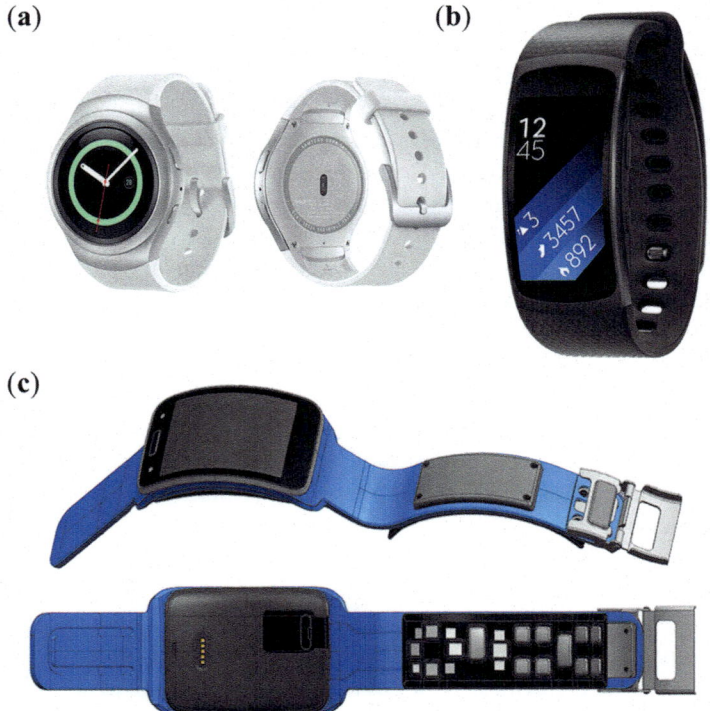

Fig. 3.7 SPMHDs developed by Samsung. (**a**) Gear S2 (front and back views), (**b**) Gear Fit2, and (**c**) Simband (top and bottom views). Reproduced with permission from Samsung

alerts to breaking down the sedentary behavior. The Gear 2 has the IP68 rating, which shows its resistance to dust, dirt, water, and sweat. It has internal memory of 4 GB, RAM of 512 MB, Dual-Core 1.0 GHz processor, 250 mAh Li-ion battery, Bluetooth v4.1, Wi-Fi (802.11 b/g/n 2.4 GHz), and NFC capability. It can be purchased online at a price range of US$299.99–449.99 based on the customized accessories.

The company has also launched Samsung Gear Fit2 [75] (Fig. 3.7b), which is a slimmer built-in GPS-based smartwatch that enables the user to track his step count, floors climbed, sleep quality, and heart rate throughout the day. The built-in GPS provides real-time stats of the physical activity of the user on the map. It automatically recognized the types of activities of the user, such as cycling, running, strength training, yoga, pilates, working out on the elliptical, and other activities. The user receives all notifications from desired apps on the phone and can also respond to calls and text. The charging is done simply by placing it on the charging cradle, and a single charge can last up to 4 days. It also has an IP68 rating and is thus resistant to dust, dirt, water, and sweat. It has 4 GB internal memory, 512 MB RAM, Dual Core (1 GHz Exynos 3250) processor, 200 mAh Li-ion battery, the weight of just 30 g, Bluetooth v4.1, and Wi-Fi. (802.11 b/g/n). This gadget can be purchased at a price of US$179.99.

Samsung has also developed an open-source reference design platform called Simband [76] (Fig. 3.7c), including an open reference sensor module that integrates various advanced sensing technologies. The product has not been commercialized but kept as an open platform, with open software, open hardware, and open mechanical architecture. It facilitates the development of new digital health solutions. The potential sensors integrated into Simband are stationed in the multi-sensor module called Simsense. These sensors are multichannel photoplethysmograph (PPG), ECG, bioimpedance (Bio-Z), galvanic skin response (GSR), accelerometer, and temperature. The multichannel PPG involves the shining of various LED lights on the skin to measure the changes in the blood flow at the microvascular level and determine the necessary physiological health parameters of BP, heart rate, and other parameters. ECG complements the working of the PPG sensor to include the pulse arrival time into the estimation of BP while bioimpedance monitors a range of parameters such as blood flow and body fat. GSR sensors monitor the electrical conductivity of the skin that could be used for the determination of stress levels. Samsung employs a shuttle battery-based unique charging mechanism for Simband, where the battery attaches magnetically to the device and charges it while the user sleeps. Simband has an empty bucket to house customized sensor modules close to the arteries in the anterior part of the wrist. This will enable the digital healthcare professionals to place their sensor module inside the Simband, thereby facilitating easy integration of the sensors that will utilize the power and a secure communication provided by Simband. The technology will enable the developers to design their sensors. It has Bluetooth and Wi-Fi communication to provide access to the Cloud and Samsung Architecture for Multimodal Interactions (SAMI) data platform. Simband has various operation modes: monitoring mode, collection mode, continuous collection mode, and fitness mode for different applications.

3.2.7 Runtastic GmbH

Runtastic GmbH [77] has developed various FDA-cleared and CE-marked global positioning system (GPS)-enabled SPMHDs for sports and fitness (Fig. 3.8), such as Runtastic Heart Rate Combo Monitor, Runtastic Libra weighing scale, Runtastic GPS Watch, and Heart Rate Monitor, and various accessories.

The Runtastic Heart Rate Combo Monitor, comprising a transmitter and a chest strap that are splash proof and powered by lithium batteries, is designed for the measurement of heart rates. The heart rate measurements are transmitted from the chest strap (transmitter) to the smartphone via a low-power Bluetooth® smart technology. The chest strap sends the heart rate signal at a transmission frequency of 5.3 kHz, which is compatible with most training devices in the gym if a separate Runtastic receiver (charged by a lithium battery) is used. Initially, the contacts of the transmitter are moistened by an ECG gel, which is then connected to the strap with the help of two push buttons. This is followed by the adjustment of the elastic strap, enabling the sensors to contact the chest below the pectoral muscles. However, the SPMHD is not intended for persons with limited physical, sensory, or mental abilities and lack experience/knowledge. The device must also be protected from an adamant magnetic field that potentially interferes with the signal and causes a decrease of accuracy. Persons with pacemakers are required to consult their doctors before they can use the device with a price tag of US$69.99.

(a)   (b)

(c)   (d)   (e)   (f)

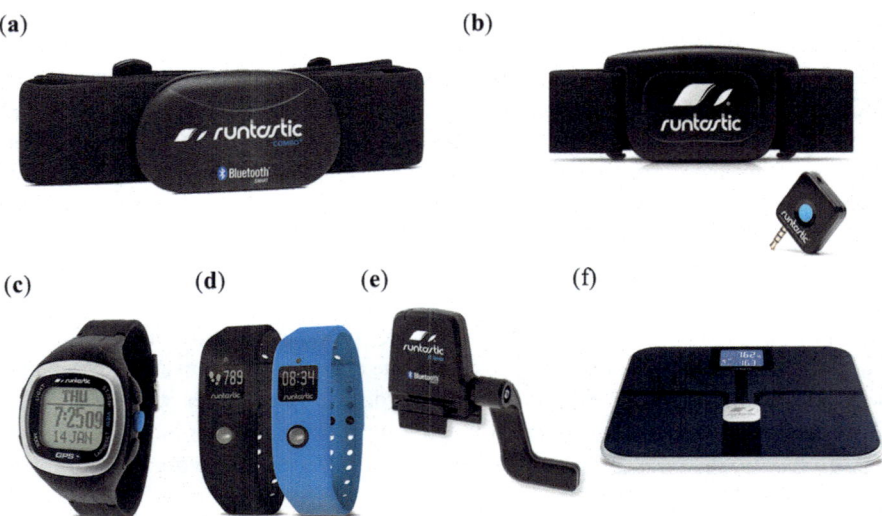

Fig. 3.8 SBMHDs developed by Runtastic GmbH. (**a**) Bluetooth Low Energy Chest Strap of Runtastic Heart Rate Combo Monitor. (**b**) Chest Strap and Dongle of Runtastic Heart Rate Monitor. (**c**) Runtastic GPS Watch. (**d**) Runtastic Orbit. (**e**) Runtastic Speed and Cadence Sensor. (**f**) Runtastic LIBRA weighing scale. Reproduced with permission from Runtastic GmbH

The Runtastic devices require the users to download the Runtastic app on their smartphone and set up their personalized account before they can use the devices and acquire the results in the smart app via Bluetooth connection. The Runtastic app in the smartphone displays the results of the heart rate in real time during the exercises. If the Runtastic receiver is plugged into the headphone jack of the smartphone, it activates the receiver to provide the real-time results from the transmitter immediately on to the smartphone after enabling the receiver ON in the smartphone settings. The receiver's battery lasts about 2.5 years if it is used daily for 1 h. However, the chest strap needs to be used with caution as it might contain latex components that trigger allergic reactions such as skin irritations and redness. It must be discontinued immediately if the person is experiencing any allergic reaction.

The Runtastic activity tracker and the Heart Rate Monitor, sold at US$149.99, tracks and monitors the pace, speed, duration, distance, lap times, training zones, burnt calories, and heart rate together with the elevation change and target heart rate training zones. It is lightweight as the watch and the monitor weight just 57.5 g and 60 g, respectively. The Watch has a battery life of up to 14 h (while using GPS), a customizable display, night light function, a reliable compass with navigation functions, and other functions. The device is charged via a USB cable containing six pins. It transfers the fitness data to the user's personal account on www.Runtastic. com, which can be assessed through a computer, cell phone, or tablet connected to the Internet. The website provides a detailed analysis of the results that is shared online with the Runtastic community. The company has launched a series of GPS activity watches. A more recent version is the Runtastic Orbit, about US$99.99. It is a 24-h activity, fitness and sleep tracker that is also equipped with time and alarm modes. This waterproof device has an integrated ambient light sensor for advanced sleep tracking. It has a wireless feature that synchronizes automatically with the smart app on the smartphone by Bluetooth® Smart technology. Other gadgets such as Fitbit [83], Garmin [84], and Nuband [85, 86] are very similar to the wearable gadgets that are described in this chapter.

The Runtastic Libra is a Bluetooth®-enabled digital body analysis scale that measures critical body metrics: the body weight (up to 180 kg), body fat, body water percentage, muscle mass, bone mass, BMI, basal metabolic rate (BMR), and active metabolic rate (AMR) (burnt calories). It can be purchased online for US$121.31. The device employs bioelectrical impedance analysis (BIA), using an imperceptible, completely harmless and safe alternating current, for the measurements of various body metrics. Muscle tissues and water have good electrical conductivity (i.e., low resistance), while bone and fat tissues exhibit low conductivity (i.e., high resistance). The scale is made up of a highly resistant glass plate coated with indium tin oxide (ITO) electrodes. It weighs 2.5 kg and runs on 3×1.5 V AAA alkaline batteries. The Bluetooth® Smart technology is used to transfer the measurements from Runtastic Libra to the smartphone/tablet that is located within 25 m via the Runtastic Libra app. The scale can be used for the automatic assessment of personal body metrics of up to eight users, who can log on to their account at www.Runtastic.com to get detailed statistics and in-depth analysis. However, Libra should not be used by persons with medical implants (e.g., pacemakers), children below 10 years old, and pregnant women. It has potential interference from strong magnetic fields, which interfere with the signal transmission.

Runtastic Speed and Cadence Sensor, sold at US$58.62, enables the cyclist to convert their smartphone into a professional cycling computer in combination with the Runtastic Road Bike or Runtastic Mountain Bike app. It records the speed, cadence, GPS position, distance, altitude, and other performance parameters. Runtastic also sells USB Power Bank with a capacity of 5600 mAh for only US$34.99. It has a rechargeable integrated LED flashlight and a mini-USB cable to recharge the power bank. The device can be used for charging of various Runtastic devices and the smartphone during extended tracking sessions.

3.2.8   Bühlmann Laboratories AG

Bühlmann Laboratories AG, Switzerland, developed the IB*Doc*® Calprotectin Home Testing system [78] (Fig. 3.9) based on the smartphone readout for the diagnosis of inflammatory bowel disease (IBD). Fecal calprotectin is a reliable indicator of inflammation, whose concentration is significantly increased in IBD patients. The test procedure requires just three simple steps. In the first step, the stool sample is extracted and then dispensed onto the test cassette using the CALEX® Valve extraction device. The second step involves the image capture of the test cassette using the CalApp® smart application inside the smartphone. The last step includes the transmission of results from the CalApp® securely into the IB*Doc*® Portal, followed by its automatic transmission to the patient's doctor for advice pertaining to the therapeutic steps that should be taken. The CalApp® requires a secure login to the

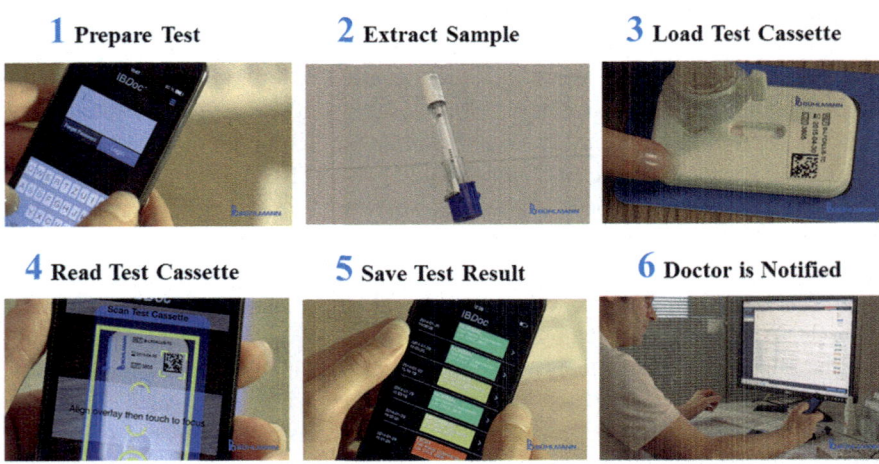

Fig. 3.9 IB*Doc*® Calprotectin Home Testing system developed by Bühlmann Laboratories AG. Reproduced with permission from Bühlmann Laboratories AG

personal account of the user. The company supplies the IB*Doc*® Camera Test card, which is used to perform the camera check before the image of the actual test cassette is acquired. The CalApp® employs state-of-the-art image processing to determine the quantitative calprotectin concentration in the sample. The test results are classified as normal, moderate, and high, similar to traffic light code, and saved locally on the phone and IB*Doc*® Portal.

3.2.9 Mobile Assay, Inc.

Mobile Assay, Inc.developed a cost-effective mobile diagnostic reader (mReader™) [79] (Fig. 3.10), which works on the principle of Mobile Image Ratiometry (MIR) and performs analysis using Instantaneous Analysis™ software. The smartphone-based mReader™ provides rapid and accurate tracking and quantification of lateral flow test strips [7, 8]. It can read multiple tests simultaneously down to 1 ppb with a high-accuracy detection and significantly higher sensitivity than the human eye. The reader requires no additional attachments and has an integrated advanced light level compensation and camera linearity to provide highly reproducible reading, unaffected by ambient light fluctuation. For processing image analysis of the dye signal on the test strips, the MIR subtracts the background noise, selects the signal bands, and provides the pixel density ratio. The bioanalytical procedure involves the dispensing of the sample at the designated area on the test strip, which

Fig. 3.10 Mobile diagnostic reader (mReader™) by Mobile Assay, Inc. Image provided by Michael Williams, Mobile Assay, Inc. Reproduced with permission from MDPI [92]

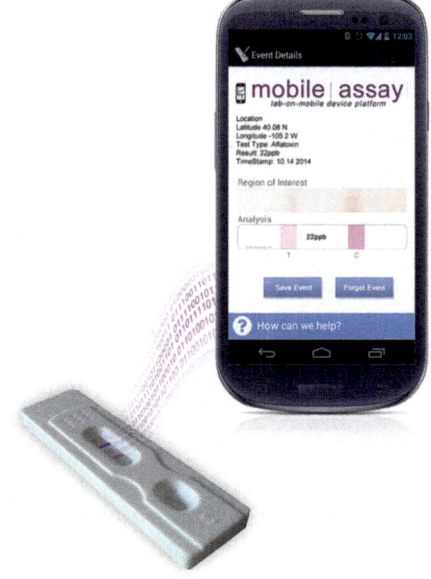

is taken by capillary action together with the dye-conjugated antibodies specific for the target analyte, across the test and control areas. The absence of the particular analyte is shown by the appearance of two bands as the dye binds at the test as well as the control lines. However, as the analyte concentration increases in the sample, the relative intensity of the test band as determined by MIR also increases.

The device is operated by the smart application that can be run on Apple-, Android-, and Windows-equipped smartphones and gadgets. The geotagged and time-stamped results are uploaded to the mobile diagnostic Cloud via Wi-Fi or a cellular network with the push of a button. The data is stored securely on the portal provided by the company using advanced encryption and data storage techniques. The stored data can be assessed by a secure "sign in" to the portal. The results stored in the Cloud are analyzed for trend analysis of the particular test. Both internal and external compliance reports can also be generated in customized formats. The Data Collection Module transfers the data in real time to the Mobile Assay Cloud™, which can be accessed locally via Tracker™. The Tracker Manager™ can also send text alerts to the clients.

The mReader™ and the rapid diagnostic assays have been used for the detection of drugs (e.g., cocaine and benzoylecgonine), food pathogens, and aflatoxin. It detects $0.1–300$ ng mL^{-1} of cocaine, $0.003–0.1$ ng mL^{-1} of benzoylecgonine, and food pathogens [10], which facilitate the rapid and efficient tracking of the origin and severity of outbreaks. The technology is indispensable to the food producers as it prevents the large-scale distribution of contaminated food by taking measures at an early stage. This could lead to tremendous savings as about 48 million foodborne illness cases are treated annually in the United States [93], which incur an annual financial burden of US$51–78 billion [94]. Moreover, it can also be used to enhance agricultural productivity by reducing the crop losses as it enables the detection and tracking of the infection by *Botrytis cinerea* fungus that causes significant damages to plants and flowers.

3.2.10 CellScope

CellScope [80] is a startup [22] in San Francisco that was founded by Erik Douglas and Amy Sheng of Prof. Daniel Fletcher's research lab at the University of California, Berkeley. The company developed two optical attachments that modify the smartphone into a diagnostic-quality imaging system for healthcare and skin-care applications.

"CellScope Oto" is a clip-on digital Otoscope that takes high-resolution images of the middle ear to probe if the subjects have an ear infection (Fig. 3.11). The device comprises a custom-designed iPhone case, an Otoscope attachment, an Otoscope case, five tip cases, and an iPhone app. The smart app transfers the images captured by the smartphone to an HIPAA-compliant website for reviewing, comparing, and transmitting the result of ear examination. The automated analysis of the results helps in minimizing the doctor visits for the parents as the smart app enables the uploading of high-resolution images of the ear canal and eardrums on

Fig. 3.11 CellScope Oto
by CellScope. Image
provided by Cori Allen,
CellScope, Inc.
Reproduced with
permission from [92]

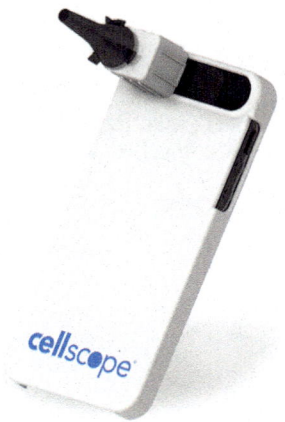

the CellScope's web platform, which can be accessed remotely by a doctor for diagnosis, treatment, and monitoring. This SPMHD will significantly reduce the healthcare costs considering about 30 million doctor visits by the parents every year in the United States. The device can screen sick children in school or daycare facilities for ear infection. The "CellScope Derm" is another clip-on Dermascope that facilitates the remote diagnosis of patient's skin conditions by capturing and transmitting highly magnified diagnostic quality images of the skin. The device has an illumination system and lower-magnification optics for capturing the images at a wider field.

3.2.11   Nonin Medical, Inc.

Nonin Medical, Inc. [81], a company that has manufactured clinically accredited pulse oximeters with high accuracy [95–97], has developed Onyx® II Model 9560 Finger Pulse Oximeter, a highly prospective SPMHD (Fig. 3.12) for US\$666. This compact and lightweight (63 g) pulse oximeter measures SpO_2 and the pulse rate of well- or poorly perfused patients, such as patients with congestive heart failure, asthma, COPD, and other cardiovascular disorders. The technology involves noninvasive pulse oximetry method [98, 99], where the red (660 nm) and infrared (910 nm) lights are passed through the perfused tissue, and the fluctuating signal due to arterial pulses is detected. The SpO_2 levels are determined from the difference in color that is analyzed by the ratio of the absorbed red and infrared light. The well-oxygenated blood is characterized by bright red color, while the poorly oxygenated blood is dark red. The device can perform the measurements on a large number of subjects with the thickness of the fingers varying from 0.8 to 2.5 cm. It can also be used in persons having light to dark skin tones and good to low perfusion. The device stores at least 20 single point measurements and transmits the results wirelessly up to 100 m. The advanced SmartPoint algorithm enables the automated determination of SpO_2 and

Fig. 3.12 Onyx® II Model
9560 Finger Pulse
Oximeter developed by
Nonin Medical, Inc.
Reproduced with
permission from [92]

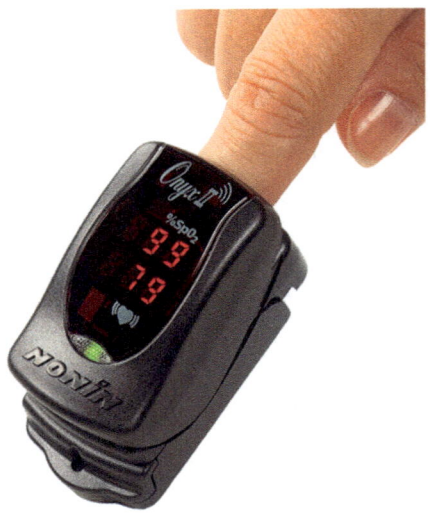

the pulse rate and employs a sophisticated power-saving feature that automatically adjusts the transmitted power based on the distance between the device and the main unit. Moreover, it uses the PureSAT signal processing technology for high precision as it effectively removes the noise, artifacts, and interferences. It uses two AAA batteries, which guarantee operations for over 1 year. It measures SpO_2 and the pulse rate in the ranges of 0–100% and 18–321 BPM, respectively. The average root mean square (RMS) accuracies for the SpO_2 range of 70–100% and the pulse rate of 20–250 BPM are ±2 and ±3, respectively. Apart from healthcare settings, the device can also be used as a personalized device.

The Bluetooth radio in Onyx® II Model 9560 complies with the Bluetooth version 2.0 Specification that supports the Serial Port Protocol (SPP), the Health Device Profile (HDP) with security mode 2 (service level enforced), IEEE11073, and Continua. Further, it is certified to Microsoft® HealthVault®, a free online platform that communicates and receives data from the device for personalized healthcare management. The device complies with the IEC 60601-1-2 for electromagnetic compatibility, part 15 of the Federal Communications Commission (FCC) Rules as a Class B digital device, and ISO 10993-1. However, the Federal Law (USA) restricts this device to sale by or on the order of a licensed practitioner.

3.2.12   Cicret

Cicret Bracelet [82], the next generation smart bracelet by Cicret, can perform different tasks on the arm of the users with all skin colors, similar to what they can do with a tablet but without any need to pick up the smartphone (Fig. 3.13). It enables the users to answer phone calls, read e-mails, play games, check weather, navigation, and many other tasks. The device is water-resistant, employs a removable

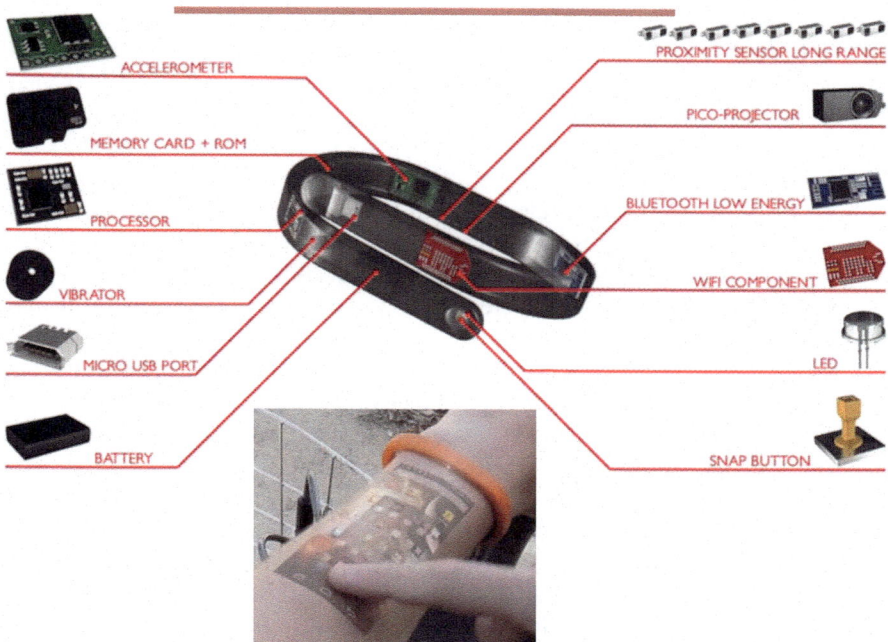

Fig. 3.13 Circlet Bracelet and the integral components. The inlet shows working of the Cicret Bracelet on the arm of the user. Reproduced with permission from Circlet

battery, functions with an Android operating system, and has an internal memory of 32 or 64 GB. Although the company has built the prototypes and intended to sell it in the market by the end of 2016, the product is currently priced at US$250. The company is currently raising US$0.5 million to go for industrial production. The device has a pico projector that projects the smartphone screen onto the arm. It has eight long-range proximity sensors, which make the user's skin as a touchscreen. When the user puts a finger on the screen that appears on the arm, one of the sensors is stopped, which sends the information back to the processor in the bracelet. The Circlet Bracelet has an accelerometer, Bluetooth, Wi-Fi component, LED, processor, vibrator, micro USB port, removable battery, memory card and ROM, and a snap button. The technology will be used in many healthcare applications, which are currently being conceptualized and investigated by many healthcare professionals and researchers.

3.3   Conclusions and Prospects

Smartphones have become ubiquitous and emerged as an ideal platform for mH and telemedicine applications. As 70% of the smartphone users are residing in developing countries, where there is a critical need for mH due to the shortage of healthcare professionals and infrastructure, SPMHDs would play an instrumental role in such countries for increased healthcare outreach and better healthcare management. SPMHDs would empower the patients and users to be the active decisionmakers in their healthcare. They will create a learning environment, where the users can analyze their healthcare results and adjust their lifestyle by implementing the simple physical activity, nutritional, and other interventions to achieve visible and sustained health benefits.

Most of the SPMHDs have already been CE marked, while FDA has further approved some. These devices have already penetrated the consumer market and are being used by millions of people worldwide. It has significantly improved the people awareness by making them more health conscious and has led to critically enhanced and sustainable health outcomes by enabling better healthcare monitoring and management. The use of SPMHDs would significantly cut down the healthcare costs and motivate the users to participate in effective prevention and management of chronic health diseases, such as diabetes, obesity, cardiovascular disorders, stress, and cancer, by implementing simple lifestyle interventions.

The development of SPMHDs has demonstrated the successful convergence of various scientific disciplines, such as engineering, biomedical sciences, medicine, chemistry, physical sciences, etc. The ongoing multidisciplinary research will further expand the applications of SPMHDs, thereby paving the way for next-generation personalized healthcare monitoring and management. However, several challenges need to be overcome, such as clinical accuracy, reproducibility, robustness, miniaturization, regulatory compliance, and adaptability to various smartphone models.

The recent years have witnessed tremendous advances in Cloud computing, which is essential for SPMHDs, as it leads to significant cost savings by minimizing the infrastructure costs [100]. However, there are potential concerns about data security and privacy [101, 102]. Most nations want to store the data physically within their national boundaries, as per their existing laws, which need to be complied with by all SPMHDs [103]. This limitation has been solved by companies such as Amazon Web Services, which now allows companies to store their data within their national boundaries. The Google's Government Cloud also allows governments to store their data in their countries as per their data security guidelines. But there is an immense need to create international Cloud computing standards, which has led to the start of several initiatives, such as EuroCloud and Google Data Liberation Front.

The personal information data in personal health records (PHRs) could be exposed to third-party servers and unauthorized parties, which is a potential concern as the ethical guidelines have given the patients full control over their PHRs. This has been counteracted by implementing effective strategies, such as employing attribute-based encryption [104] and using a trusted third party [103]. Several Cloud computing models have also been developed to deal with the regulatory requirements of security and privacy [105].

The benefits of electronic health records (EHRs) in improving caregivers' decisions and patients' outcomes have been widely demonstrated [106]. The Health Information Technology for Economic and Clinical Health (HITECH) Act in the United States has further authorized incentive payments via insurance agencies to the healthcare practitioners, who would use EHRs to achieve specified improvements in care delivery [107]. The smartphone-based mobile Cloud computing [108], being employed in the SPMHDs, would facilitate next generation of personalized mH [109]. The next decade will witness the SPMHD-based next-generation healthcare boom based on the great increase of smartphone's features, increased functionality of mobile Cloud computing, and critically improved mH enabling technologies. These developments enable much better healthcare in the developing countries, a primary focus of healthcare researchers and professionals for a long time.

References

1. Ozcan A. Mobile phones democratize and cultivate next-generation imaging, diagnostics and measurement tools. Lab Chip. 2014.
2. Thilakanathan D, Chen S, Nepal S, Calvo R, Alem L. A platform for secure monitoring and sharing of generic health data in the Cloud. Futur Gener Comput Syst. 2014;35:102–13.
3. Portfolio Research Mobile Facebook. 2013. http://www.portioresearch.com/media/3986/Portio%20Research%20Mobile%20Factbook%202013pdf.
4. Vashist SK, Mudanyali O, Schneider EM, Zengerle R, Ozcan A. Cellphone-based devices for bioanalytical sciences. Anal Bioanal Chem. 2014;406(14):3263–77.
5. You DJ, Park TS, Yoon JY. Cell-phone-based measurement of TSH using Mie scatter optimized lateral flow assays. Biosens Bioelectron. 2013;40(1):180–5.
6. Mudanyali O, Dimitrov S, Sikora U, Padmanabhan S, Navruz I, Ozcan A. Integrated rapid-diagnostic-test reader platform on a cellphone. Lab Chip. 2012;12(15):2678–86.
7. Tseng D, Mudanyali O, Oztoprak C, Isikman SO, Sencan I, Yaglidere O, et al. Lensfree microscopy on a cellphone. Lab Chip. 2010;10(14):1787–92.
8. Cooper DC, Callahan B, Callahan P, Burnett L. Mobile image ratiometry: a new method for instantaneous analysis of rapid test strips. Nat Preced. 2012. https://doi.org/10.1038/npre201268271.
9. Cadle BA, Rasmus KC, Varela JA, Leverich LS, O'Neill CE, Bachtell RK, et al. Cellular phone-based image acquisition and quantitative ratiometric method for detecting cocaine and benzoylecgonine for biological and forensic applications. Subst Abus. 2010;4:21–33.
10. Cooper DC. Mobile image ratiometry for the detection of Botrytis cinerea (Gray Mold). Nat Preced. 2012. https://doi.org/10.1038/npre201269891.
11. Mudanyali O, Tseng D, Oh C, Isikman SO, Sencan I, Bishara W, et al. Compact, light-weight and cost-effective microscope based on lensless incoherent holography for telemedicine applications. Lab Chip. 2010;10(11):1417–28.
12. Bishara W, Sikora U, Mudanyali O, Su TW, Yaglidere O, Luckhart S, et al. Holographic pixel super-resolution in portable lensless on-chip microscopy using a fiber-optic array. Lab Chip. 2011;11(7):1276–9.
13. Zhu H, Yaglidere O, Su TW, Tseng D, Ozcan A. Cost-effective and compact wide-field fluorescent imaging on a cell-phone. Lab Chip. 2011;11(2):315–22.
14. Smith ZJ, Chu K, Espenson AR, Rahimzadeh M, Gryshuk A, Molinaro M, et al. Cell-phone-based platform for biomedical device development and education applications. PLoS One. 2011;6(3):e17150.
15. Breslauer DN, Maamari RN, Switz NA, Lam WA, Fletcher DA. Mobile phone based clinical microscopy for global health applications. PLoS One. 2009;4(7):e6320.
16. Lillehoj PB, Huang MC, Truong N, Ho CM. Rapid electrochemical detection on a mobile phone. Lab Chip. 2013;13(15):2950–5.

17. Wireless Smart Gluco-Monitoring System. http://www.ihealthlabs.com/glucometer/wireless-smart-gluco-monitoring-system/.
18. Geiger GE, Oberding JW, Ward RN, White KD. Blood glucose meter/modem interface arrangement. 2007. U.S. Patent No. 7,181,350. 20 Feb 2007.
19. Peeters JP. Diagnostic radio frequency identification sensors and applications thereof. 2011. U.S. Patent No. 8,077,042. 13 Dec 2011.
20. Shen L, Hagen JA, Papautsky I. Point-of-care colorimetric detection with a smartphone. Lab Chip. 2012;12(21):4240–3.
21. Lu Y, Shi W, Qin J, Lin B. Low cost, portable detection of gold nanoparticle-labeled microfluidic immunoassay with camera cell phone. Electrophoresis. 2009;30(4):579–82.
22. Coskun AF, Wong J, Khodadadi D, Nagi R, Tey A, Ozcan A. A personalized food allergen testing platform on a cellphone. Lab Chip. 2013;13(4):636–40.
23. Zhu H, Sikora U, Ozcan A. Quantum dot enabled detection of Escherichia coli using a cellphone. Analyst. 2012;137(11):2541–4.
24. Thomas MA, Narayan PR, Christian C. Mitigating gaps in reproductive health reporting in outlier communities of Kerala, India—A mobile phone-based health information system. Health Policy Technol. 2012;1(2):69–76.
25. McGeough CM, O'Driscoll S. Camera phone-based quantitative analysis of C-reactive protein ELISA. IEEE Trans Biomed Circ Syst. 2013;7(5):655–9.
26. Preechaburana P, Gonzalez MC, Suska A, Filippini D. Surface plasmon resonance chemical sensing on cell phones. Angew Chem. 2012;51(46):11585–8.
27. Zhu H, Mavandadi S, Coskun AF, Yaglidere O, Ozcan A. Optofluidic fluorescent imaging cytometry on a cell phone. Anal Chem. 2011;83(17):6641–7.
28. Zhu H, Sencan I, Wong J, Dimitrov S, Tseng D, Nagashima K, et al. Cost-effective and rapid blood analysis on a cell-phone. Lab Chip. 2013;13(7):1282–8.
29. Benhamou PY, Melki V, Boizel R, Perreal F, Quesada JL, Bessieres-Lacombe S, et al. One-year efficacy and safety of Web-based follow-up using cellular phone in type 1 diabetic patients under insulin pump therapy: the PumpNet study. Diabetes Metab. 2007;33(3):220–6.
30. Botsis T, Hartvigsen G. Current status and future perspectives in telecare for elderly people suffering from chronic diseases. J Telemed Telecare. 2008;14(4):195–203.
31. Carrera PM, Dalton AR. Do-it-yourself healthcare: the current landscape, prospects and consequences. Maturitas. 2014;77(1):37–40.
32. Carter MC, Burley VJ, Nykjaer C, Cade JE. Adherence to a smartphone application for weight loss compared to website and paper diary: pilot randomized controlled trial. J Med Internet Res. 2013;15(4):e32.
33. Coulter A. Engaging patients in healthcare. McGraw-Hill International; 2011.
34. Donker T, Petrie K, Proudfoot J, Clarke J, Birch MR, Christensen H. Smartphones for smarter delivery of mental health programs: a systematic review. J Med Internet Res. 2013;15(11):e247.
35. Duffy MB. Humanizing the healthcare experience: the key to improved outcomes. Gastrointest Endosc. 2014;79(3):499–502.
36. Fiordelli M, Diviani N, Schulz PJ. Mapping mHealth research: a decade of evolution. J Med Internet Res. 2013;15(5):e95.
37. Franc S, Borot S, Ronsin O, Quesada JL, Dardari D, Fagour C, et al. Telemedicine and type 1 diabetes: is technology per se sufficient to improve glycaemic control? Diabetes Metab. 2014;40(1):61–6.
38. Free C, Phillips G, Galli L, Watson L, Felix L, Edwards P, et al. The effectiveness of mobile-health technology-based health behaviour change or disease management interventions for health care consumers: a systematic review. PLoS Med. 2013;10(1):e1001362.
39. Free C, Phillips G, Watson L, Galli L, Felix L, Edwards P, et al. The effectiveness of mobile-health technologies to improve health care service delivery processes: a systematic review and meta-analysis. PLoS Med. 2013;10(1):e1001363.
40. Honka A, Kaipainen K, Hietala H, Saranummi N. Rethinking health: ICT-enabled services to empower people to manage their health. IEEE Rev Biomed Eng. 2011;4:119–39.

41. Joe J, Demiris G. Older adults and mobile phones for health: a review. J Biomed Inform. 2013;46(5):947–54.
42. Kaplan RM, Stone AA. Bringing the laboratory and clinic to the community: mobile technologies for health promotion and disease prevention. Annu Rev Psychol. 2013;64:471–98.
43. Luxton DD, McCann RA, Bush NE, Mishkind MC, Reger GM. mHealth for mental health: integrating smartphone technology in behavioral healthcare. Prof Psychol-Res Pr. 2011;42(6):505–12.
44. O'Reilly GA, Spruijt-Metz D. Current mHealth technologies for physical activity assessment and promotion. Am J Prev Med. 2013;45(4):501–7.
45. Pagoto S. The current state of lifestyle intervention implementation research: where do we go next? Transl Behav Med. 2011;1(3):401–5.
46. Price M, Yuen EK, Goetter EM, Herbert JD, Forman EM, Acierno R, et al. mHealth: a mechanism to deliver more accessible, more effective mental health care. Clin Psychol Psychother. 2013.
47. Stephens J, Allen J. Mobile phone interventions to increase physical activity and reduce weight: a systematic review. J Cardiovasc Nurs. 2013;28(4):320–9.
48. Martínez-Pérez B, de la Torre-Díez I, López-Coronado M. Mobile health applications for the most prevalent conditions by the World Health Organization: review and analysis. J Med Internet Res. 2013;15(6).
49. Phillips G, Felix L, Galli L, Patel V, Edwards P. The effectiveness of M-health technologies for improving health and health services: a systematic review protocol. BMC Res Notes. 2010;3(1):250.
50. Mosa AS, Yoo I, Sheets L. A systematic review of healthcare applications for smartphones. BMC Med Inform Decis Mak. 2012;12(1):67.
51. Bellina L, Missoni E. Mobile cell-phones (M-phones) in telemicroscopy: increasing connectivity of isolated laboratories. Diagn Pathol. 2009;4:19.
52. Dayer L, Heldenbrand S, Anderson P, Gubbins PO, Martin BC. Smartphone medication adherence apps: potential benefits to patients and providers. J Am Pharm Assoc. 2013;53(2):172.
53. Hasvold PE, Wootton R. Use of telephone and SMS reminders to improve attendance at hospital appointments: a systematic review. J Telemed Telecare. 2011;17(7):358–64.
54. Lester RT, Ritvo P, Mills EJ, Kariri A, Karanja S, Chung MH, et al. Effects of a mobile phone short message service on antiretroviral treatment adherence in Kenya (WelTel Kenya1): a randomised trial. Lancet. 2010;376(9755):1838–45.
55. Montes JM, Medina E, Gomez-Beneyto M, Maurino J. A short message service (SMS)-based strategy for enhancing adherence to antipsychotic medication in schizophrenia. Psychiatry Res. 2012;200(2–3):89–95.
56. Tripp N, Hainey K, Liu A, Poulton A, Peek M, Kim J, et al. An emerging model of maternity care: smartphone, midwife, doctor? Women Birth. 2014;27(1):64–7.
57. Demidowich AP, Lu K, Tamler R, Bloomgarden Z. An evaluation of diabetes self-management applications for Android smartphones. J Telemed Telecare. 2012;18(4):235–8.
58. Rao A, Hou P, Golnik T, Flaherty J, Vu S. Evolution of data management tools for managing self-monitoring of blood glucose results: a survey of iPhone applications. J Diabetes Sci Technol. 2010;4(4):949–57.
59. Migliore M. Smartphones or tablets for a better communication and education between residents and consultant in a teaching hospital. J Surg Educ. 2013;70(4):437–8.
60. Payne KFB, Wharrad H, Watts K. Smartphone and medical related App use among medical students and junior doctors in the United Kingdom (UK): a regional survey. BMC Med Inform Decis Mak. 2012;12(1):121.
61. Lunny C, Taylor D, Memetovic J, Warje O, Lester R, Wong T, et al. Short message service (SMS) interventions for the prevention and treatment of sexually transmitted infections: a systematic review protocol. Syst Rev. 2014;3(1):7.
62. Muessig KE, Pike EC, Legrand S, Hightow-Weidman LB. Mobile phone applications for the care and prevention of HIV and other sexually transmitted diseases: a review. J Med Internet Res. 2013;15(1):e1.

63. Lee AWM, Ng JKY, Wong EYW, Tan A, Lau AKY, Lai SFY. Lecture Rule No. 1: Cell phones ON, please! A low-cost personal response system for learning and teaching. J Chem Educ. 2013;90(3):388–9.
64. Wallace S, Clark M, White J. 'It's on my iPhone': attitudes to the use of mobile computing devices in medical education, a mixed-methods study. BMJ Open. 2012;2(4).
65. Lau JK, Lowres N, Neubeck L, Brieger DB, Sy RW, Galloway CD, et al. iPhone ECG application for community screening to detect silent atrial fibrillation: a novel technology to prevent stroke. Int J Cardiol. 2013;165(1):193–4.
66. Peck JL, Stanton M, Reynolds GE. Smartphone preventive health care: parental use of an immunization reminder system. J Pediatr Health Care. 2014;28(1):35–42.
67. Lwin MO, Vijaykumar S, Fernando ON, Cheong SA, Rathnayake VS, Lim G, et al. A 21st century approach to tackling dengue: crowdsourced surveillance, predictive mapping and tailored communication. Acta Trop. 2013;130C:100–7.
68. Doyle GJ, Garrett B, Currie LM. Integrating mobile devices into nursing curricula: opportunities for implementation using Rogers' Diffusion of Innovation model. Nurse Educ Today. 2014;34(5):775–82.
69. http://www.ihealthlabs.com/.
70. Xie L, Wang T, Huang T, Hou W, Huang G, Du Y. Dew inspired breathing-based detection of genetic point mutation visualized by naked eye. Sci Rep. 2014;4:6300.
71. http://www.alivecor.com/home.
72. http://gentag.com/.
73. http://www.apple.com/watch/.
74. http://www.samsung.com/global/galaxy/gear-s2/.
75. http://www.samsung.com/global/galaxy/gear-fit2/.
76. http://www.samsung.com/us/ssic/pdf/Samsung_Simband_Backgrounderpdf.
77. Yang Y, Zhang H, Liu Y, Lin ZH, Lee S, Lin Z, et al. Silicon-based hybrid energy cell for self-powered electrodegradation and personal electronics. ACS Nano. 2013;7(3):2808–13.
78. http://www.ibdoc.net/?lang=en.
79. Woolley CF, Hayes MA. Emerging technologies for biomedical analysis. Analyst. 2014;139(10):2277–88.
80. Wu WH, Bui AA, Batalin MA, Au LK, Binney JD, Kaiser WJ. MEDIC: medical embedded device for individualized care. Artif Intell Med. 2008;42(2):137–52.
81. http://www.nonin.com/PulseOximetry/Finger/Onyx9560.
82. https://cicret.com/wordpress/.
83. https://www.fitbit.com/us.
84. http://www.garmin.com/en-GB/.
85. http://www.nubandsports.com/nuband01/.
86. http://www.nubandsports.com/nuband-active/.
87. http://www.cellmic.com/.
88. Vashist SK, Zheng D, Al-Rubeaan K, Luong JHT, Sheu FS. Technology behind commercial devices for blood glucose monitoring in diabetes management: a review. Anal Chim Acta. 2011;703(2):124–36.
89. Vashist SK. Non-invasive glucose monitoring technology in diabetes management: a review. Anal Chim Acta. 2012;750:16–27.
90. Vashist SK. Continuous glucose monitoring systems: a review. Diagnostics. 2013;3(4):385–412.
91. Gudmundsson J, Besenbacher S, Sulem P, Gudbjartsson DF, Olafsson I, Arinbjarnarson S, et al. Genetic correction of PSA values using sequence variants associated with PSA levels. Sci Transl Med. 2010;2(62):62ra92.
92. Vashist SK, Schneider EM, Luong JHT. Commercial smartphone-based devices and smart applications for personalized healthcare monitoring and management. Diagnostics (Basel). 2014;4(3):104–28.
93. Incidence and trends of foodborne illness. 2011. http://www.cdc.gov/features/dsfoodnet/.

94. Scharff RL. Economic burden from health losses due to foodborne illness in the United States. J Food Prot. 2012;75(1):123–31.
95. Bickler PE, Feiner JR, Severinghaus JW. Effects of skin pigmentation on pulse oximeter accuracy at low saturation. Anesthesiology. 2005;102(4):715–9.
96. Macnab AJ, Smith M, Phillips N, Smart P. Oximeter reliability in a subzero environment. Aviat Space Environ Med. 1996;67(11):1053–6.
97. Schermer T, Leenders J, in 't Veen H, van den Bosch W, Wissink A, Smeele I, et al. Pulse oximetry in family practice: indications and clinical observations in patients with COPD. Fam Pract. 2009;26(6):524–31.
98. Jubran A. Pulse oximetry. Crit Care. 1999;3(2):R11–7.
99. Sinex JE. Pulse oximetry: principles and limitations. Am J Emerg Med. 1999;17(1):59–67.
100. Marston S, Li Z, Bandyopadhyay S, Zhang J, Ghalsasi A. Cloud computing — The business perspective. Decis Support Syst. 2011;51(1):176–89.
101. Subashini S, Kavitha V. A survey on security issues in service delivery models of cloud computing. J Netw Comput Appl. 2011;34(1):1–11.
102. Sun DW, Chang GR, Sun LN, Wang XW. Surveying and analyzing security, privacy and trust issues in cloud computing environments. Proc Eng. 2011;15:2852–6.
103. Zissis D, Lekkas D. Addressing cloud computing security issues. Futur Gener Comput Syst. 2012;28(3):583–92.
104. Li M, Yu SC, Zheng Y, Ren K, Lou WJ. Scalable and secure sharing of personal health records in cloud computing using attribute-based encryption. IEEE Trans Parall Distr. 2013;24(1):131–43.
105. Schweitzer EJ. Reconciliation of the cloud computing model with US federal electronic health record regulations. J Am Med Inform Assoc. 2012;19(2):161–5.
106. Blumenthal D, Tavenner M. The "meaningful use" regulation for electronic health records. N Engl J Med. 2010;363(6):501–4.
107. Blumenthal D. Launching HITECH. N Engl J Med. 2010;362(5):382–5.
108. Dinh HT, Lee C, Niyato D, Wang P. A survey of mobile cloud computing: architecture, applications, and approaches. Wirel Commun Mob Comput. 2013;13(18):1587–611.
109. Boulos MN, Wheeler S, Tavares C, Jones R. How smartphones are changing the face of mobile and participatory healthcare: an overview, with example from eCAALYX. Biomed Eng Online. 2011;10(1):24.

Chapter 4
Point-of-Care Diabetes Management Softwares and Smart Applications

Sandeep Kumar Vashist

Contents

4.1 Introduction

Diabetes is a major healthcare concern worldwide, which affects more than 422 million people worldwide and is prevalent in about 8.5% of adults over 18 years of age. Therefore, the management of diabetes is of critical importance as it enables the diabetics to have a normal lifestyle by avoiding costly and lethal diabetic complications. The developing nations don't have the desired number of healthcare professionals and the infrastructure that could effectively monitor and manage the substantially increasing number of diabetics. Therefore, there is need for the diabetics for personalized healthcare so that they can take charge of their own health by acquiring the desired skills, awareness, tools, and technologies. Several advanced diabetic management softwares have been developed by the big companies for the

© Springer Nature Switzerland AG 2019
S. K. Vashist, J. H. T. Luong, *Point-of-Care Technologies Enabling Next-Generation Healthcare Monitoring and Management*, https://doi.org/10.1007/978-3-030-11416-9_4

home BGM market, which have enabled the diabetics to effectively read and ana-
lyze their glucose measurements, predict the trend in glucose, and assess the BGM
data history. The most prominent diabetic management softwares are FreeStyle
CoPilot Health Management System by Abbott [1], ACCU-CHEK® 360° Diabetes
Management System by Roche [2], Dexcom Studio software by Dexcom [3],
OneTouch® Diabetes Management Software by LifeScan [4], and CareLink®
Personal Therapy Management software by Medtronic [5].

The mobile healthcare (mH) equipped smartphones, smart wearable gadgets,
and smart devices have revolutionized the diabetic healthcare and have penetrated
the market rapidly, as evident from the enormous users worldwide. This has led to
the evolving trend toward personalized and integrated mH, which would be a
major healthcare delivery concept in the near future. The mH market is estimated
to reach US$ 26 billion by 2017 [6]. The iHealth Align is the smallest FDA-
approved and CE-certified SP-based blood glucose meter [7], which has started a
new trend in SP-based personalized BGM. SPs are the ideal point-of-care (POC)
mH device [8–11], which are being used by billions of users worldwide. A large
number of smart applications for the diabetic BGM and monitoring of basic physiological parameters have also been developed [12], such as GluCoMo™ by
Artificial Life, Inc. [13] and iHealth Gluco-Smart [14] by iHealth Labs. These
smart applications empower the diabetics to live a healthy lifestyle by providing
them not only the educational modules and tips but also monitor their blood glucose and/or insulin or other medications to effectively manage their diabetes.
They have all the desired features that enable the meticulous planning of routine
tasks that the diabetics have to follow. This has led to increased compliance of
diabetics to medical and lifestyle interventions, thereby enabling better health
outcomes with significantly reduced diabetes healthcare management costs that
accounts for most of the healthcare expenditure worldwide. The increased diabetes self-management via the emerging smart applications motivates the diabetics
to maintain a healthy lifestyle via frequent monitoring and lifestyle intervention,
which results in reduced diabetic complications [15–17]. This has resulted in the
recommendation provided by the American Diabetes Association (ADA) for the
integration of data and information from the self-monitoring of blood glucose into
clinical and self-management plans [17].

The emerging trend is toward the smart gadget-based wearable healthcare technologies such as smart watches that monitors the basic physiological parameters,
such as physical activity and pulse, in real time. The coming years will witness
many of the diabetic blood glucose monitoring devices and smart applications for
diabetic management being successfully adapted to the smart watches. An example
is the iHealth Gluco-Smart application that has already been adapted to be used in
the smart watch.

The chapter describes the main commercial POC diabetes management smart
applications. The emerging trend and challenges of big data, mH, and smart wearable devices in diabetes management are also discussed.

4.2   Diabetes Management Softwares and Smart Applications

4.2.1   FreeStyle CoPilot Health Management System

The FreeStyle CoPilot Health Management System [1] is an advanced diabetic data management tool developed by Abbott. It allows diabetics, caregivers, and healthcare professionals to effectively manage their diabetes by considering the guided insights from the software reports. The software interfaces with the supported blood glucose monitoring devices from Abbott Diabetes Care, thereby enabling the recorded glucose test results to be uploaded into the software for comprehensive analysis and interpretation. Further, it enables the users to record relevant information about their meals, carbohydrate intake, medication, exercise, physical activities, ketones, insulin, medical exams, and lab results. Apart from displaying the glucose trends and patterns, insulin dosage, and carbohydrate intake, the software provides easy-to-read and easy-to-understand visual graphs, charts, and reports that enable diabetics to more effectively manage their diabetes. The guided insights provided by the software empower the diabetics to fully understand their blood glucose measurements and their diabetic management plan or interventions.

The software provides 12 reports for the glucose readings, i.e., diary list, logbook, glucose average, glucose modal day, glucose line, glucose histogram, glucose pie chart, statistics, lab and exam record, daily combination view, weekly pump view, and healthcare provider (HCP) group analysis. It allows the printing of reports and sending them to the desired HCP or caretakers. It provides the 2-week glucose summary with logbook report, thereby providing the diabetics a consolidated view of glucose modal day, glucose pie, statistics, and logbook reports during the specified 2 weeks. The glucose modal day and the glucose line reports provide the daily pattern of glucose levels and the trends in glucose levels, respectively. The glucose average report provides the blood glucose averages during the pre- and post-meal times of the day. It is useful for identifying the specific day times when there is need for more glucose testing. The glucose histogram and pie chart reports show the histogram and pie chart views, respectively, of all glucose readings into the designated target zones. The statistics report provides the pre- and post-meal glucose readings, carbohydrate intake, and insulin dosages during the stated period in a tabular format. On the other hand, the logbook report shows in a table the glucose readings, carbohydrate intake, and insulin doses taken during the day. The glucose statistics table reports the glucose readings taken during a day with the highest and lowest readings in each time periods together with the average glucose and standard deviations within and across various time periods. Further, the insulin statistics report provides a tabular representation of average insulin dosages over the specified period. Moreover, the pump statistics report will provide the insulin pump statistics if insulin is being administered by the diabetic using an insulin pump. The lab and exam record report shows a tabular representation of data from the lab tests and medical exams during the mentioned period. Lastly, the HCP group analysis report is available to the HCPs and enables them to view the data of all the patients managed by them.

The FreeStyle CoPilot Health Management System has two modes, i.e., Home User for diabetics and HCP for healthcare professionals. Each diabetic and healthcare professional has a unique profile that is protected by a secure password. The software allows multiple home users, family members, and multiple HCPs to share the use of the software. It enables the users to share their data and recorded health information with their HCPs.

4.2.2   ACCU-CHEK® 360° Diabetes Management System

The ACCU-CHEK® 360° Diabetes Management System [2] developed by Roche is a PC-based software, which collects all the glucose measurements made using Roche blood glucose meters by the diabetics. It is compatible with ACCU-CHEK Aviva Expert meter, ACCU-CHEK Aviva Combo meter, ACCU-CHEK Spirit Combo insulin pump, and ACCU-CHEK Spirit insulin pump. The software offers diabetics a simplified visualization of the blood glucose results via easy-to-read and easy-to-understand comprehensive graphs that enables them to effectively manage their diabetes by taking timely actions. It provides the users considerable flexibility as they can customize the reports based on their needs and can even create express reports for immediate use. As the blood glucose meter measurements and the insulin pump information can be downloaded and integrated on a single graph, the detailed information is very useful to the users for more effective diabetes management. The analysis of the trend in the blood glucose measurements enables the diabetics to visualize the effects of nutritional, dietary, physical activity and other lifestyle interventions, and/or medications on their blood glucose readings. The customizable reports are very helpful to the diabetic HCPs as they provide very useful information about their patients, which enables them to devise a more effective treatment plan.

4.2.3   OneTouch® Diabetes Management Software

The OneTouch® Diabetes Management Software [4] from LifeScan gathers the glucose measurement data from any OneTouch® blood glucose meter developed by LifeScan using the data port. The software provides an easy-to-read and easy-to-understand comprehensive visual picture of blood glucose measurement data together with 11 reports that simplifies the identification of glucose trends, such as nighttime and daytime highs and lows, the best daytime, and the meal-related patterns, daily, weekly, monthly, or quarterly. The reports include the logbook, glucose trend, 14-day summary, standard day, data list, average reading, pie chart, histogram, insulin, exception, and health checks. They provide an analysis of the blood glucose results, considering the various factors and highlighting the out-of-target range results. The users can view their results and print, fax, or share them with their HCPs, carers, or family members. Further, the software enables the addition and editing of information to a patient record.

The logbook report provides the glucose levels, glucose trends, and analysis of health-related data that can impact the glucose readings, while the pie chart report shows the percentage of glucose measurements within, above, and below the target range. The glucose trend report provides an analysis of track changes in glucose readings from one day to another, while the standard day report provides the pattern of glucose measurements during the day. The 14-day summary report provides a graphical summary of the logbook, pie chart, and glucose trend reports for a specific 14-day period. The average reading report monitors the average blood glucose measurements and analyzes the impact of exercise, physical activities, and meal on the measurements. The histogram report provides the pre- and post-meal patterns in glucose values. The data list report depicts a sequential view of all data provided by the software, such as glucose, exercise, physical activities, and medications. Of interest is the exception report that ranks patients based on the key diabetic glucose management measures and screens out the patients that require closer diabetes management. Further, the insulin report analyzes the relation between glucose levels, carbohydrate intake in meals, and the insulin doses, while the health checks report analyzes the effects of diabetes on other health factors, such as blood pressure, weight, HbA1c level, and doctor visits.

The OneTouch® Diabetes Management Software is no longer being distributed by the company. It has been replaced by OneTouch Reveal® App for mobiles and the Internet, which can perform all the functions and has some additional features for diabetes monitoring and management.

4.2.4   CareLink® Personal Therapy Management Software

The CareLink® Personal Therapy Management software [5] by Medtronic collects and analyzes the glucose measurement and insulin delivery data from Medtronic glucose meters, continuous glucose monitoring systems, and insulin pumps. It enables users to determine the desired insulin intake based on their blood glucose levels and analyze the effect of physical activity and meals on the glucose levels. It has been observed that the users of CareLink® Personal Therapy Management software have improved control of glycated hemoglobin (HbA1c) level, which is an indicator of long-term average of blood glucose levels, w.r.t. diabetics, using insulin pump without any software [18]. The software acts as a virtual logbook of all glucose measurements performed by the diabetics and provides them with thorough analysis of measurements and easy-to-read and easy-to-understand visual charts and graphs. The blood glucose measurements are stored in the software in the form of tables. The data analysis and the reports generated by the CareLink®software enable the HCP and the diabetic to understand the glucose patterns and the associated problems. It empowers the HCPs to make appropriate adjustments in therapy of diabetics and manage their diabetes more effectively. The HCPs can remotely access and review the CareLink® data of their patients for getting critical insights into their glucose patterns. Further, the analysis of glucose patterns also guides the diabetics to prevent the dangerous hypoglycemic episodes at night and maintain strict glycemic control within the euglycemic range. Moreover, the diabetics can also analyze the effects of taking the specific foods and portion sizes on their blood glucose levels, which empower them to manage their diabetes more effectively.

4.2.5 Dexcom STUDIO Software

Dexcom has developed the Dexcom STUDIO [3] diabetes management software that downloads the glucose measurement data after interfacing with the Dexcom glucose meters, such as Dexcom G4 Platinum Continuous Glucose Monitor. The software provides glucose distribution, glucose trends, hourly and daily statistics, and daily trends along with the Success Report and Dexcom PORTRAIT summary report. But Dexcom STUDIO is only available on Windows operating systems. Dexcom provides another software, i.e., Dexcom CLARITY™, for Mac users, which has similar features, and a Dexcom Clarity's Dashboard that provides the essential information and most relevant insights for diabetes management.

The Dexcom PORTRAIT summary report is a one-page summary of the critical bioanalytical parameters about diabetic glucose management. It facilitates the identification of clinically significant glucose patterns and their prioritization with the pattern map. Further, it identifies the most significant glucose patterns that should be targeted together with an insightful summary. Apart from this, the report provides the prospective strategies for diabetic glucose management along with possible considerations and interpretation. The hourly and daily statistics report provides an assessment of the hourly and daily glycemic patterns and variability, while the trends report provides an assessment of the glycemic patterns. The glucose distribution report shows the percent time high, low, and in-target glucose ranges, the overall glucose distribution, and the assessment of pre- and post-prandial control. On the other hand, the success report illustrates the glycemic control during a week, month, or quarter. It allows diabetics to track their glycemic control and achieve and sustain tight glycemic control for better diabetes management. Of interest is the pattern map report that provides the visual graphic representation of clinically significant glycemic excursions, i.e., nighttime and daytime highs and lows, along with the possible considerations to avoid such excursions. Moreover, it highlights the most significant hyper- and hypoglycemic excursions and their frequency of occurrence. Further, it provides the summary of glucose statistics and calibration frequency along with therapy considerations and suggestions for better glycemic control.

4.2.6   iHealth Gluco-Smart

An innovative FDA-approved and CE-compliant smartphone (SP)-based blood glucose meter, known as iHealth Align, has been developed by iHealth Labs Inc. It plugs directly into the 3.5 mm audio jack of the SP and transfers the glucose measurement results in real time to the iHealth Gluco-Smart [14] (Fig. 4.1) that works with the iHealth Align and another glucose meter, i.e., iHealth Gluco-Monitoring System, developed by iHealth Inc. The iHealth Gluco-Monitoring System interfaces to the iOS and Android operating systems-based SPs via low-energy Bluetooth transfer. The iHealth Gluco-Smart application automatically handles all the glucose monitoring tasks, such as digital logging of glucose measurements, coding, and counting of the test strips, which critically reduces the manual handling time and eliminates manual errors. All the glucose measurements data is saved to the secure personalized iHealth Cloud service that is free to access for the users provided they have set up their personal account. The personalized iHealth Cloud can be accessed at any place and time via Internet or Wi-Fi connection. The smart application provides an easy analysis and visualization of glucose test results and enables the user to measure, record, manage, and share their glucose measurements results. The measuring mode allows users to view their glucose measurement results on their SP in real time. The results can then be tagged with further details by the users, such as physical activities, meals taken, and voice memo, for more insights and better understanding. The smart application also enables the uploading of the offline glucose test measurements and enables the scanning of the new glucose test strips via smart tracking. On the other hand, the record mode of the smart applications enables the users to get an easy-to-read and easy-to-understand graphical summary of their blood glucose measurements stored securely in their iHealth Cloud personal account for up to past 3 months. Of interest is the managing mode in the iHealth Gluco-Smart, which provides a review of the personal digital logbook. The logbook contains the complete details of glucose measurements, such as time and date stamp of the measurements, meals taken, carbohydrates consumed, physical activity performed, and voice memo of the user. The users can visualize their glucose trends and statistics during the day, based on which they can effectively manage the hypo- or hyperglycemic episodes during the specific times predicted by the glucose trend curve. The managing mode also enables the user to set up alarm alerts and reminders for when they need to perform the glucose measurements and take insulin and/ or other medication. A smart application has also been developed by the iHealth, Inc., for the Apple Watch that provides the users a summary of their previous week's glucose measurements with trends and statistics without any need for opening the iHealth Gluco-Smart application on their SP. The users also receive notifications for the reminders that are set on their SP. Further, iHealth, Inc., has developed a dedicated smart application for the HCPs, known as iHealth Pro. It contains all the functions of iHealth Gluco-Smart application with the additional features such as enabling the HCPs to visualize the glucose measurements data of all the patients registered in their clinical practice. It enables the HCPs and patients to communicate with each other via the messenger in iHealth Pro.

(A)

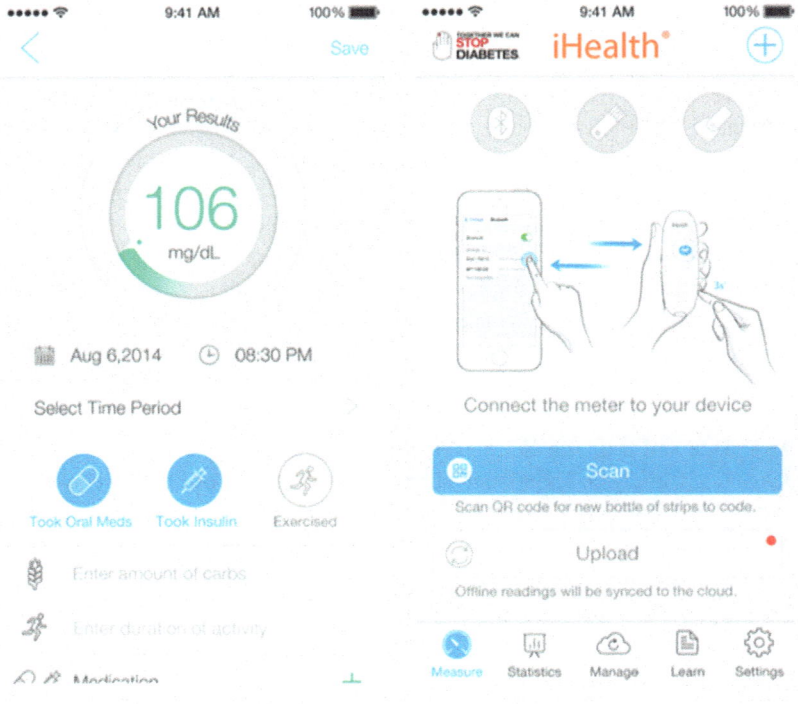

(B)

Apple Watch

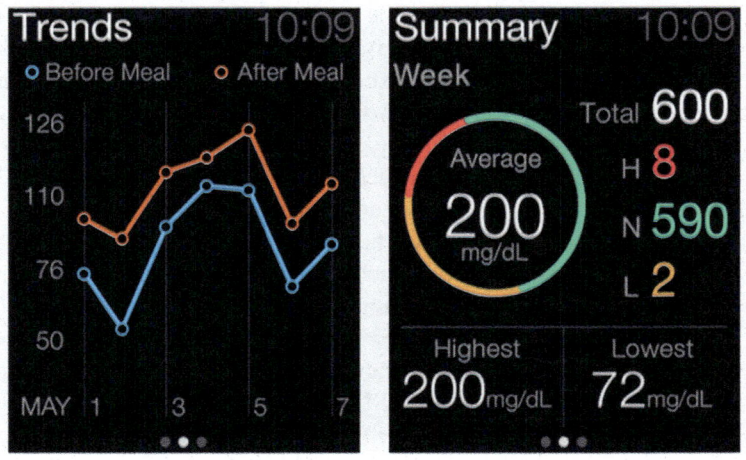

Fig. 4.1 iHealth Gluco-Smart. Screenshots of the smart application on (**a**) iPhone and (**b**) Apple Watch. Images are copyright of iHealth Labs, Inc. Reproduced with permission from iHealth Labs Inc.

4.2.7 Glooko™ App

Roche has developed a diabetic management smart application called Glooko™ app [19] which can be downloaded on iPhone- and Android-based SPs and smart devices. The smart application can collect the blood glucose measurements data from any ACCU-CHEK blood glucose meter and view it. The ACCU-CHEK Aviva Connect meter connects to the Glooko™ app after automatic synchronization of blood glucose measurements. But other ACCU-CHEK meters require a Glooko MeterSync Blue device to upload the blood glucose measurements data from the glucose meter to the smart application. The Glooko™ app provides an easy-to-read and easy-to-understand glucose trend and analysis of the blood glucose measurements. It empowers the diabetics to effectively manage their blood glucose level via effective lifestyle and nutritional or medical intervention. The users can share their glucose measurements and reports with their HCPs and set up reminders with push notifications on a SP for the desired blood glucose measurements and insulin injections or medications, thereby increasing their compliance. They can also use Glooko ProConnect to share their blood glucose measurements data with other websites or online dashboards. The Glooko™ app enables the users to add pre- and post-meal notes about their carbohydrate intake, physical activity, and insulin doses. The users can also analyze the effect of diet, activity, and insulin on their blood glucose profile. Moreover, there is an inbuilt database of more than 200,000 foods inside the Glooko™ app, which guides the users to determine their relative glucose values and facilitates more precise insulin dosing.

4.2.8 ACCU-CHEK® Connect

ACCU-CHEK®Connect diabetes management app [20] is an innovative smart application by Roche that is available for download on iOS and Android-equipped smart devices having Bluetooth® Smart technology. It interfaces to the ACCU-CHEK Aviva Connect glucose meter wirelessly by Bluetooth® Smart technology and receives the glucose measurements data. The users have to create their personal ACCU-CHEK Connect online portal account in order to be able to review and visualize their glucose measurements data, generate reports, and share the data and information with their doctors and HCPs. ACCU-CHEK® Connect application can also be customized for sending texts to the caregiver, parent, or HCP about the new blood glucose measurements performed by the diabetic. The glucose measurements received by the ACCU-CHEK® Connect application are stored automatically in the Cloud and can be accessed via ACCU-CHEK Connect online portal at any place and time. The smart application further enables the users to calculate the precise insulin dose via the inbuilt ACCU-CHEK Bolus Advisor [21] but only after activation by the doctor, which makes the determination of mealtime insulin easier. The application also contains a 3-day profile tool for the visualization of glucose trend curve and analysis of the effects of activity, food, and insulin on the blood glucose levels. Further, it has the Testing in Paris tool to determine the effect of meals, stress, or activity on the blood glucose. The extensive information data and information provided by the smart application enables the doctors to make better and informed decisions for improved diabetic management.

4.2.9 GluCoMo™

GluCoMo™ [13] is a prospective smart application from Artificial Life, Inc. (Fig. 4.2), that can be downloaded from the iTunes store at a nominal price of US$ 0.99. It facilitates the management of diabetic monitoring and provides patient coaching. The application acts as an electronic diary and a reminder system for diabetics and has a well-developed telematics feature compatible with various platforms, such as iOS, Android, Symbian, Windows Phone 7, and Java. It allows diabetics to monitor and manage their blood glucose levels, diet, insulin intake, physical

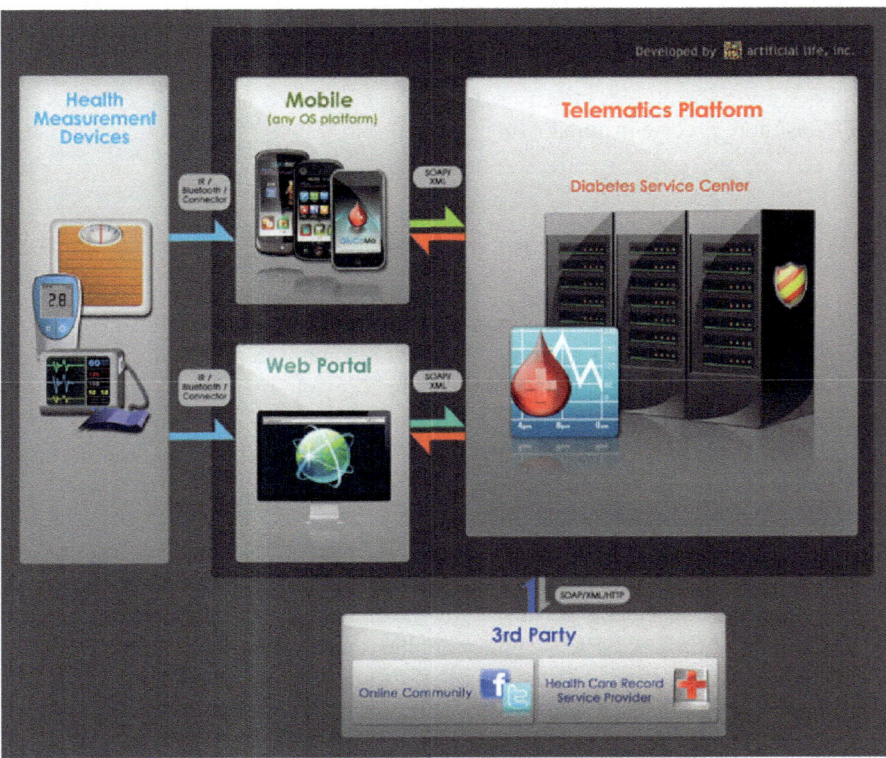

Fig. 4.2 GluCoMo™ developed by Artificial Life, Inc. Reproduced with permission from Artificial Life, Inc.

activities, and basic physiological parameters, such as blood pressure, pulse, and weight, which are critical for effective diabetes management. The application has customized mobile client applications, an interactive web portal, and a secure telematics platform, which enables the transfer of data and information to the patients, doctors, hospitals, administrators, and authorized healthcare professionals. The data is securely stored and transferred via the smart application that employs advanced data encryption. The Internet or Wi-Fi connectivity updates the glucose measurement data on a central database via the client application. Only the certified doctors and authorized HCPs are given the access to the data. Apart from this, the smart application facilitates real-time communication between doctors and patients and also among various hospitals. It enables the doctors to share advice and provide medical opinions and diagnostics for better healthcare. GluCoMo™ issues warnings to the diabetics when dangerous trends are detected in their glucose measurements. It alerts the diabetics to pursue lifestyle interventions, such as increased physical activity, to keep their blood glucose under control. Moreover, diabetics can set up alarmed automated alerts for engaging in various physical activities based on their glucose trend after analyzing the effect of various physical activities on their blood glucose. It empowers diabetics to devise more effective personalized lifestyle intervention. Further, the diabetics can engage in online interactions and share via built-in forums. They have access to an informative diabetes handbook, which acts as an educational tool to guide them with the diabetic facts, prevalence, monitoring, and management. However, the smart application is not being distributed by the developer.

4.3 Critiques and Outlook

There is an immense need for highly effective diabetes management softwares and smart applications for empowering the diabetics and enabling them to be active decision makers in their healthcare. It is apparent from numerous peer-reviewed reports and manuscripts that the use of such softwares and smart applications critically improve the diabetic monitoring and management, and lead to better and sustained health outcomes and significantly reduced healthcare costs. They improve the knowledge, behavior, and efficacy of diabetics that enables more effective diabetes management [22]. The blood glucose measurement data of diabetics can be accessed by users and doctors at any place and time, which enables the HCPs to monitor and manage the health of their patients by developing effective healthcare strategies in real time. The options for telemedicine and communication in diabetes management softwares and smart applications are further providing the desired means of healthcare delivery as doctors can communicate with their patients and provide them the desired advice to manage and control their diabetes. These developments illustrate the successful convergence of various scientific disciplines to develop innovative mH technologies. The developments in smart systems, mH, and telemedicine will further lead to next generation of diabetes management softwares and smart applications for personalized diabetic monitoring and management. The significant rise in funding for mH, rapidly growing public interest for improved healthcare, and an evolving trend toward empowering the users to effectively manage their health are providing an impetus to develop novel health solutions. The FDA-approved and CE-accredited iHealth Align, which is the smallest SP-based blood glucose meter, is a remarkable achievement in diabetes healthcare and will inspire the development of innovative devices. However, there are still pending concerns about the rapidly evolving SP models, data security, and regulatory compliance and achieving the high analytical performance for clinically-viable POC devices. The ongoing efforts are specifically targeted to tackle these technical challenges and provide effective healthcare solutions for diabetes management.

The diabetic management softwares and smart applications are being used by numerous diabetics worldwide. The major health benefits include more effective diabetic monitoring and management, improved compliance, decreased hyperglycemic and hypoglycemic episodes, sustained health, and better health outcomes. The enhanced understanding of the glucose measurements and effect of physical activity, diet, and other lifestyle interventions on the glucose readings empower the diabetics to maintain their glucose level within the normal physiological range and avoid costly diabetic complications. It has resulted in significantly reduced number of visits of diabetics to their doctors, thereby leading to critical reduction in healthcare costs. The globally-evolving trend toward mH and Cloud computing would provide surplus opportunities for big data, which could be used for predictive healthcare monitoring.

The rapid advances in Cloud computing are facilitating the development of diabetes smart applications and paving way to improved and affordable healthcare [23]. It also results in additional cost savings due to reduced infrastructure and operational costs for diabetes monitoring and management. But, on the other hand, it has led to increased concerns about the data security and privacy of personal information [24–26]. The national laws and guidelines of most countries substantiate the physical storing of data within their national boundaries, which requires tremendous research and development efforts to establish Cloud computing capability that complies with the stringent regulatory and national norms [27]. Amazon and Google have effectively counteracted this limitation and provided adequate solutions. Google's Government Cloud product enables the nations to store their data within their national boundary, as desired by their national data security guidelines. Amazon Web Services also permits businesses to store data physically within the national boundary. There is a need to create international Cloud computing standards, as substantiated by the enormous striking developments in Cloud computing that have resulted in several initiatives, such as EuroCloud and Google's Data Liberation Front. The main focus of such initiatives is to establish the international standards in Cloud computing.

The protection of personal information in personal electronic health records (PEHRs) is a major concern at present as the international ethical guidelines state that the patients are the owner and have complete control of their PEHRs. But there is a need for guidelines about the ownership of the medical data and the responsibility to safeguard the private information in healthcare [28]. The personal information of the patients should never be provided to the third-party servers and unauthorized parties. Presently, it is addressed via attribute-based encryption strategies [29], engaging an authorized and trusted third party [27] and employing advanced Cloud computing models that ensure security and privacy of personal data [30]. Moreover, the Cloud is providing advanced information security, which is better than the security standards being employed by the companies and government agencies [31, 32]. Undoubtedly, the use of PEHRs leads to critical improvements in caregivers' decisions and patients' health outcomes [33], which are well known to HCPs, community, and patients. It has led to the Health Information Technology for Economic and Clinical Health Act (HITECH) in the United States, which offers authorized incentive payments via the insurance agencies to the HCPs that use PEHRs to achieve specified improvements in the healthcare delivery [34]. The emerging diabetic smart applications using the smartphone-based mobile Cloud computing [35] are equipped with advanced features that are enabling the personalized mH monitoring and management [36].

Most diabetic smart applications don't employ stringent clinical validation studies or involve HCPs' feedback during development. Therefore, they are lacking in intelligent coaching and behavioral management, which substantiates the need for robust, systematic, regulated, and clinically-validated diabetes management softwares and smart applications in the near future. They should be peer-reviewed and clinically evaluated, and patients should be informed about the trustful diabetic softwares and smart applications together with their utility [37]. The guidelines and procedures to regulate mobile medical applications, including those for diabetes management [38], have been issued recently by the US Food and Drug Administration (FDA). Similarly, the European Union has revised the guidelines for the regulation of smart applications for healthcare under the EU medical devices directive 93/42/EEC [39]. But there are still many pending concerns that need to be tackled, such as ethical issues, personal privacy issues, data ownership, data processing, clinical efficacy, and regulatory compliance.

The diabetics experience several frustrations daily, pertaining to their diabetes monitoring and management, as shown by a recent survey [40]. Most of the diabetics need to be empowered and engaged to effectively manage their health and keep their blood glucose level under control via frequent testing and lifestyle interventions. But they require daily care and more frequent visits to their HCPs. The major frustrations of diabetics are the lack in interactions and timely communications with HCPs, difficulties in scheduling appointments with them, and challenging diabetes management. The survey suggested a set of recommendations for more effective diabetes care and management. There is a need for centralized real-time access of patients' medical records that can be readily accessed by the HCPs via a nationwide PEHR system. Further, there is a requirement for timely electronic access to expected and completed lab results, which is only feasible if each HCP adopts an online reservation system. The diabetics can also schedule their appointments with HCP, get confirmations and reminders, and have access to their lab results. An example is the prospective smart application called MyQuest that has been developed by Quest

Diagnostics [41]. The patients become more aware of their health and ask much better questions when they have access to their lab results [42]. The survey has also highlighted the need for an online scheduling system that will enable patients to search HCPs near them and schedule an appointment with them. An example of such a system is the Zocdoc [43]. Lastly, the survey recommended better tools for diabetes management, i.e., improved blood glucose monitoring and medication reminders, alerts for low insulin volume in the insulin pump and need to manually check the blood glucose level, text messaging from healthcare team members, and intelligent and interactive PEHR system. The text messaging to poorly controlled diabetics encourages them for improved glycemic control, as shown by a recent study [44]. Further, a personalized treatment plan and advice, taking into account the need and preferences of diabetics, can also be provided via a text message.

Most insurance plans do not cover the diabetic management softwares and smart applications [45]. Therefore, reimbursement and costs of such softwares and smart applications will play a critical role in diabetes management. The mH-equipped software and smart applications and interactive learning tools should be used by HCPs [46] to effectively manage the health of diabetics. However, considering the risk about the authenticity of information provided and the provider, the online social networking services should be used with care in diabetes management [47].

The coming years will witness innovative and advanced diabetic management softwares and smart applications that would be clinically-acceptable and regulatory compliant. They would employ next-generation Cloud computing, advanced contributing technologies, and cost-effective smart wearable gadgets with remarkable features. The emerging smart devices will have several advanced features for the monitoring and management of general health in addition to GPRS tracking, text alerts, simplified communications, easy-to-understand visual data, personalized healthcare suggestions, and a dedicated Healthbook application.

4.4 Conclusions

Diabetes management softwares and smart applications are essential for more effective diabetes management. They empower the diabetics to keep their blood glucose level sustained within the normal physiological range by maintaining an active lifestyle and healthy diet. The visualization of blood glucose measurement data and the prediction of glucose trend during the day enable the diabetics to effectively manage their diabetes. They can set up automated alarmed alerts, if their blood glucose level goes outside the normal range, and automated reminders for frequent monitoring of their blood glucose and engaging in physical activities. Smart watches and other smart wearable devices are providing an integrated healthcare solution for continuous monitoring of the physical activity and basic physiological parameters of diabetics, which are equally critical for diabetes management. They also show the data, alerts, and reminders issued by the smart application, which increases the compliance of diabetics for diabetes monitoring and management, treatment, and lifestyle interventions.

References

1. FreeStyle CoPilot Health Management System. https://www.myfreestyle.com/copilot-software. Accessed 11 Nov 2018.
2. ACCU-CHEK® 360° diabetes management system. https://www.accu-chek.com/apps-and-software/360deg-diabetes-management-system/support. Accessed 11 Nov 2018.
3. Dexcom Studio. https://www.dexcom.com/dexcom-studio. Accessed 11 Nov 2018.
4. OneTouch® Diabetes Management Software. https://www.onetouch.ca/products/softwares-and-apps/onetouch-diabetes-management-software#manuals-and-downloads. Accessed 11 Nov 2018.
5. CareLink® Personal Therapy Management Software. http://www.medtronicdiabetes.com/products/carelink-personal-diabetes-software. Accessed 11 Nov 2018.
6. 1.7B to download health apps by 2017. https://www.mobihealthnews.com/20814/report-1-7b-to-download-health-apps-by-2017. Accessed 11 Nov 2018.
7. iHealth Align. https://ihealthlabs.com/glucometer/ihealth-align/. Accessed 11 Nov 2018.
8. Kwon L, Long KD, Wan Y, Yu H, Cunningham BT. Medical diagnostics with mobile devices: comparison of intrinsic and extrinsic sensing. Biotechnol Adv. 2016;34(3):291–304.
9. Vashist SK, Luppa PB, Yeo LY, Ozcan A, Luong JHT. Emerging technologies for next-generation point-of-care testing. Trends Biotechnol. 2015;33(11):692–705.
10. Vashist SK, Mudanyali O, Schneider EM, Zengerle R, Ozcan A. Cellphone-based devices for bioanalytical sciences. Anal Bioanal Chem. 2014;406(14):3263–77.
11. Vashist SK, Schneider EM, Luong JHT. Commercial smartphone-based devices and smart applications for personalized healthcare monitoring and management. Diagnostics. 2014;4(3):104–28.
12. Diabetes app market report 2016–2021. https://www.giiresearch.com/report/r2g569222-diabetes-app-market-report.html. Accessed 11 Nov 2018.
13. GluCoMo™. http://www.diabetesincontrol.com/glucomo/. Accessed 11 Nov 2018.
14. iHealth Gluco-Smart. https://ihealthlabs.eu/de/54-ihealth-gluco-smart.html. Accessed 11 Nov 2018.
15. Eng DS, Lee JM. The promise and peril of mobile health applications for diabetes and endocrinology. Pediatr Diabetes. 2013;14(4):231–8.
16. Schütt M, Kern W, Krause U, Busch P, Dapp A, Grziwotz R, et al. Is the frequency of self-monitoring of blood glucose related to long-term metabolic control? Multicenter analysis including 24,500 patients from 191 centers in Germany and Austria. Exp Clin Endocrinol Diabetes. 2006;114(7):384–8.
17. Association AD. Standards of medical care in diabetes—2015. Diabetes Care. 2015;38:S33–40.
18. Corriveau EA, Durso PJ, Kaufman ED, Skipper BJ, Laskaratos LA, Heintzman KB. Effect of Carelink, an internet-based insulin pump monitoring system, on glycemic control in rural and urban children with type 1 diabetes mellitus. Pediatr Diabetes. 2008;9(4 Pt 2):360–6.
19. Glooko™ app. https://www.accu-chek.com/apps-and-software/glookotm-app-iphoner-and-android/support. Accessed 11 Nov 2018.
20. ACCU-CHEK® Connect diabetes management app. https://www.accu-chek.com/apps-and-software/connect-app. Accessed 11 Nov 2018.
21. Barnard K, Parkin C, Young A, Ashraf M. Use of an automated bolus calculator reduces fear of hypoglycemia and improves confidence in dosage accuracy in patients with type 1 diabetes mellitus treated with multiple daily insulin injections. J Diabetes Sci Technol. 2012;6(1):144–9.
22. Guo SH-M, Chang H-K, Lin C-Y. Impact of mobile diabetes self-care system on patients' knowledge, behavior and efficacy. Comput Ind. 2015;69:22–9.
23. Marston S, Li Z, Bandyopadhyay S, Zhang J, Ghalsasi A. Cloud computing—the business perspective. Decis Support Syst. 2011;51(1):176–89.
24. Subashini S, Kavitha V. A survey on security issues in service delivery models of cloud computing. J Netw Comput Appl. 2011;34(1):1–11.

25. Sun D, Chang G, Sun L, Wang X. Surveying and analyzing security, privacy and trust issues in cloud computing environments. Procedia Eng. 2011;15:2852–6.
26. Istepanian RS. Mobile applications for diabetes management: efficacy issues and regulatory challenges. Lancet Diabetes Endocrinol. 2015;3(12):921–3.
27. Zissis D, Lekkas D. Addressing cloud computing security issues. Future Gener Comput Syst. 2012;28(3):583–92.
28. Khansa L, Cook DF, James T, Bruyaka O. Impact of HIPAA provisions on the stock market value of healthcare institutions, and information security and other information technology firms. Comput Secur. 2012;31(6):750–70.
29. Li M, Yu S, Zheng Y, Ren K, Lou W. Scalable and secure sharing of personal health records in cloud computing using attribute-based encryption. IEEE Trans Parallel Distrib Syst. 2013;24(1):131–43.
30. Schweitzer EJ. Reconciliation of the cloud computing model with US federal electronic health record regulations. J Am Med Inform Assoc. 2012;19(2):161–5.
31. Khansa L, Zobel CW. Assessing innovations in cloud security. J Comput Inf Syst. 2014;54(3):45–56.
32. Khansa L, Zobel CW, Goicochea G. Creating a taxonomy for mobile commerce innovations using social network and cluster analyses. Int J Electron Commer. 2012;16(4):19–52.
33. Blumenthal D, Tavenner M. The "meaningful use" regulation for electronic health records. N Engl J Med. 2010;363(6):501–4.
34. Blumenthal D. Launching HITECH. N Engl J Med. 2010;362(5):382–5.
35. Dinh HT, Lee C, Niyato D, Wang P. A survey of mobile cloud computing: architecture, applications, and approaches. Wirel Commun Mob Comput. 2013;13(18):1587–611.
36. Boulos MN, Wheeler S, Tavares C, Jones R. How smartphones are changing the face of mobile and participatory healthcare: an overview, with example from eCAALYX. Biomed Eng Online. 2011;10(1):24.
37. Basilico A, Marceglia S, Bonacina S, Pinciroli F. Advising patients on selecting trustful apps for diabetes self-care. Comput Biol Med. 2016;71:86–96.
38. Administration UFaD. Mobile medical applications: guidance for industry and Food and Drug Administration staff. https://www.fda.gov/medicaldevices/digitalhealth/mobilemedicalapplications/default.htm. Accessed 11 Nov 2018.
39. The new regulations on medical devices. https://ec.europa.eu/growth/sectors/medical-devices/regulatory-framework_en. Accessed 11 Nov 2018.
40. Khansa L, Davis Z, Davis H, Chin A, Irvine H, Nichols L, et al. Health information technologies for patients with diabetes. Technol Soc. 2016;44:1–9.
41. Get Your Results On Your Mobile Phone. https://myquest.questdiagnostics.com/web/home. Accessed 11 Nov 2018.
42. HHS strengthens patients' right to access lab test reports. https://www.hhs.gov/hipaa/for-professionals/special-topics/clia/index.html. Accessed 11 Nov 2018.
43. ZocDoc. https://www.zocdoc.com/. Accessed 11 Nov 2018.
44. Dobson R, Carter K, Cutfield R, Hulme A, Hulme R, McNamara C, et al. Diabetes text-message self-management support program (SMS4BG): a pilot study. JMIR Mhealth Uhealth. 2015;3(1):e32.
45. Practice Transformation for Physicians and Health Care Teams. https://www.niddk.nih.gov/health-information/communication-programs/ndep/health-professionals/practice-transformation-physicians-health-care-teams. Accessed 11 Nov 2018.
46. Rider BB, Lier SC, Johnson TK, Hu DJ. Interactive web-based learning: translating health policy into improved diabetes care. Am J Prev Med. 2016;50(1):122–8.
47. Toma T, Athanasiou T, Harling L, Darzi A, Ashrafian H. Online social networking services in the management of patients with diabetes mellitus: systematic review and meta-analysis of randomised controlled trials. Diabetes Res Clin Pract. 2014;106(2):200–11.

Chapter 5
Paper-Based Point-of-Care Immunoassays

Sandeep Kumar Vashist

Contents

5.1 Introduction

The detection of clinical analytes is critically important for the diagnosis, monitoring, and management of diseases in healthcare. Various IA formats, such as enzyme-linked immunosorbent assay (ELISA), radioimmunoassay, and automated analyzer-based IA, have already been developed and are being used for the reliable detection of analytes [1]. They involve the highly specific biomolecular interactions between the antibody (Ab) and antigen (Ag), where the Ag is detected via a sandwich or competitive IA depending on whether it is a large or small molecule, respectively. However, despite superior analytical performance, the conventional IAs have

© Springer Nature Switzerland AG 2019
S. K. Vashist, J. H. T. Luong, *Point-of-Care Technologies Enabling Next-Generation Healthcare Monitoring and Management*,
https://doi.org/10.1007/978-3-030-11416-9_5

several limitations for POCT. The manual IAs require highly-skilled analysts, prolonged analysis time, multiple process steps, and expensive instruments. On the other hand, the automated IAs require a very costly analyzer, additional infrastructure, and operational costs. Therefore, the existing IA formats are inappropriate for POCT in remote settings.

PIAs address this emerging need for simple and cost-effective IAs for remote settings [2–11]. Paper can be mass-produced at a very low cost [12] and is easy to functionalize, use, and read. They could be easily modified for the intended use by changing their physical and chemical properties [13–15], such as surface area, porosity, strength, durability, hydrophilicity/hydrophobicity, biocompatibility, etc. The most common paper substrates in PIAs are filter paper, chromatography paper [9], nitrocellulose membrane [16], paper-polymer composite [17], and paper-nanomaterial composites [18–20]. The porosity, surface chemistry, and optical properties of the paper substrates play a critical role in the bioanalytical applications [9].

During the last two decades, several prospective microfluidic paper-based analytical devices (μPADs) have been demonstrated by researchers [7, 21–35]. A wide range of manufacturing technologies, such as cutting [36–38], wax printing [39–42], and photolithography [7, 43]), have also been developed for the preparation of PADs. The porosity of the paper enables the PADs to drive the liquid via capillary force and provides a large surface area for the immobilization of IA reagents and detection of analytes via specific biomolecular reactions.

The most widely used PIA format was dipstick that was first used in 1950s [44]. It paved the way to various paper-based assay devices for different applications [15]. Subsequently, the PIA that was driven by capillary force was developed [45] followed by the radioimmunoassay for human chorionic gonadotropin (hCG) [46]. These developments led to the development of the first lateral flow assay (LFA) for hCG in 1980s [47], which was a big commercial success as it enabled the home pregnancy testing. Thereafter, the μPADs were developed and used for protein detection [43]. Finally, various paper-based IA devices have been demonstrated for a wide range of bioanalytical applications, such as in healthcare, food safety, environmental monitoring, etc. [5, 6, 8, 15, 48].

We describe here various PIAs together with the advances made, future trends, pending concerns, prospects, and future directions. The rapidly increasing number of peer-reviewed publications during the last four decades shows the continuously growing interest in researchers for the development of prospective PIAs.

5.2 Paper-Based Immunoassay Formats

A large number of PIAs have been reported [49], which can be categorized into dipstick, paper-based enzyme-linked immunosorbent assay (P-ELISA), LFAs, and μPADs. Dipstick test strips have been mainly used for the measurement of pH in solution, urine, or saliva [50]. They have also been used for the measurement of lead acetate, potassium iodide, and other chemicals and metabolites in urine. The diagnostic procedure involves the dipping of a strip into an analyte solution and visualizing/quantifying the change in color.

The P-ELISA employs the paper-based plate instead of the conventional 96-well microtiter plate, which is cost-effective, easy to manufacture, and requires less sample [51, 52]. However, all IA steps are similar to that of conventional ELISA [53, 54]. On the other hand, LFAs are rapid PIAs that are successfully used in a wide range of bioanalytical applications [55, 56] due to their low-cost, rapid sample-to-answer time, simplicity, and visual readout without the need for expensive instruments. LFAs employ test strips fabricated from a nitrocellulose membrane along which the sample, which is first dispensed on a sample pad, laterally flows over a conjugate pad, where the analyte binds to conjugate particles (e.g., gold nanoparticles (AuNPs) [57] and upconversion nanoparticles [58]) due to the capillary action with the aid of an absorbent pad (Fig. 5.1A). The capture of complexes at the test line occurs due to the binding of the target molecules to pre-conjugated capture molecules [16], whereas unbound conjugated particles are captured at the control line by binding to other capture molecules. One of the most widely used paper-based LFAs is the home pregnancy test strip, which detects the urine hormone human chorionic gonadotropin (hCG) through the binding of anti-hCG antibody-conjugated colored particles to hCG in urine, followed by the binding of hCG and anti-hCG antibody to the monoclonal anti-hCG antibody and IgG, respectively. The test has been extended to primary hepatic carcinoma biomarkers [62], diagnosis of acquired immunodeficiency syndrome (AIDS) [63], and other target analytes. Various sandwich and competitive LFAs for analytes, i.e., antigens and antibodies, have been developed [8, 55, 64]. Although most of the LFAs are qualitative and provide a simple positive or negative confirmation for a disease, they could also be semi-quantitative or quantitative.

Further, µPADs are the most recent PIA formats that have been widely used for multifarious bioanalytical applications [7, 32, 65, 66]. Two-dimensional (2D) or even three-dimensional (3D) µPADs are created by patterning paper with a variety of assay designs [7, 67] (Fig. 5.1B). The aqueous fluid movement is driven mainly by capillary stresses [7] confined within virtual microchannels formed on paper by patterning physical (e.g., by cutting, inkjet etching, plasma etching, wax printing, photolithography, plotting, etc.) or chemical hydrophobic boundaries [68]. 3D µPADs are obtained by stacking layers of the 2D patterned paper, offering potential advantages for additional assay complexity, and multiplexing capability [69]. Other fabrication strategies for 3D µPADs are spray adhesives [70], thermal adhesives (toner) [71], cutting and lamination [68], and origami, i.e., folding [72], techniques. A variety of assays have been developed for paper, such as sandwich ELISAs [51, 73, 74]. The µPADs have been used to develop microfluidic paper-based electrochemical devices (µPEDs) by printing electrodes on paper for the detection of glucose, lactate, uric acid, cholesterol, alcohol, and nucleic acid [75, 76] (Fig. 5.1C). Of interest is the ongoing development of a novel paper-based biosensor [61] (Fig. 5.1D).

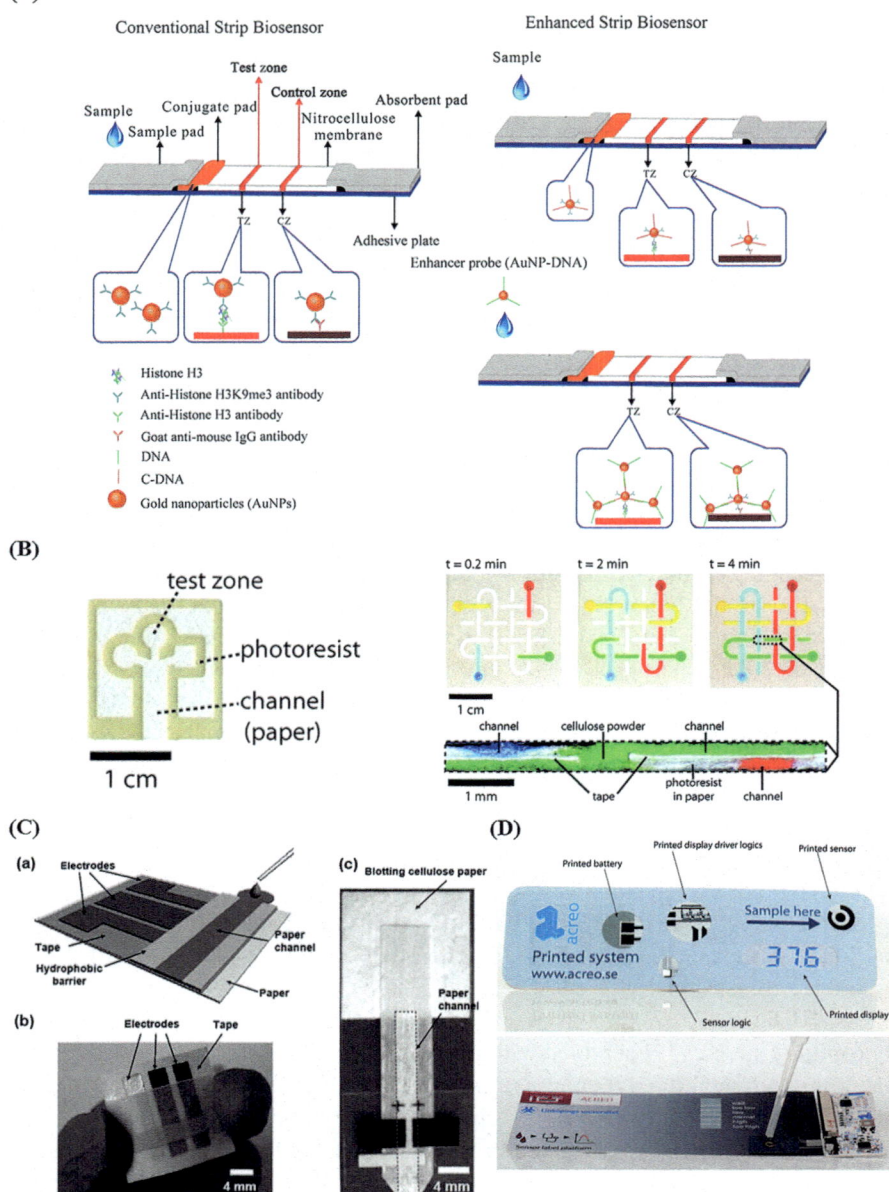

Fig. 5.1 Paper-based emerging technologies for POCT [49]. (**A**) Conventional and enhanced lateral flow immunoassays (LFIAs) for the visual detection of trimethylated lysine 9 of histone H3 (H3K9me3) in 20 ng of histone extract from HeLa cells within 15 min [59]. (**B**) A typical 2D [7] (left) and 3D [28] (right) microfluidic paper-based analytical device (μPAD). (**C**) Microfluidic paper-based electrochemical devices (μPEDs) [60]: (*a*) schematic view, (*b*) actual image of a μPED for the analysis of blood glucose, (*c*) the μPED, which has two printed carbon electrodes, i.e., the working and counter electrodes and a printed Ag/AgCl electrode as the pseudo-reference electrode. The fluidic channel was fabricated by patterning SU-8 as a hydrophobic barrier to the aqueous solution. (**D**) Conceptual rendering (top) and image (bottom) of a completely printed paper-based amperometric biosensor [61]. Reproduced with permission from the Elsevier B.V

5.3 Detection Principles Employed in Paper-Based Immunoassays

PIAs enable the detection of analytes by employing different detection principles, such as colorimetric, thermal, electronic, and magnetic nanoparticles. The pros and cons of each detection principle are discussed below.

5.3.1 Colorimetric Detection

The colorimetric detection of analytes using PIAs has been the most widely used detection principle as the colorimetric signal could be visually analyzed by the analysts without the need of any expensive reader [77]. Varying labels, such as AuNPs, enzymes, carbon NPs (CNPs), and magnetic NPs (MNPs), have been used to develop colorimetric PIAs with high sensitivity [55] (Fig. 5.2).

Enzymes are the most commonly used labels for the detection of analytes in conventional microtiter plate-based ELISAs. However, P-ELISAs employ the same process steps, but they are low-cost, rapid, and simple w.r.t. conventional ELISA [51, 74, 81]. P-ELISA platforms have been developed by various mass-manufacturing methods. The wax-patterned paper microzone plates were used for multistep P-ELISAs [48, 51, 81]. An automated P-ELISA has been developed using magnetic particle-based IA and the control of magnetic particles via a magnet [82]. Another prospective format involves the use of microfluidics for automated P-ELISAs on patterned paper [74].

AuNPs, ruby red, are conjugated to detection Ab in colorimetric PIAs [83], especially LFIAs [78] or μPADs [43]. They have been widely used for colorimetric PIAs as they are low cost, easy to synthesize, biocompatible, stable, and easy to functionalize [64, 84]. However, it is critical to select AuNPs of appropriate size, concentration, and pH for a PIA as it can impact its analytical performance [85]. The analytical performances of AuNPs-based PIAs are improved by employing various AuNPs composites with enzymes [86], other AuNPs [87], silica nanorods [88], MNPs [89], or silver nanoparticles [90]. Similarly, CNPs could also improve the analytical performance of PIAs as they have a large surface area that leads to higher binding capacity and thus higher signal [79, 84, 91, 92]. They can be prepared by various physical and chemical methods [79]. Moreover, they are low-cost, easy to synthesize, non-toxic, stable, and have good optical and electrical properties [93].

Various MNPs and MNP composites have also been used for developing high-sensitivity colorimetric PIAs [94–97]. They have a small size, excellent colloidal stability, strong magnetism, high biomolecular binding, intense color, and ability to functionalize with various functional groups [98]. They are easy to synthesize by various synthetic procedures, such as the conventional solvothermal reaction [99].

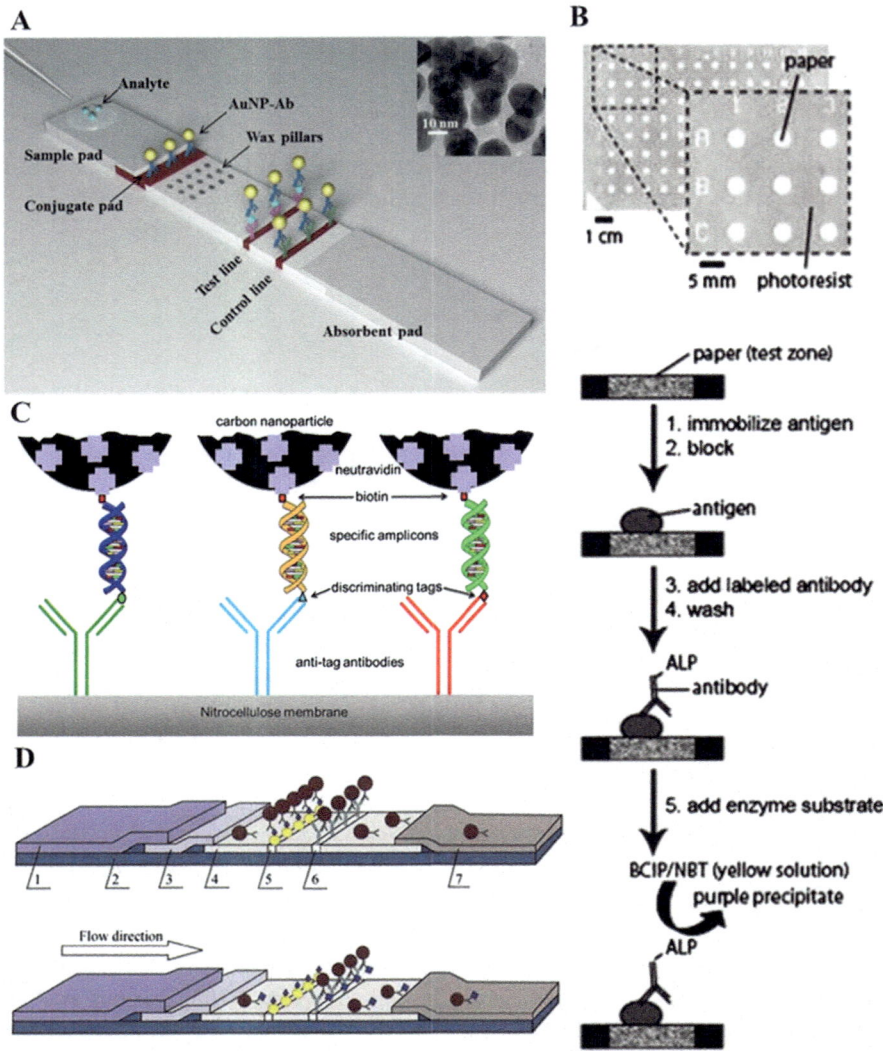

Fig. 5.2 Colorimetric detection-based PIAs based on the use of (**a**) AuNPs in LFAs [78], (**b**) enzymes in P-ELISA [51], (**c**) CNPs in LFAs [79], (**d**) MNPs in LFAs [80]. Reproduced with permission from Elsevier B.V

5.3.2 Thermal Detection

The thermal detection method in PIAs is highly sensitive and could lead to a many-fold increase in the analytical performance of PIAs w.r.t. visual detection by the naked eye [5, 100, 101] (Fig. 5.3). It is based on the photothermal effects of metal NPs, such as AuNPs [102, 103]. The method requires a laser to heat the test zone of PIAs for over a min, which is followed by the recording and analysis of thermal signal by a thermal contrast reader. However, the limitation of this detection method is the requirement for additional instruments, complex operation steps, and skilled analysts.

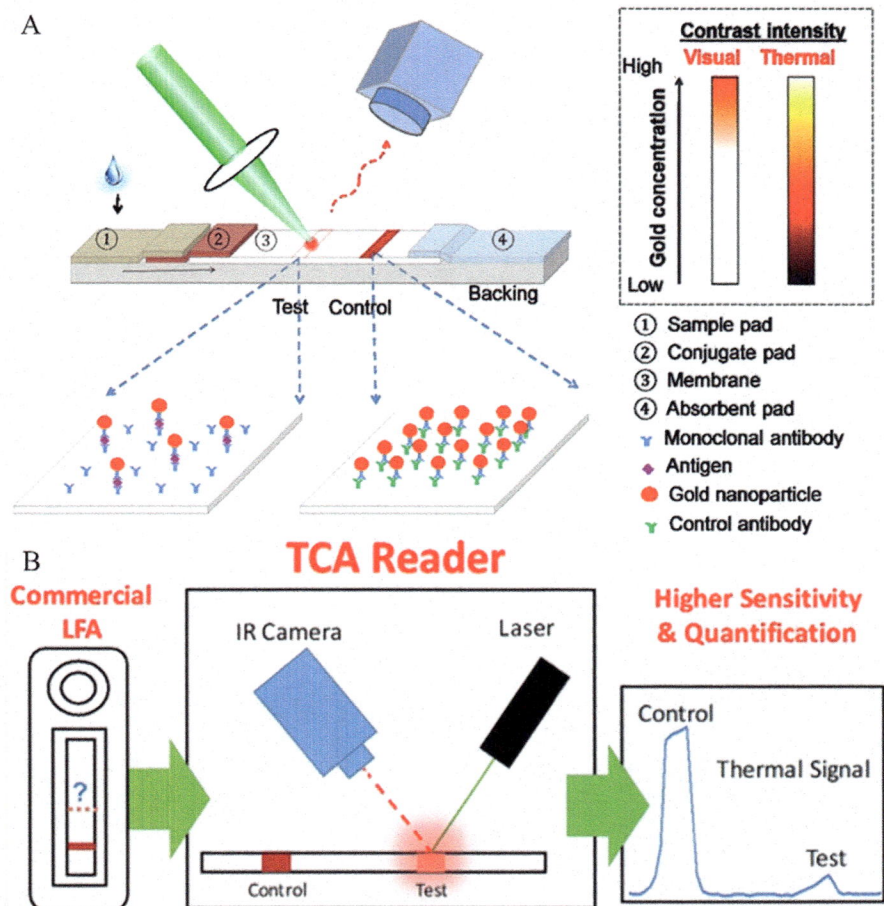

Fig. 5.3 Thermal detection-based PIA. Schematics of (**a**) thermal contrast method for LFAs [100] and (**b**) thermal contrast amplification principle [101]. Reproduced with permission from Elsevier B.V

5.3.3 Electrochemical Detection

The electrochemical detection has been widely used in PIAs due to its considerable simplicity, ease of manufacture, label-free detection, low-cost readers, and high sensitivity [84, 104–106]. As it is predominantly used in the commercial blood glucose monitoring, a wide range of technologies are available for the fabrication of electrodes on papers, such as sputtering, coating, screen printing, ink-jet printing, 3D printing, handwriting, etc. [107–110]. The electrochemical PIAs have been widely used for POCT in healthcare, food safety, environmental monitoring, and

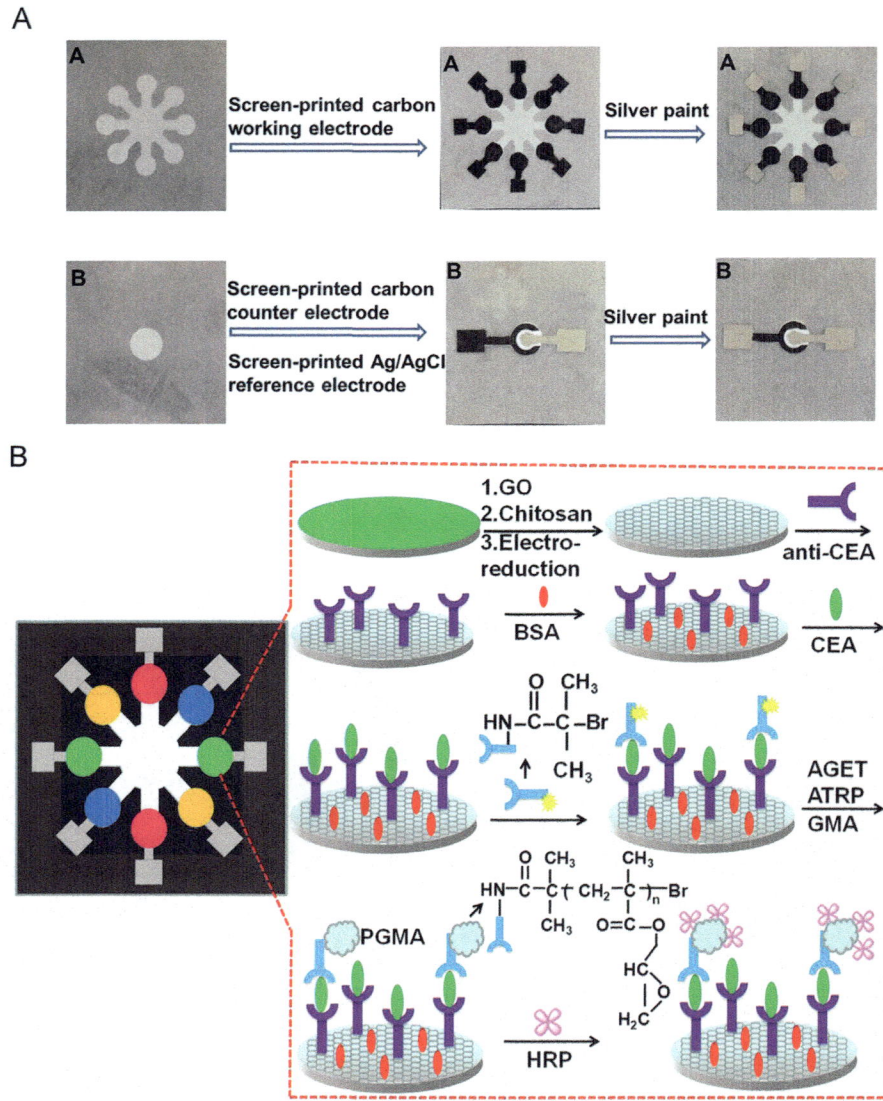

Fig. 5.4 (**a**) Fabrication of the microfluidic electrochemical PIA device and (**b**) schematic of the fabrication of paper device and the IA procedure for carcinoembryonic antigen (CEA) as an example [33]. The developed PIA device was employed for the multiplex detection of CEA, alphafetoprotein, cancer antigen 125, and carbohydrate antigen 153. Reproduced with permission from Elsevier B.V

veterinary sciences [111]. Of interest is the electrochemical PIAs for the multiplex detection of cancer biomarkers using a paper-based microfluidic electrochemical device and a controlled radical polymerization reaction [33] (Fig. 5.4). They have also been used for the detection of other analytes [112–115].

5.3.4 Magnetic Detection

The magnetic detection-based PIAs are prospective as MNPs provides a stable magnetic signal and are easy to control and functionalize [64]. A magnetic reader is needed to excite the MNPs and measure the magnetic field from MNPs in the entire detection zone of PIAs [80, 84, 95, 116] (Fig. 5.5). It is different from conventional LFAs that measure the colorimetric signal from the top few micrometers of nitrocellulose paper. Magnetic PIAs show superior analytical performance, which are easy to adapt to meet the assay specifications by selecting the appropriate size, concentration, and type of MNPs [95].

5.3.5 Chemiluminescence and Electrochemiluminescence Detection

Various chemiluminescent [34, 81, 117–119] and electrochemiluminescent [120–122] PIAs have been developed by researchers as chemiluminescence detection provides a very high analytical sensitivity. The chemiluminescent IA is very similar to that of colorimetric IA except the enzyme substrate provided at the end.

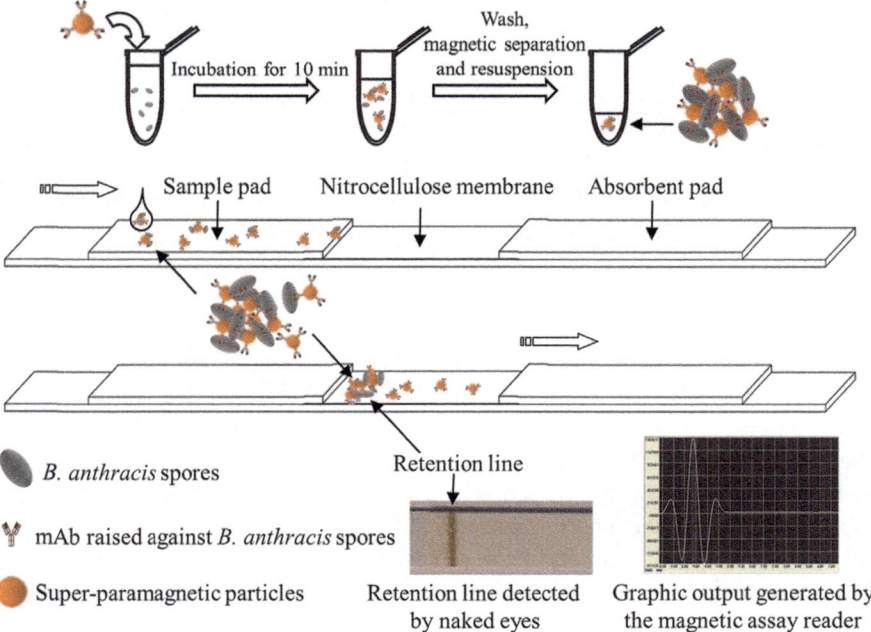

Fig. 5.5 Schematic of the magnetic detection-based LFA for *Bacillus anthracis* spores [116]. Reproduced with permission from Elsevier B.V

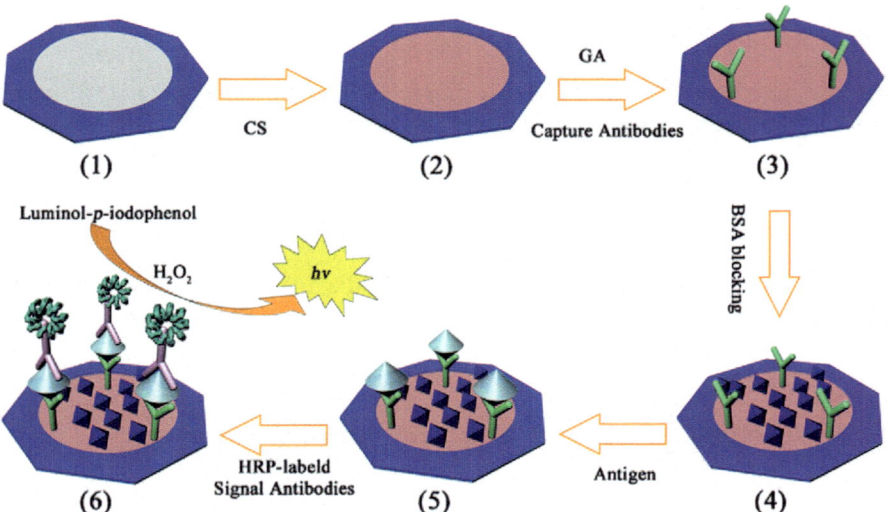

Fig. 5.6 Schematic of the fabrication and IA procedure for a paper-based chemilumines-cent ELISA [81]. (1) Wax-screen-printed paper zone, (2) chitosan-modified paper zone, (3) cap-ture antibodies immobilized paper zone through glutaraldehyde cross-linking, (4) BSA blocked paper zone, (5) paper zone after incubation with antigen solution, (6) paper zone after incubation with HRP-labeled signal antibodies and triggering CL reaction. CS, GA, BSA, and HRP represent chitosan, glutaraldehyde, bovine serum albumin, and horseradish peroxidase, respectively. Reproduced with permission from Elsevier B.V

The luminol-p-iodophenol combined with H_2O_2 is the most widely used substrate for chemiluminescent PIAs [81]. On the other hand, the electrochemiluminescent PIAs employ specific labels, such as green-luminescent graphene quantum dots functionalized with Au@Pt core-shell NPs [120], tris-(bipyridine)–ruthenium [Ru $(bpy)3^{2+}$]–tri-n-propylamine [122], etc. A specific chemiluminescent detector-based readout device measures the signal in the dark (Fig. 5.6).

5.4   Advances in Paper-Based Immunoassays

The conventional PIAs have low sensitivity and specificity with most of them enabling only the qualitative detection of analytes [49]. Therefore, there is a need to improve the bioanalytical performance of PIAs by advances in chemistry, nanopar-ticles, signal enhancement, readers, new biosensor approaches, and complementary technologies. The most prominent advances in PIAs along with the future trends are discussed here.

5.4.1   Increase in Analytical Sensitivity

The decrease in the limit of detection (LOD) of PIAs is desired for bioanalytical applications that demand high analytical sensitivity. Various strategies have been developed to increase the sensitivity of PIAs. The most prominent strategy is the use of nanocomposite labels (Fig. 5.7a) with increased surface area that enables higher

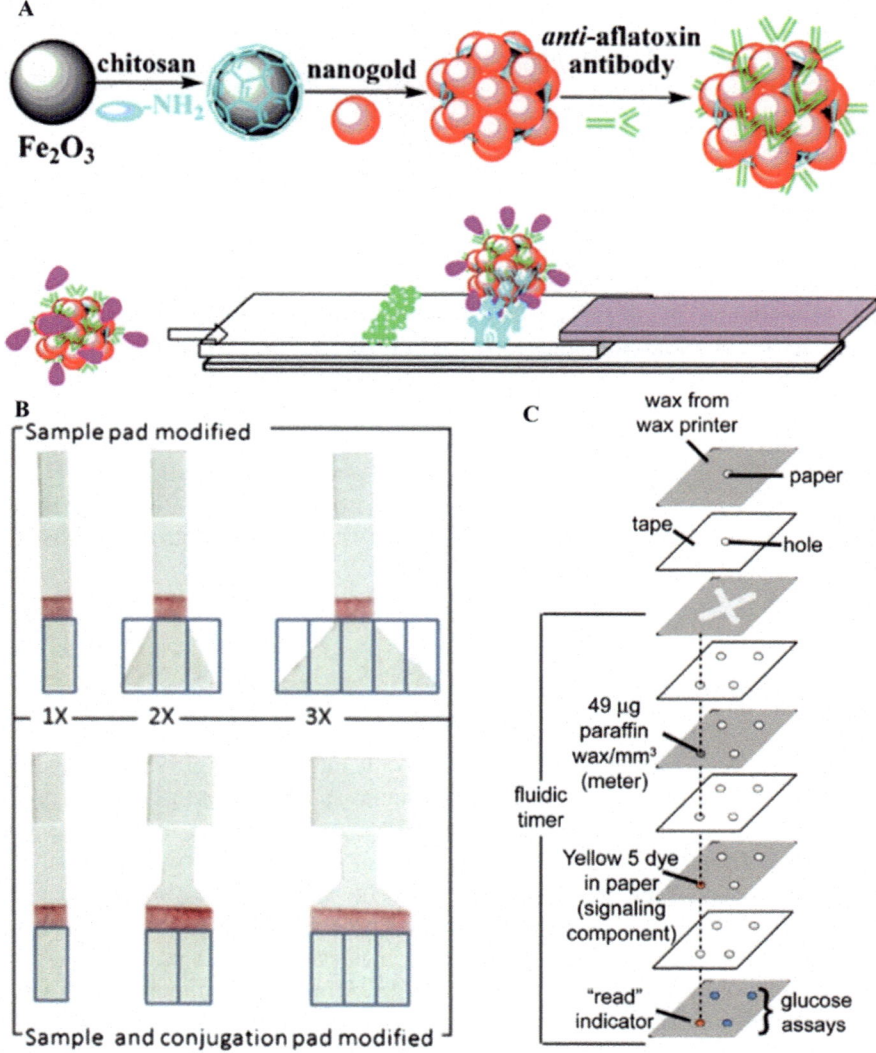

Fig. 5.7 Approaches to increase the sensitivity of PIAs. (**a**) Use of nanocomposite labels such as MNPs decorated with AuNPs [89], (**b**) microfluidics and modification of architecture [123], and (**c**) microfluidics with hydrophobic boundaries in μPAD [39]. Reproduced with permission from Elsevier B.V

biomolecular binding, which leads to greater signal in PIAs [124]. The use of optimal NP label, capture Ab, and other reagents used in PIAs [85, 125] can also increase the IA sensitivity. Another prospective approach is the use of improved architecture and design of PIA devices, such as the use of varied strip width [123] and the addition of a pad [126] in LFA (Fig. 5.7b). Of interest is the use of microfluidic technologies that increases the sensitivity and performance of PIAs by enabling the multiple process steps and mixing of IA reagents [127]. The microfluidic channels are constructed by providing hydrophobic barriers via waxing [39] or photolithography [43] and/or by cutting boundaries [37, 38] (Fig. 5.7c). They provide the direction to the liquid flow in PIAs. The reaction time can be increased to facilitate the specific IA by employing the barriers, such as trehalose [32] or wax pillars [78], which decrease the flow of reagents.

5.4.2 Automated Microfluidic Operations

The conventional PIAs that operate based on the principle of ELISA are limited in their bioanalytical applications as they require complex multiple process steps [128, 129]. The advent of microfluidics have led to PIAs for POCT by enabling the automation of multiple steps in PIA, such as sample treatment, immune reaction, and detection of signal [130], using the capillary action of paper and various types of paper-based platforms (two- or three-dimensional). An interesting development is the use of the paper-based device to separate plasma from whole blood [131]. Further, various strategies, such as the use of a dissolvable film [132] and flap value [133], can provide the adequate microfluidic flow rate for the controlled release of reagents in microfluidic channels.

5.4.3 Multiplex Detection

The conventional paper-based device can only detect a single analyte, while many analytes need to be detected in a particular sample in routine clinical practice. This can be achieved by multiplex PIAs. An interesting approach is the multiplexed LFA that involves the integration of several LFA strips into a single device, where each LFA strip can detect a specific analyte [15]. Another prospective multiplex format is the barcode competitive LFA for the detection of three pesticides in a single step [134]. However, it is essential to analyze the cross-reactivity of analytes in such formats critically. Of interest is the multiplex LFA format for the simultaneous detection of antibodies against human immunodeficiency virus (HIV), hepatitis B virus (HBV), and hepatitis C virus (HCV) [135] (Fig. 5.8).

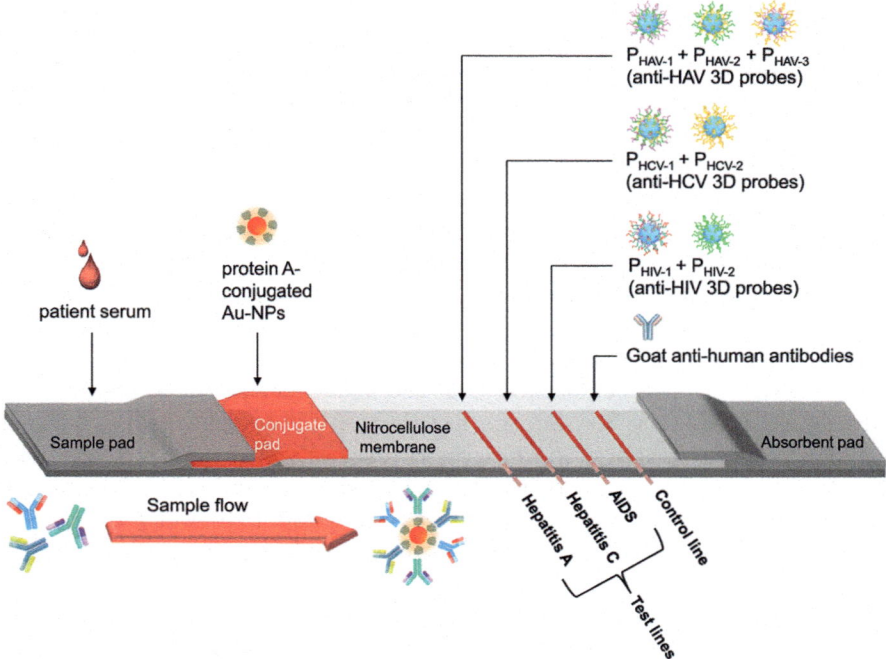

Fig. 5.8 Multiplex lateral flow immunoassay for the detection of anti-HIV, anti-HCV, and anti-HAV antibodies [135]. The control line contains goat anti-human secondary antibodies. HIV, HCV, and HAV represent human immunodeficiency virus, hepatitis C virus, and hepatitis B virus, respectively. Reproduced with permission from Elsevier B.V

5.4.4 Quantitative Determination of Analytes

The conventional PIAs, based on the visual detection of analytes via naked eyes, enable only the qualitative analyte detection. They can only analyze the presence or absence of analyte. However, there is an extensive need for semi-quantitative or quantitative PIAs for various bioanalytical applications. Several prospective strategies have been reported by researchers for semi-quantitative PIA, such as the barcode-style LFA strip based on competitive IA [136–138] and the three-line LFA strip (i.e., test, antigen, and control lines) based on sandwich IA [139]. However, the semi-quantitative PIAs are inappropriate for clinical diagnostic applications that require quantitative determination of target analyte concentration.

Several strategies have been reported for the quantitative PIAs based on the use of advanced readers and image analysis system. The colorimetric, chemiluminescent, thermal contrast, electrochemical, and magnetic readers have been used by various researchers to measure the specific IA signal. The advanced image analysis system can then determine the concentration of the analyte. The digital cameras and LFA strip scanners have been used for taking the pictures of LFA strip [5, 104], but the recent trend is the fully integrated smartphone-based reader that can capture the images and analyze them instantaneously to provide the concentration of the analyte [140–144].

With the advent of low-cost and widespread accessibility of SP technology, the current trend has now shifted to highly precise quantification using SP-based image analysis [145]. A compact and lightweight integrated rapid diagnostic test reader [146] employs an SP-based optomechanical attachment for real-time detection and quantification of target analytes using LFAs. Cellmic (previously Holomic LLC) has developed various commercial SP-based POC readers for the readout of LFA, i.e., Holomic Rapid Diagnostic Test Reader (HRDR-200) and HRDR-300 [147] (Fig. 5.9a). The prototype and working of the device concept used in HRDR-200 are available elsewhere [8]. HRDR-200 is a compact, low-cost, and lightweight hand-held SP reader that reads chromatographic and fluorescent assays in various assay formats, i.e., lateral flow, flow-through, and dipstick. The device comprises an integrated reader housing and an SP, which comes together with a smart application and access to secure Cloud Services and Test Developer. The company has also developed an SP-based fluorescent reader, i.e., HRDR-300 (Fig. 5.9b), which employs an advanced image processing algorithm for the multicolor imaging readout of the control and test lines of LFA. The users can select the excitation in the range of 350–700 nm and the emission in the range of 300–800 nm. The rest of the device features is similar to that of HRDR-200. The rapid diagnostic test (RDT) reader prototype [8] used for HRDR-200 is a compact and lightweight (~65 g) device comprising a plano-convex lens, a microcontroller, and three LED arrays. Two LED arrays are positioned underneath the RDT tray for the reflection imaging of RDT, while one LED array is located at the top for the transmission imaging of RDT. The device enables the quantitative determination of an analyte by reflection or transmission imaging modes of RDT under diffused LED illumination. It is powered by

(A)   **(B)**

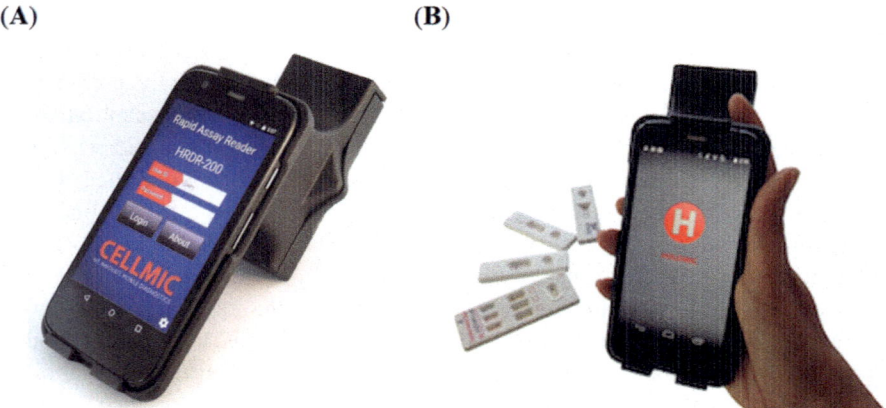

Fig. 5.9 Smartphone-based readers for rapid diagnostic tests developed by Cellmic. (**a**) Holomic Rapid Diagnostic Test Reader (HRDR-200) (**b**) HRDR-300. Reproduced with permission from Cellmic

external batteries or the SP's internal battery via USB connection. The raw images captured by the SP's camera are processed by a smart application in less than 0.2 s, and the results are shared with a central server that could be assessed by a remote computer using web browsers.

A more recent advance is the development of a µPAD with fluidic batteries integrated directly into the microfluidic channels [148–150], which provide power to on-chip devices such as LEDs and electrochromic displays for POC diagnostics. Ongoing research efforts focus on multiplex detection of analytes [147, 151, 152] and the development of fully integrated platforms that incorporate sample pretreatment and separation [153]. An innovative development is the completely printed paper-based amperometric biosensor [61].

5.5 Critiques and Outlook

There is a need to demonstrate the batch-to-batch consistency of paper-based platforms, which is one of the major challenges for the development of clinically-viable PIAs [154, 155]. As the paper-based platforms are prone to high non-specific binding, there is a need to employ appropriate blocking buffers and check for interference from potential non-specific physiological and pharmacological substances. Despite the numerous research papers and demonstrations of PIAs for various bioanalytical applications, the robust clinical validation and alignment with clinically-accredited predicate IAs are still pending [156]. It remains to be seen whether the PIAs can match the precision, accuracy, sensitivity, specificity, reproducibility, and robustness of established technologies that are being used routinely in clinical diagnostics and bioanalytical settings. Therefore, there is an extensive need for regulatory-compliant PIAs that address the requirements of healthcare.

There is an immense need to develop fully integrated paper-based platforms that can perform POCT without any or minimal requirement for refrigeration, ancillary equipment, or additional process steps. The developments in SP-based readers and smart readers have circumvented the need for bulky and expensive detection instruments that are used in the central laboratory. However, there are growing concerns about the security of patients' data in such mobile health devices that are based on cloud computing and involve data storage and transmission via Bluetooth and wireless networks. Therefore, there is a need for mobile health companies to employ advanced encryption algorithms to secure the confidential data and patients' personal health records. There are numerous ongoing efforts toward the establishment of an international Cloud computing standard, such as the creation of EuroCloud and Google Data Liberation Front [157].

The health insurance companies play a critical role in clinical diagnostics as they provide the reimbursement for the use of IAs. Therefore, there is an extensive need for IVD developers to demonstrate the clinical utility, affordability, benefits, and features of PIAs. The developers should consult the health insurance companies from the early stages of product development.

The IVD manufacturer should consider the end-user scenario and conditions for the development of PIAs. As most IAs are developed in the standard bioanalytical labs under controlled ambient conditions, there is a lack of understanding about how the developed PIA might perform in various end-user settings. These factors should be incorporated into the design and development plan of a PIA and should be checked during the development of the product.

5.6   Conclusions

PIAs are ideal for POCT in developing countries and remote settings as they are cheap, simple, easy-to-use, and easy-to-understand. They can be used at any place and time without any need for highly-skilled analysts, expensive readers, and continuous power supply. Various PIAs have been developed for multifarious applications. Moreover, there have been tremendous advances in PIAs, which have not only increased their analytical sensitivity but also led to automated microfluidic operations and development of prospective multiplex PIAs. The emerging trend is strongly focused on the development of quantitative PIAs employing fully-integrated smart readers, such as those based on SPs. But the analytical performance of PIAs is not yet adequate for realistic applications in clinical diagnostics, food safety, environmental monitoring, agriculture, and veterinary sciences. Further, PIAs have significant non-specific binding that considerably increases the non-reproducibility of assays. Therefore, there is a need for novel IA chemistries, better blocking strategies, and improved signal detection. However, the ongoing research efforts and the advances in complementary technologies will pave the way to robust, reproducible, and analytically superior PIAs in the coming years.

References

1. Vashist SK, Luong JHT. Handbook of immunoassay technologies: approaches, performances, and applications. London: Academic Press; 2018.
2. Ahmed S, Bui MP, Abbas A. Paper-based chemical and biological sensors: engineering aspects. Biosens Bioelectron. 2016;77:249–63.
3. Chen Y-H, Kuo Z-K, Cheng C-M. Paper–a potential platform in pharmaceutical development. Trends Biotech. 2015;33(1):4–9.
4. Ge L, Yu J, Ge S, Yan M. Lab-on-paper-based devices using chemiluminescence and electro-generated chemiluminescence detection. Anal Bioanal Chem. 2014;406(23):5613–30.
5. Hu J, Wang S, Wang L, Li F, Pingguan-Murphy B, Lu TJ, et al. Advances in paper-based point-of-care diagnostics. Biosens Bioelectron. 2014;54:585–97.
6. Liana DD, Raguse B, Gooding JJ, Chow E. Recent advances in paper-based sensors. Sensors. 2012;12(9):11505–26.
7. Martinez AW, Phillips ST, Whitesides GM, Carrilho E. Diagnostics for the developing world: microfluidic paper-based analytical devices. Anal Chem. 2009;82(1):3–10.

8. Parolo C, Merkoci A. Paper-based nanobiosensors for diagnostics. Chem Soc Rev. 2013;42(2):450–7.
9. Pelton R. Bioactive paper provides a low-cost platform for diagnostics. Trends Anal Chem. 2009;28(8):925–42.
10. Rolland JP, Mourey DA. Paper as a novel material platform for devices. MRS Bull. 2013;38(04):299–305.
11. Then WL, Garnier G. Paper diagnostics in biomedicine. Rev Anal Chem. 2013;32(4):269–94.
12. Li X, Ballerini DR, Shen W. A perspective on paper-based microfluidics: current status and future trends. Biomicrofluidics. 2012;6(1):11301–1130113.
13. Jaganathan S, Vahedi Tafreshi H, Pourdeyhimi B. Modeling liquid porosimetry in modeled and imaged 3-D fibrous microstructures. J Colloid Interface Sci. 2008;326(1):166–75.
14. Pan N. On uniqueness of fibrous materials. WIT Trans Ecol Environ. 2004;73:10. https://doi.org/10.2495/DN040491.
15. Yetisen AK, Akram MS, Lowe CR. Paper-based microfluidic point-of-care diagnostic devices. Lab Chip. 2013;13(12):2210–51.
16. Wong R, Tse H. Lateral flow immunoassay. New York: Humana Press; 2009.
17. Han YL, Wang W, Hu J, Huang G, Wang S, Lee WG, et al. Benchtop fabrication of three-dimensional reconfigurable microfluidic devices from paper-polymer composite. Lab Chip. 2013;13(24):4745–9.
18. Park S, Mohanty N, Suk JW, Nagaraja A, An J, Piner RD, et al. Biocompatible, robust free-standing paper composed of a TWEEN/graphene composite. Adv Mater. 2010;22(15):1736–40.
19. Nanomaterials SB. Paper powers battery breakthrough. Nat Nanotechnol. 2007;2(10):598–9.
20. Wang DW, Li F, Zhao J, Ren W, Chen ZG, Tan J, et al. Fabrication of graphene/polyaniline composite paper via *in situ* anodic electropolymerization for high-performance flexible electrode. ACS Nano. 2009;3(7):1745–52.
21. Chen X, Chen J, Wang F, Xiang X, Luo M, Ji X, et al. Determination of glucose and uric acid with bienzyme colorimetry on microfluidic paper-based analysis devices. Biosens Bioelectron. 2012;35(1):363–8.
22. He M, Liu Z. Paper-based microfluidic device with upconversion fluorescence assay. Anal Chem. 2013;85(24):11691–4.
23. Lei KF, Yang S-I, Tsai S-W, Hsu H-T. Paper-based microfluidic sensing device for label-free immunoassay demonstrated by biotin–avidin binding interaction. Talanta. 2015;134:264–70.
24. Li X, Tian J, Shen W. Quantitative biomarker assay with microfluidic paper-based analytical devices. Anal Bioanal Chem. 2010;396(1):495–501.
25. Liu F, Zhang C. A novel paper-based microfluidic enhanced chemiluminescence biosensor for facile, reliable and highly-sensitive gene detection of Listeria monocytogenes. Sens Actuators B Chem. 2015;209:399–406.
26. Mao X, Huang TJ. Microfluidic diagnostics for the developing world. Lab Chip. 2012;12(8):1412–6.
27. Martinez AW, Phillips ST, Carrilho E, Thomas SW 3rd, Sindi H, Whitesides GM. Simple telemedicine for developing regions: camera phones and paper-based microfluidic devices for real-time, off-site diagnosis. Anal Chem. 2008;80(10):3699–707.
28. Martinez AW, Phillips ST, Whitesides GM. Three-dimensional microfluidic devices fabricated in layered paper and tape. Proc Natl Acad Sci U S A. 2008;105(50):19606–11.
29. Mu X, Zhang L, Chang S, Cui W, Zheng Z. Multiplex microfluidic paper-based immunoassay for the diagnosis of hepatitis C virus infection. Anal Chem. 2014;86(11):5338–44.
30. Noiphung J, Songjaroen T, Dungchai W, Henry CS, Chailapakul O, Laiwattanapaisal W. Electrochemical detection of glucose from whole blood using paper-based microfluidic devices. Anal Chim Acta. 2013;788:39–45.
31. Rattanarat P, Dungchai W, Cate DM, Siangproh W, Volckens J, Chailapakul O, et al. A microfluidic paper-based analytical device for rapid quantification of particulate chromium. Anal Chim Acta. 2013;800:50–5.

32. Schilling KM, Lepore AL, Kurian JA, Martinez AW. Fully enclosed microfluidic paper-based analytical devices. Anal Chem. 2012;84(3):1579–85.
33. Wu Y, Xue P, Hui KM, Kang Y. A paper-based microfluidic electrochemical immunodevice integrated with amplification-by-polymerization for the ultrasensitive multiplexed detection of cancer biomarkers. Biosens Bioelectron. 2014;52:180–7.
34. Yu J, Wang S, Ge L, Ge S. A novel chemiluminescence paper microfluidic biosensor based on enzymatic reaction for uric acid determination. Biosens Bioelectron. 2011;26(7):3284–9.
35. Zhao C, Thuo MM, Liu X. A microfluidic paper-based electrochemical biosensor array for multiplexed detection of metabolic biomarkers. Sci Technol Adv Mater. 2013;14(5):054402.
36. Hu J, Wang L, Li F, Han YL, Lin M, Lu TJ, et al. Oligonucleotide-linked gold nanoparticle aggregates for enhanced sensitivity in lateral flow assays. Lab Chip. 2013;13(22):4352–7.
37. Fu E, Ramsey SA, Kauffman P, Lutz B, Yager P. Transport in two-dimensional paper networks. Microfluid Nanofluidics. 2011;10(1):29–35.
38. Song MB, Joung HA, Oh YK, Jung K, Ahn YD, Kim MG. Tear-off patterning: a simple method for patterning nitrocellulose membranes to improve the performance of point-of-care diagnostic biosensors. Lab Chip. 2015;15(14):3006–12.
39. Noh H, Phillips ST. Fluidic timers for time-dependent, point-of-care assays on paper. Anal Chem. 2010;82(19):8071–8.
40. Carrilho E, Martinez AW, Whitesides GM. Understanding wax printing: a simple micropatterning process for paper-based microfluidics. Anal Chem. 2009;81(16):7091–5.
41. Zhong Z, Wang Z, Huang G. Investigation of wax and paper materials for the fabrication of paper-based microfluidic devices. Microsyst Technol. 2012;18(5):649–59.
42. Lu Y, Shi W, Qin J, Lin B. Fabrication and characterization of paper-based microfluidics prepared in nitrocellulose membrane by wax printing. Anal Chem. 2009;82(1):329–35.
43. Martinez AW, Phillips ST, Butte MJ, Whitesides GM. Patterned paper as a platform for inexpensive, low-volume, portable bioassays. Angew Chem Int Ed. 2007;46(8):1318–20.
44. Free AH, Adams EC, Kercher ML, Free HM, Cook MH. Simple specific test for urine glucose. Clin Chem. 1957;3(3):163–8.
45. Glad C, Grubb AO. Immunocapillary migration—a new method for immunochemical quantitation. Anal Biochem. 1978;85(1):180–7.
46. Vaitukaitis JL, Braunstein GD, Ross GT. A radioimmunoassay which specifically measures human chorionic gonadotropin in the presence of human luteinizing hormone. Am J Obstet Gynecol. 1972;113(6):751–8.
47. Hawkes R, Niday E, Gordon J. A dot-immunobinding assay for monoclonal and other antibodies. Anal Biochem. 1982;119(1):142–7.
48. Le S, Zhou H, Nie J, Cao C, Yang J, Pan H, et al. Fabrication of paper devices via laser-heating-wax-printing for high-tech enzyme-linked immunosorbent assays with low-tech pen-type pH meter readout. Analyst. 2017;142(3):511–6.
49. Vashist SK, Luppa PB, Yeo LY, Ozcan A, Luong JHT. Emerging technologies for next-generation point-of-care testing. Trends Biotechnol. 2015;33(11):692–705.
50. Young RO, Young SR. The pH miracle: balance your diet, reclaim your health. New York: Hachette UK; 2008.
51. Cheng CM, Martinez AW, Gong J, Mace CR, Phillips ST, Carrilho E, et al. Paper-based ELISA. Angew Chem Int Ed Engl. 2010;49(28):4771–4.
52. Tian J, Li X, Shen W. Printed two-dimensional micro-zone plates for chemical analysis and ELISA. Lab Chip. 2011;11(17):2869–75.
53. Avrameas S, Ternynck T. Enzyme-linked immunosorbent assay (ELISA). 1998.
54. O'Connor EF, Paterson S, De La Rica R. Naked-eye detection as a universal approach to lower the limit of detection of enzyme-linked immunoassays. Anal Bioanal Chem. 2016;408(13):3389–93.
55. Bahadır EB, Sezgintürk MK. Lateral flow assays: principles, designs and labels. Trends Anal Chem. 2016;82:286–306.
56. Koczula KM, Gallotta A. Lateral flow assays. Essays Biochem. 2016;60(1):111–20.

57. Daniel MC, Astruc D. Gold nanoparticles: assembly, supramolecular chemistry, quantum-size-related properties, and applications toward biology, catalysis, and nanotechnology. Chem Rev. 2004;104(1):293–346.

58. Lin M, Zhao Y, Wang S, Liu M, Duan Z, Chen Y, et al. Recent advances in synthesis and surface modification of lanthanide-doped upconversion nanoparticles for biomedical applications. Biotechnol Adv. 2012;30(6):1551–61.

59. Ge C, Yu L, Fang Z, Zeng L. An enhanced strip biosensor for rapid and sensitive detection of histone methylation. Anal Chem. 2013;85(19):9343–9.

60. Nie Z, Nijhuis CA, Gong J, Chen X, Kumachev A, Martinez AW, et al. Electrochemical sensing in paper-based microfluidic devices. Lab Chip. 2010;10(4):477–83.

61. Turner AP. Biosensors: sense and sensibility. Chem Soc Rev. 2013;42(8):3184–96.

62. Yang Q, Gong X, Song T, Yang J, Zhu S, Li Y, et al. Quantum dot-based immunochromatography test strip for rapid, quantitative and sensitive detection of alpha fetoprotein. Biosens Bioelectron. 2011;30(1):145–50.

63. van den Berk GE, Frissen PH, Regez RM, Rietra PJ. Evaluation of the rapid immunoassay determine HIV 1/2 for detection of antibodies to human immunodeficiency virus types 1 and 2. J Clin Microbiol. 2003;41(8):3868–9.

64. Sajid M, Kawde A-N, Daud M. Designs, formats and applications of lateral flow assay: a literature review. J Saudi Chem Soc. 2015;19(6):689–705.

65. Liu W, Cassano CL, Xu X, Fan ZH. Laminated paper-based analytical devices (LPAD) with origami-enabled chemiluminescence immunoassay for cotinine detection in mouse serum. Anal Chem. 2013;85(21):10270–6.

66. Xia Y, Si J, Li Z. Fabrication techniques for microfluidic paper-based analytical devices and their applications for biological testing: a review. Biosens Bioelectron. 2016;77:774–89.

67. Nilghaz A, Wicaksono DH, Gustiono D, Majid FAA, Supriyanto E, Kadir MRA. Flexible microfluidic cloth-based analytical devices using a low-cost wax patterning technique. Lab Chip. 2012;12(1):209–18.

68. Cassano CL, Fan ZH. Laminated paper-based analytical devices (LPAD): fabrication, characterization, and assays. Microfluidic Nanofluidics. 2013;15(2):173–81.

69. Martinez AW, Phillips ST, Whitesides GM. Three-dimensional microfluidic devices fabricated in layered paper and tape. Proc Natl Acad Sci. 2008;105(50):19606–11.

70. Lewis GG, DiTucci MJ, Baker MS, Phillips ST. High throughput method for prototyping three-dimensional, paper-based microfluidic devices. Lab Chip. 2012;12(15):2630–3.

71. Schilling KM, Jauregui D, Martinez AW. Paper and toner three-dimensional fluidic devices: programming fluid flow to improve point-of-care diagnostics. Lab Chip. 2013;13(4):628–31.

72. Liu H, Crooks RM. Three-dimensional paper microfluidic devices assembled using the principles of origami. J Am Chem Soc. 2011;133(44):17564–6.

73. Liu X, Cheng C, Martinez A, Mirica K, Li X, Phillips S, et al., editors. A portable microfluidic paper-based device for ELISA. Micro Electro Mechanical Systems (MEMS), 2011 IEEE 24th International Conference on. IEEE; 2011.

74. Apilux A, Ukita Y, Chikae M, Chailapakul O, Takamura Y. Development of automated paper-based devices for sequential multistep sandwich enzyme-linked immunosorbent assays using inkjet printing. Lab Chip. 2013;13(1):126–35.

75. Nie Z, Deiss F, Liu X, Akbulut O, Whitesides GM. Integration of paper-based microfluidic devices with commercial electrochemical readers. Lab Chip. 2010;10(22):3163–9.

76. Lu J, Ge S, Ge L, Yan M, Yu J. Electrochemical DNA sensor based on three-dimensional folding paper device for specific and sensitive point-of-care testing. Electrochim Acta. 2012;80:334–41.

77. Huang X, Aguilar ZP, Xu H, Lai W, Xiong Y. Membrane-based lateral flow immunochromatographic strip with nanoparticles as reporters for detection: a review. Biosens Bioelectron. 2016;75:166–80.

78. Rivasa L, Medina-Sáncheza M, de la Escosura-Muñiza A, Merkoçi A. Improving sensitivity of gold nanoparticles-based lateral flow assays by using wax-printed pillars as delay barriers of microfluidics. Lab Chip. 2014;14:4406–14.

79. Posthuma-Trumpie GA, Wichers JH, Koets M, Berendsen LB, van Amerongen A. Amorphous carbon nanoparticles: a versatile label for rapid diagnostic (immuno)assays. Anal Bioanal Chem. 2012;402(2):593–600.
80. Wang D-B, Tian B, Zhang Z-P, Deng J-Y, Cui Z-Q, Yang R-F, et al. Rapid detection of *Bacillus anthracis* spores using a super-paramagnetic lateral-flow immunological detection-system. Biosens Bioelectron. 2013;42:661–7.
81. Wang S, Ge L, Song X, Yu J, Ge S, Huang J, et al. Paper-based chemiluminescence ELISA: lab-on-paper based on chitosan modified paper device and wax-screen-printing. Biosens Bioelectron. 2012;31(1):212–8.
82. Li X, Zwanenburg P, Liu X. Magnetic timing valves for fluid control in paper-based micro-fluidics. Lab Chip. 2013;13(13):2609–14.
83. Zhou W, Gao X, Liu D, Chen X. Gold nanoparticles for *in vitro* diagnostics. Chem Rev. 2015;115(19):10575–636.
84. Quesada-Gonzalez D, Merkoci A. Nanoparticle-based lateral flow biosensors. Biosens Bioelectron. 2015;73:47–63.
85. Safenkova I, Zherdev A, Dzantiev B. Factors influencing the detection limit of the lateral-flow sandwich immunoassay: a case study with potato virus X. Anal Bioanal Chem. 2012;403(6):1595–605.
86. Parolo C, de la Escosura-Muniz A, Merkoci A. Enhanced lateral flow immunoassay using gold nanoparticles loaded with enzymes. Biosens Bioelectron. 2013;40(1):412–6.
87. Shen G, Zhang S, Hu X. Signal enhancement in a lateral flow immunoassay based on dual gold nanoparticle conjugates. Clin Biochem. 2013;46(16–17):1734–8.
88. Xu H, Chen J, Birrenkott J, Zhao JX, Takalkar S, Baryeh K, et al. Gold-nanoparticle-decorated silica nanorods for sensitive visual detection of proteins. Anal Chem. 2014;86(15):7351–9.
89. Tang D, Sauceda JC, Lin Z, Ott S, Basova E, Goryacheva I, et al. Magnetic nanogold microspheres-based lateral-flow immunodipstick for rapid detection of aflatoxin B2 in food. Biosens Bioelectron. 2009;25(2):514–8.
90. Fu Q, Liu HL, Wu Z, Liu A, Yao C, Li X, et al. Rough surface Au@Ag core–shell nanoparticles to fabricating high sensitivity SERS immunochromatographic sensors. J Nanobiotech. 2015;13(1):81.
91. Blažková M, Rauch P, Fukal L. Strip-based immunoassay for rapid detection of thiabenda-zole. Biosens Bioelectron. 2010;25(9):2122–8.
92. Linares EM, Kubota LT, Michaelis J, Thalhammer S. Enhancement of the detection limit for lateral flow immunoassays: evaluation and comparison of bioconjugates. J Immunol Methods. 2012;375(1–2):264–70.
93. Suarez-Pantaleon C, Wichers J, Abad-Somovilla A, van Amerongen A, Abad-Fuentes A. Development of an immunochromatographic assay based on carbon nanoparticles for the determination of the phytoregulator forchlorfenuron. Biosens Bioelectron. 2013;42:170–6.
94. Huang Y-M, Dao-Feng L, Wei-Hua L, Xiong Y-H, Wan-Chun Y, Kun L, et al. Rapid detection of aflatoxin M1 by immunochromatography combined with enrichment based on immuno-magnetic nanobead. Chin J Anal Chem. 2014;42(5):654–9.
95. Wang Y, Xu H, Wei M, Gu H, Xu Q, Zhu W. Study of superparamagnetic nanoparticles as labels in the quantitative lateral flow immunoassay. Mater Sci Eng C. 2009;29(3):714–8.
96. Liu C, Jia Q, Yang C, Qiao R, Jing L, Wang L, et al. Lateral flow immunochromatographic assay for sensitive pesticide detection by using Fe3O4 nanoparticle aggregates as color reagents. Anal Chem. 2011;83(17):6778–84.
97. Yan J, Liu Y, Wang Y, Xu X, Lu Y, Pan Y, et al. Effect of physiochemical property of Fe3O4 particle on magnetic lateral flow immunochromatographic assay. Sens Actuators B Chem. 2014;197:129–36.
98. Tang Y, Li Z, He N, Zhang L, Ma C, Li X, et al. Preparation of functional magnetic nanoparticles mediated with PEG-4000 and application in Pseudomonas aeruginosa rapid detection. J Biomed Nanotechnol. 2013;9(2):312–7.
99. Xu X, Deng C, Gao M, Yu W, Yang P, Zhang X. Synthesis of magnetic microspheres with immobilized metal ions for enrichment and direct determination of phosphopeptides by matrix-assisted laser desorption ionization mass spectrometry. Adv Mater. 2006;18(24):3289–93.

100. Qin Z, Chan WC, Boulware DR, Akkin T, Butler EK, Bischof JC. Significantly improved analytical sensitivity of lateral flow immunoassays by using thermal contrast. Angew Chem Int Ed. 2012;51(18):4358–61.
101. Wang Y, Qin Z, Boulware DR, Pritt BS, Sloan LM, Gonzalez IJ, et al. Thermal contrast amplification reader yielding 8-fold analytical improvement for disease detection with lateral flow assays. Anal Chem. 2016;88(23):11774–82.
102. Shen S, Henry A, Tong J, Zheng R, Chen G. Polyethylene nanofibres with very high thermal conductivities. Nat Nanotech. 2010;5(4):251.
103. Govorov AO, Richardson HH. Generating heat with metal nanoparticles. Nano Today. 2007;2(1):30–8.
104. Cate DM, Adkins JA, Mettakoonpitak J, Henry CS. Recent developments in paper-based microfluidic devices. Anal Chem. 2015;87(1):19–41.
105. Luo S, Xiao H, Yang S, Liu C, Liang J, Tang Y. Ultrasensitive detection of pentachlorophenol based on enhanced electrochemiluminescence of Au nanoclusters/graphene hybrids. Sens Actuators B Chem. 2014;194:325–31.
106. Xu Y, Lou B, Lv Z, Zhou Z, Zhang L, Wang E. Paper based solid-state electrochemilumines-cence sensor using poly (sodium 4-styrenesulfonate) functionalized graphene/nafion com-posite film. Anal Chim Acta. 2013;763:20–7.
107. Li Z, Liu H, Ouyang C, Hong Wee W, Cui X, Jian Lu T, et al. Recent advances in pen-based writing electronics and their emerging applications. Adv Funct Mater. 2016;26(2):165–80.
108. Li Z, Li F, Hu J, Wee WH, Han YL, Pingguan-Murphy B, et al. Direct writing electrodes using a ball pen for paper-based point-of-care testing. Analyst. 2015;140(16):5526–35.
109. Siegel AC, Phillips ST, Wiley BJ, Whitesides GM. Thin, lightweight, foldable thermochro-mic displays on paper. Lab Chip. 2009;9(19):2775–81.
110. Matsuda Y, Shibayama S, Uete K, Yamaguchi H, Niimi T. Electric conductive pattern ele-ment fabricated using commercial inkjet printer for paper-based analytical devices. Anal Chem. 2015;87(11):5762–5.
111. Li Z, Hu J, Xu F, Li F. Recent developments of three-dimensional paper-based electrochemi-cal devices for cancer cell detection and anticancer drug screening. Curr Pharm Biotechnol. 2016;17(9):802–9.
112. Wang P, Ge L, Yan M, Song X, Ge S, Yu J. Paper-based three-dimensional electrochemical immunodevice based on multi-walled carbon nanotubes functionalized paper for sensitive point-of-care testing. Biosens Bioelectron. 2012;32(1):238–43.
113. Ge L, Yan J, Song X, Yan M, Ge S, Yu J. Three-dimensional paper-based electrochemilu-minescence immunodevice for multiplexed measurement of biomarkers and point-of-care testing. Biomaterials. 2012;33(4):1024–31.
114. Li W, Li L, Li M, Yu J, Ge S, Yan M, et al. Development of a 3D origami multiplex electro-chemical immunodevice using a nanoporous silver-paper electrode and metal ion functional-ized nanoporous gold–chitosan. Chem Commun. 2013;49(83):9540–2.
115. Ma C, Li W, Kong Q, Yang H, Bian Z, Song X, et al. 3D origami electrochemical immuno-device for sensitive point-of-care testing based on dual-signal amplification strategy. Biosens Bioelectron. 2015;63:7–13.
116. Wang DB, Tian B, Zhang ZP, Wang XY, Fleming J, Bi LJ, et al. Detection of Bacillus anthra-cis spores by super-paramagnetic lateral-flow immunoassays based on "Road Closure". Biosens Bioelectron. 2015;67:608–14.
117. Ge L, Wang S, Song X, Ge S, Yu J. 3D origami-based multifunction-integrated immunode-vice: low-cost and multiplexed sandwich chemiluminescence immunoassay on microfluidic paper-based analytical device. Lab Chip. 2012;12(17):3150–8.
118. Li W, Ge S, Wang S, Yan M, Ge L, Yu J. Highly sensitive chemiluminescence immunoassay on chitosan membrane modified paper platform using TiO2 nanoparticles/multiwalled car-bon nanotubes as label. Luminescence. 2013;28(4):496–502.
119. Wang S, Ge L, Song X, Yan M, Ge S, Yu J, et al. Simple and covalent fabrication of a paper device and its application in sensitive chemiluminescence immunoassay. Analyst. 2012;137(16):3821–7.

120. Li L, Li W, Ma C, Yang H, Ge S, Yu J. Paper-based electrochemiluminescence immunodevice for carcinoembryonic antigen using nanoporous gold-chitosan hybrids and graphene quantum dots functionalized Au@Pt. Sens Actuators B Chem. 2014;202:314–22.
121. Li W, Li M, Ge S, Yan M, Huang J, Yu J. Battery-triggered ultrasensitive electrochemiluminescence detection on microfluidic paper-based immunodevice based on dual-signal amplification strategy. Anal Chim Acta. 2013;767:66–74.
122. Yan J, Ge L, Song X, Yan M, Ge S, Yu J. Paper-based electrochemiluminescent 3D immunodevice for lab-on-paper, specific, and sensitive point-of-care testing. Chem Eur J. 2012;18(16):4938–45.
123. Parolo C, Medina-Sanchez M, de la Escosura-Muniz A, Merkoci A. Simple paper architecture modifications lead to enhanced sensitivity in nanoparticle based lateral flow immunoassays. Lab Chip. 2013;13(3):386–90.
124. Shan S, Lai W, Xiong Y, Wei H, Xu H. Novel strategies to enhance lateral flow immunoassay sensitivity for detecting foodborne pathogens. J Agric Food Chem. 2015;63(3):745–53.
125. Qian S, Bau HH. A mathematical model of lateral flow bioreactions applied to sandwich assays. Anal Biochem. 2003;322(1):89–98.
126. Toley BJ, McKenzie B, Liang T, Buser JR, Yager P, Fu E. Tunable-delay shunts for paper microfluidic devices. Anal Chem. 2013;85(23):11545–52.
127. Liu Z, Hu J, Zhao Y, Qu Z, Xu F. Experimental and numerical studies on liquid wicking into filter papers for paper-based diagnostics. Appl Therm Eng. 2015;88:280–7.
128. Lutz B, Liang T, Fu E, Ramachandran S, Kauffman P, Yager P. Dissolvable fluidic time delays for programming multi-step assays in instrument-free paper diagnostics. Lab Chip. 2013;13(14):2840–7.
129. Whitesides GM. Viewpoint on "Dissolvable fluidic time delays for programming multi-step assays in instrument-free paper diagnostics". Lab Chip. 2013;13(20):4004–5.
130. Li C, Boban M, Snyder SA, Kobaku SP, Kwon G, Mehta G, et al. Paper-based surfaces with extreme wettabilities for novel, open-channel microfluidic devices. Adv Funct Mater. 2016;26(33):6121–31.
131. Sun Y, Kharaghani A, Tsotsas E. Micro-model experiments and pore network simulations of liquid imbibition in porous media. Chem Eng Sci. 2016;150:41–53.
132. Jahanshahi-Anbuhi S, Henry A, Leung V, Sicard C, Pennings K, Pelton R, et al. Paper-based microfluidics with an erodible polymeric bridge giving controlled release and timed flow shutoff. Lab Chip. 2014;14(1):229–36.
133. Jahanshahi-Anbuhi S, Chavan P, Sicard C, Leung V, Hossain SM, Pelton R, et al. Creating fast flow channels in paper fluidic devices to control timing of sequential reactions. Lab Chip. 2012;12(23):5079–85.
134. Wang L, Cai J, Wang Y, Fang Q, Wang S, Cheng Q, et al. A bare-eye-based lateral flow immunoassay based on the use of gold nanoparticles for simultaneous detection of three pesticides. Microchim Acta. 2014;181(13–14):1565–72.
135. Lee J-H, Seo HS, Kwon J-H, Kim H-T, Kwon KC, Sim SJ, et al. Multiplex diagnosis of viral infectious diseases (AIDS, hepatitis C, and hepatitis A) based on point of care lateral flow assay using engineered proteinticles. Biosens Bioelectron. 2015;69:213–25.
136. Zhang D, Li P, Liu W, Zhao L, Zhang Q, Zhang W, et al. Development of a detector-free semi-quantitative immunochromatographic assay with major aflatoxins as target analytes. Sens Actuators B Chem. 2013;185:432–7.
137. Zhang D, Li P, Zhang Q, Li R, Zhang W, Ding X, et al. A naked-eye based strategy for semi-quantitative immunochromatographic assay. Anal Chim Acta. 2012;740:74–9.
138. Fang Q, Wang L, Cheng Q, Cai J, Wang Y, Yang M, et al. A bare-eye based one-step signal amplified semiquantitative immunochromatographic assay for the detection of imidacloprid in Chinese cabbage samples. Anal Chim Acta. 2015;881:82–9.
139. Oh YK, Joung HA, Han HS, Suk HJ, Kim MG. A three-line lateral flow assay strip for the measurement of C-reactive protein covering a broad physiological concentration range in human sera. Biosens Bioelectron. 2014;61:285–9.

140. Chen A, Wang R, Bever CR, Xing S, Hammock BD, Pan T. Smartphone-interfaced lab-on-a-chip devices for field-deployable enzyme-linked immunosorbent assay. Biomicrofluidics. 2014;8(6):064101.
141. Li B, Li L, Guan A, Dong Q, Ruan K, Hu R, et al. A smartphone controlled handheld microfluidic liquid handling system. Lab Chip. 2014;14(20):4085–92.
142. Vatsyayan P. Recent advances in the study of electrochemistry of redox proteins, Trends in Bioelectroanalysis bioanalytical reviews, vol. 6. Cham: Springer; 2016. p. 223–62.
143. Zhang D, Liu Q. Biosensors and bioelectronics on smartphone for portable biochemical detection. Biosens Bioelectron. 2016;75:273–84.
144. Breslauer DN, Maamari RN, Switz NA, Lam WA, Fletcher DA. Mobile phone based clinical microscopy for global health applications. PLoS One. 2009;4(7):e6320.
145. Vashist SK, Mudanyali O, Schneider EM, Zengerle R, Ozcan A. Cellphone-based devices for bioanalytical sciences. Anal Bioanal Chem. 2014;406(14):3263–77.
146. Mudanyali O, Dimitrov S, Sikora U, Padmanabhan S, Navruz I, Ozcan A. Integrated rapid-diagnostic-test reader platform on a cellphone. Lab Chip. 2012;12(15):2678–86.
147. Pollock NR, Rolland JP, Kumar S, Beattie PD, Jain S, Noubary F, et al. A paper-based multiplexed transaminase test for low-cost, point-of-care liver function testing. Sci Transl Med. 2012;4(152):152ra29.
148. Thom NK, Yeung K, Pillion MB, Phillips ST. "Fluidic batteries" as low-cost sources of power in paper-based microfluidic devices. Lab Chip. 2012;12(10):1768–70.
149. Thom NK, Lewis GG, DiTucci MJ, Phillips ST. Two general designs for fluidic batteries in paper-based microfluidic devices that provide predictable and tunable sources of power for on-chip assays. RSC Adv. 2013;3(19):6888–95.
150. Liu H, Crooks RM. Paper-based electrochemical sensing platform with integral battery and electrochromic read-out. Anal Chem. 2012;84(5):2528–32.
151. Dineva MA, Candotti D, Fletcher-Brown F, Allain JP, Lee H. Simultaneous visual detection of multiple viral amplicons by dipstick assay. J Clin Microbiol. 2005;43(8):4015–21.
152. Vella SJ, Beattie P, Cademartiri R, Laromaine A, Martinez AW, Phillips ST, et al. Measuring markers of liver function using a micropatterned paper device designed for blood from a fingerstick. Anal Chem. 2012;84(6):2883–91.
153. Yang X, Forouzan O, Brown TP, Shevkoplyas SS. Integrated separation of blood plasma from whole blood for microfluidic paper-based analytical devices. Lab Chip. 2012;12(2):274–80.
154. Abe K, Kotera K, Suzuki K, Citterio D. Inkjet-printed paperfluidic immuno-chemical sensing device. Anal Bioanal Chem. 2010;398(2):885–93.
155. Li CZ, Vandenberg K, Prabhulkar S, Zhu X, Schneper L, Methee K, et al. Paper based point-of-care testing disc for multiplex whole cell bacteria analysis. Biosens Bioelectron. 2011;26(11):4342–8.
156. Vashist SK, Venkatesh AG, Mitsakakis K, Czilwik G, Roth G, von Stetten F, et al. Nanotechnology-based biosensors and diagnostics: technology push versus industrial/healthcare requirements. BioNanoSci. 2012;2(3):115–26.
157. Vashist SK, Schneider EM, Luong JHT. Commercial smartphone-based devices and smart applications for personalized healthcare monitoring and management. Diagnostics. 2014;4(3):104–28.

Chapter 6
Lab-on-a-Chip-Based Point-of-Care Immunoassays

Sandeep Kumar Vashist

Contents

6.1 Introduction

There is a critical need for adequate resources, infrastructure, professionals, and in vitro diagnostic (IVD) technologies in the developing nations for the low-cost but reliable diagnosis of diseases. The use of such low-cost and easy-to-use and easy-to-understand IVD technologies will significantly increase the outreach of healthcare. POC testing (POCT) [1] enables rapid and cost-effective clinical diagnosis using minimal sample volumes at the point-of-need, i.e., bedside of a patient, in a physician's office, at home, or in paramedical support vehicles, as well as secondary and tertiary care settings. It provides the test results just within a few minutes using a simple protocol with minimal process steps. LOC-based POC IAs are the most prospective development in this regard as they would enable POCT at the point-of-need, which is more often the case in developing countries and remote settings. The numerous developments in LOC platforms, POCT, and complementary technologies, such as mobile healthcare (mH) technologies, have considerably improved the healthcare monitoring and management. The current generation of LOC-based POC

© Springer Nature Switzerland AG 2019
S. K. Vashist, J. H. T. Luong, *Point-of-Care Technologies Enabling*
Next-Generation Healthcare Monitoring and Management,
https://doi.org/10.1007/978-3-030-11416-9_6

IAs employ novel immunobiosensing concepts, microfluidic protocols, innovative platforms, novel reagent storage and release mechanisms, and advanced readers.

The breathtaking advances in CP technologies during the last decade and their use for various bioanalytical applications have started a new era of digital health, which is providing the tools for personalized healthcare monitoring and management. The most prospective developments are the use of CPs for the readout of various LOC-based POC IAs, which is an evolving international trend that would revolutionize POCT. CP is an ideal POC device considering their availability with more than 95% of world's population, i.e., over 7 billion CP users. Most interesting is the fact that more than 70% CP users are actually in the developing countries only, where there is a critical need for cost-effective clinical diagnostics. CPs would provide spatiotemporal tagged data and the desired communication and telemedicine tools, which would considerably improve the healthcare monitoring and management in the developing countries. The mobile health solutions market is growing at a rapid pace and is expected to reach USD 90.5 billion by 2022 [2]. The POC diagnostics' global market will reach USD 37 billion by 2021 [3], where India and China would account for a major market share due to their enormous populations and increased prevalence of chronic and infectious diseases.

Several LOC-based POC IAs have been successfully implemented in central laboratories and physician office laboratories (POLs) in the developing countries. They would be highly useful POCT tools for the primary healthcare workers in epidemics and emergencies. Therefore, LOC-based POC IAs must be affordable, robust, rapid, and reliable. This chapter provides an overview of LOC-based POC IAs together with the recent advances in complementary technologies that are paving way to next-generation POC technologies. The challenges and future trends in POCT are also discussed. The key features of various LOC-based POC IA formats are shown in Table 6.1.

6.2 Lab-on-a-Chip-Based Point-of-Care Immunoassay Formats

6.2.1 Microfluidics

A wide range of automated microfluidic LOC platforms have been developed for the rapid and highly sensitive detection of clinical analytes [5]. The blood glucose sensing strips are microfluidics-based LOC devices that are extensively employed worldwide billions of times per year, thereby contributing to the predominant market share of global biosensor market [6].

Centrifugal microfluidics-based LabDisk platform (CML) is one such microfluidic LOC platform, which has been used by many companies to develop prospective semi- or fully-automated IAs inside analyzers. Piccolo Xpress™ whole blood chemistry analyzer from Abaxis Inc., USA is an innovative POC device [7] (Fig. 6.1A), which employs a CML platform to perform up to 14 tests on a single reagent LabDisk (8 cm diameter, barcoded) (Fig. 6.1A). Abaxis has developed

Table 6.1 The conceptual potential of emerging technologies for next-generation LOC-based POC IAs for POCT. Reproduced with permission from Elsevier B.V [4]

Parameters	CP (1)	Paper (2)	LOC (3)	Next-generation LOC-based POC IAs for POCT[a] (1 + 2 + 3)
Performance				
Suitability for POCT	🟢	🟢	🟢	🟢
Technology penetration	🟢	🔴	🔴	N.A.[b]
Utility in epidemics and emergencies	🟢	🟢	🟩	🟢
Prerequisite of prolonged storage of reagents	✓	✓	✓	✓
Prerequisite of rapid assay	✓	✓	✓	✓
Portability	🟢	🟢	🟩	🟢
Cost-effectiveness of consumables	🟢	🟢	🟩	🟢
Overall cost-effectiveness	🟢	🟢	🟩	🟢
Quantitative	✓	✗	✓	✓
Sensitivity	🟢	🔴	🟩	🟢
Specificity	🟢	🟩	🟩	🟢
Throughput	🟢	🟢	🟩	🟢
Precision	🟢	🔴	🟢	🟢
Reproducibility	🟢	🔴	🟩	🟢
Capable of mass production	✓	✓	✓	✓
Compliance with regulatory guidelines	✓	✗	✓	✓
Ease of operation				
Ease of operation	🟢	🟢	🟢	🟢
Labor intensiveness	🟩	🔴	🔴	🔴
Need for power supply	✗	✓	✓	✗
Need for readout instruments	✗[c]	✗	✓	✗[c]
Standalone analysis	✓	✓	✓	✓
Personalized	✓	✗	✗	✓
Accessibility of POCT results anytime anywhere	✓	✗	✗	✓
Basic skillset required for operation	✓	✓	✗	✓
Connectivity				
Connectivity to Cloud	✓	✗	✗	✓
Smart applications & portal services	✓	✗	✗	✓
Test history and data patterns	✓	✗	✓ (Limited)	✓
Spatiotemporal mapping	✓	✗	✗	✓
Demographic data and statistics	✓	✗	✗	✓
Telemedicine support	✓	✗	✗	✓

(continued)

Table 6.1 (continued)

Parameters	CP (1)	Paper (2)	LOC (3)	Next-generation LOC-based POC IAs for POCT[a] (1 + 2 + 3)
Text alerts	✓	✗	✗	✓
Preventive healthcare tools	✓	✗	✗	✓

(High ●; medium ●; low ●)

[a]This column has been computed conceptually considering the characteristics of the component technologies

[b]N.A. not applicable

[c]A CP attachment or interfaced instrument would be required for non-optical signal detection, such as in the case of electrochemical readout

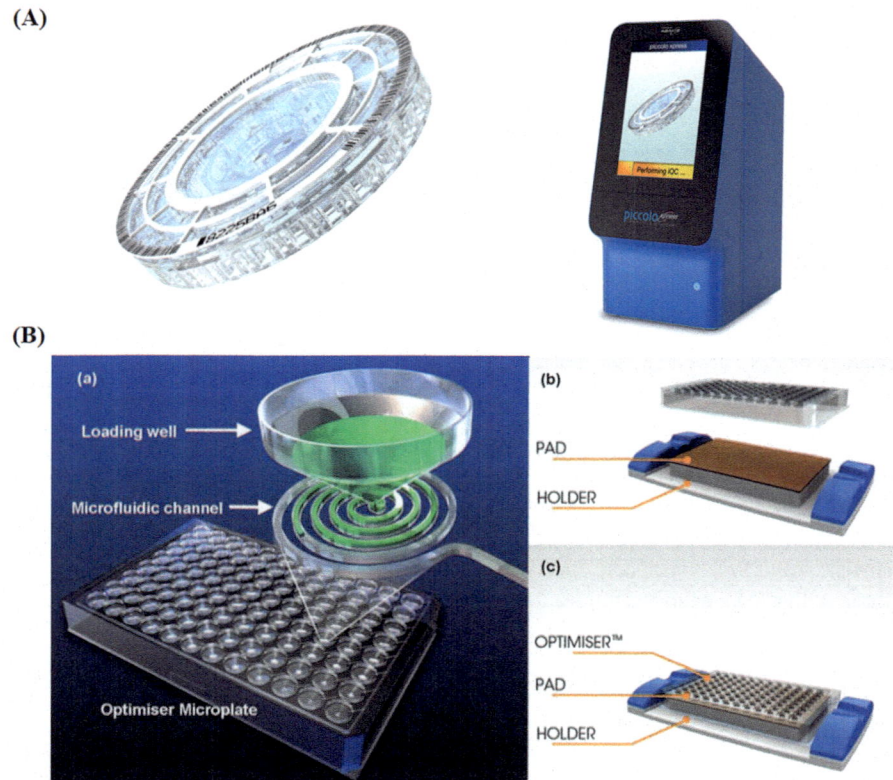

Fig. 6.1 (**A**) (left) Fully automated LOC-based IA on a centrifugal microfluidics-based LabDisk (CML) platform; (right) Piccolo Xpress chemistry analyzer. Reproduced with permission from Elsevier B.V [4]. (**B**) Optimiser™ microplates developed by Siloam Biosciences Inc., USA. Reproduced with permission from the Royal Society of Chemistry [8]

many Clinical Laboratory Improvement Amendments (CLIA) waived tests. Similar CML platforms (Gyrolab Bioaffy CDs) [9] and analyzers have been developed by Gyros Protein Technologies, Sweden. Gyrolab xPlore™ performs a single CD-based IA, while Gyrolab™ xP workstation performs up to five CDs simultaneously [10]. CML-based LOC IAs have been developed for a wide range of analytes, i.e., biomarkers, toxins, nucleic acid, pathogens, and other analytes [11]. Of interest is the rapid CML-based sandwich EIA that detects C-reactive protein (CRP) with a sample-to-answer time of just 25 min [12]. It involves the capture of CRP by anti-human CRP Ab-coated superparamagnetic Dynabeads® (M-280 tosyl activated) and HRP-labeled anti-human CRP Ab in an IA chamber of CML. The sandwich immune complexes are formed in the presence of CRP, which are transferred subsequently to the wash chambers and the detection chamber in the CML. Finally, an enzyme-substrate reaction triggers the chemiluminescent signal in the detection chamber, which is measured by a miniaturized chemiluminescent detector integrated into a portable LabDisk reader.

A novel microfluidic LOC IA is the Optimiser™ ELISA from Siloam Biosciences Inc. [8], USA, which employs an innovative microfluidic MTP (Fig. 6.1B). As the Optimiser™ ELISA requires only 4.5 µL of the sample and minimal number of process steps, it has a critically reduced sample-to-answer time of just a few minutes. The Optimiser™ MTP is a standard 96-well polystyrene MTP, where each MTP well is connected to a spiral microfluidic channel via a hole at the bottom. The IA is performed in consecutive microfluidic process steps, where the liquid dispensed into the MTP is drawn into the microchannel by capillary forces exerted by the absorbent pad at the other end of the microchannel. The sequential steps involve the dispensing of capture Ab, blocking buffer, target analyte, fluorescently-labeled detection Ab, and wash buffer, which is followed by the fluorescence readout of Optimiser™ MTP in a plate reader.

6.2.2   Cellphone

CP-based devices have been developed for the POC readout of colorimetric, fluorescent, and chemiluminescent IAs [13]. Additionally, several CP-based LOC IAs have also been demonstrated. The comprehensive descriptions of CP-based devices and IAs are not provided in this section as they are discussed in more depth in another chapter of this book. The CP-based POC reader usually employs an optically opaque attachment equipped with LEDs and diffusers, a sample chamber [14–16], and apertures in addition to a plano-convex lens in front of the CP's back camera to adjust spatial resolution and field of view [15]. The setup can be customized for fluorescent, chemiluminescent, and colorimetric readout [17].

An interesting development is the CP-based fluorimeter [18] (Fig. 6.2) that measures the full emission spectrum of a light emitter using a cradle and the CP's camera as a spectrometer [19]. Another prospective approach was the use of the CP's back camera for the colorimetric readout of microchip ELISA, via image capture

a

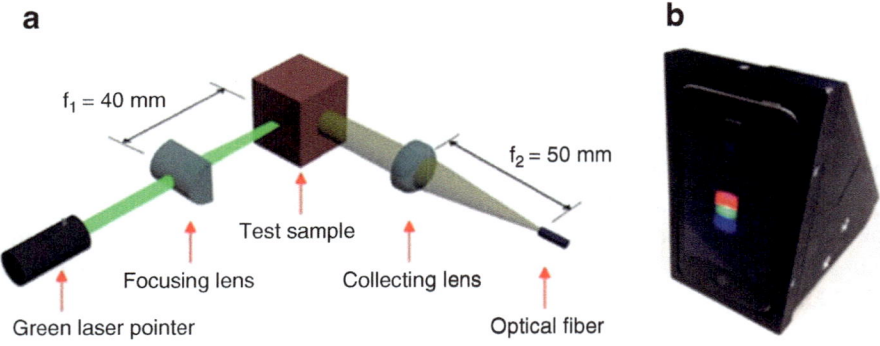

b

c

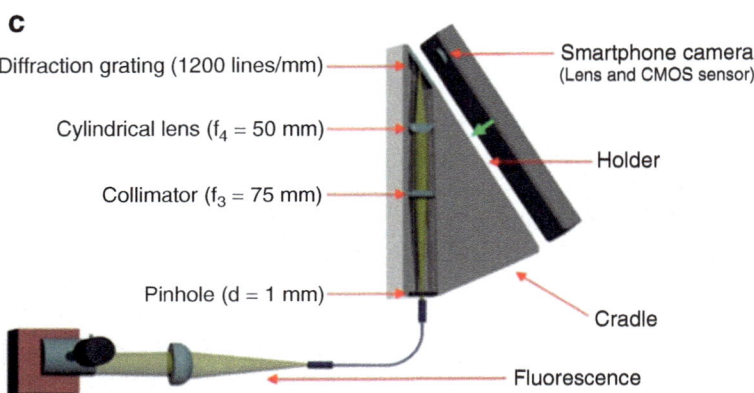

Diffraction grating (1200 lines/mm) ——————— Smartphone camera
                                              (Lens and CMOS sensor)

Cylindrical lens (f_4 = 50 mm) ———————

Collimator (f_3 = 75 mm) ——————— ——————— Holder

Pinhole (d = 1 mm) ———————

                                              Cradle

——————— Fluorescence

Fig. 6.2 An illustration of a CP-based fluorimeter system. (**a**) Schematic illustrating the optical setup; (**b**) optical cradle installed on the CP; and (**c**) fluorescent detection scheme. Reproduced with permission from the American Chemical Society [18]

and analysis, to detect HE4 cancer biomarker in urine [20]. A striking development was the CP-based colorimetric reader for 96-well MTP, which employs the smart devices' screen for the bottom illumination of the MTP inside a dark hood and CP-based imaging [13, 21] (Fig. 6.3). The reader was employed for the highly sensitive detection of CRP via one-step kinetics-based rapid sandwich ELISA [13]. It was also used for the bicinchoninic acid assay for protein estimation and some other IAs. Of interest is a CP-based colorimetric reader involving an optomechanical CP attachment to detect peanut concentrations in commercial cookies in the range of 1–25 part per million with a LOD of ~1 ppm and sample-to-response time of ~20 min [22].

LOC-based POC IAs using CP for colorimetric readout have also been developed for 25-hydroxyvitamin D [23] and total blood cholesterol [24]. Similarly, colorimetric detection-based IA using a QD-based assay and CP readout has been used to determine the activity of trypsin, chymotrypsin, and enterokinase [17]. In

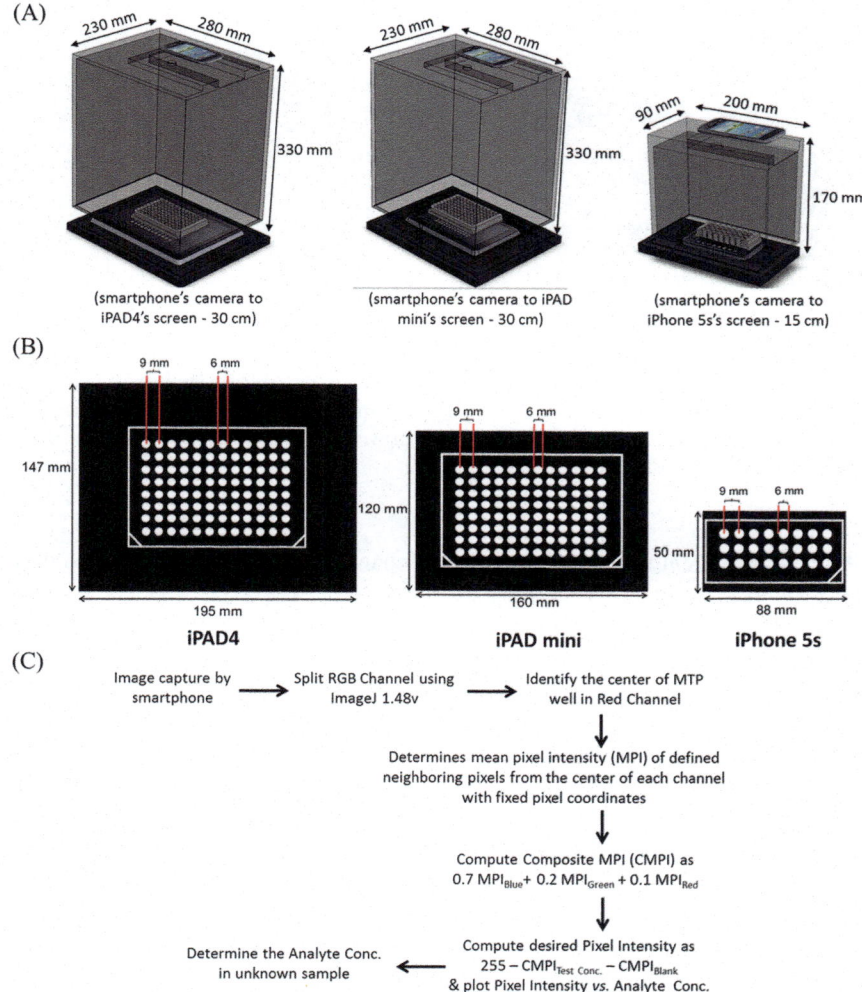

Fig. 6.3 (**a**) CP-based colorimetric readers developing using the gadgets' (iPad4, iPad mini, or iPhone 5s) screen-based bottom illumination, Samsung Galaxy SIII mini's back camera (5 MP)-based imaging, and a custom-made polyamide dark hood and polyamide base holder assembly. (**b**) Screensavers used for the screen-based bottom illumination of the 96-well microtiter plate (MTP) in gadgets. (**c**) Image processing algorithm employed for the analysis of smartphone-captured colorimetric images. Reproduced with permission from Springer Nature [21]

another investigation, biochemiluminescent detection-based IA using an LFIA mini-cartridge format and CP-based luminescence readout was used for the detection of total bile acid [25], total cholesterol [25], and salivary cortisol [26].

Commercial IAs employing CP-based readout are also available for various analytes [27, 28]. Cellmic, USA pioneered the development of several CP-based readers for low-cost readout of LFAs, ELISAs, and other assay formats. The most

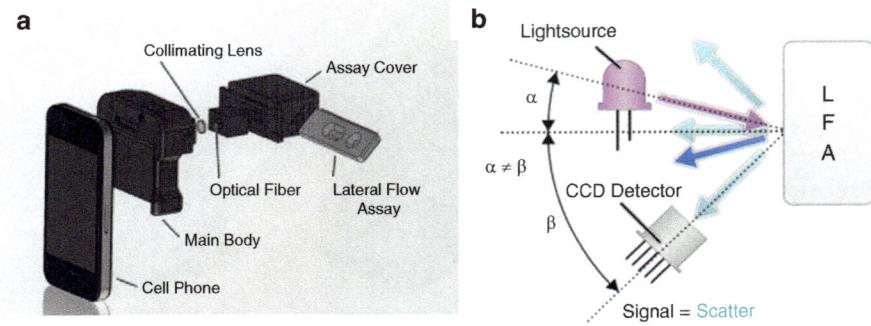

Fig. 6.4 (**a**) CP-based LFIA reader showing the placement of collimating lens and an optical fiber set at specific angles in reference to the LFA cassette [32]. (**b**) The detector is oriented at an angle, β, optimized for decreased light scattering from a nitrocellulose membrane, which differs from the angle of the light source to surface, α, providing an improved signal-to-noise ratio [32]. Reproduced with permission from Elsevier B.V

striking development was a compact optomechanical attachment-based rapid diagnostic test reader for colorimetric and fluorometric LFAs [29, 30]. A low-cost SP-based Holomic Rapid Diagnostic Test Reader (HRDR-200) [31] was developed for the readout of LFAs. It comprised of a SP, an integrated reader housing, smart application, and access to secure Cloud Services and Test Developer. Another interesting product was the recently developed HRDR-300, which enables the multicolor imaging-based fluorescence readout of LFAs with a very high accuracy based on the use of an advanced image processing algorithm. The company is further developing HRDR-400, which is a forthcoming product that could read both chromatographic and fluorescent LFAs.

An innovative development was the CP-based LFIA (Fig. 6.4), which employs the illumination provided by the SP's flash via an optical fiber and a collimating lens. The signal is detected at an optimized angle that maximizes the Mie scattering from a nitrocellulose membrane [17], thereby resulting in maximal Rayleigh scattering from AuNPs in the LFIA bands. The CP-based LFIA detected thyroid-stimulating hormone (TSH) in just 15 min with a LOD of 0.31 mIU L^{-1}, which is lower than the minimum accepted TSH concentration of 0.4 mIU L^{-1} for hyperthyroidism.

Other important advances include the development of a quantum dot (QD)-based sandwich IA, which detects *E.coli* O157: H7 employing an anti-*E.coli* O157: H7 Ab-functionalized capillary array and CP-based readout [33] with a detection limit of ~5–10 CFU/mL in water and milk samples. Of interest is the angle-resolved surface plasmon resonance (SPR) system that employs the CP's screen-based illumination and detection of the SPR signal by CP's camera [34]. The device detected β_2 microglobulin, a biomarker for cancer, kidney disease, and inflammatory disorders, in humans with a limit of detection of ~0.1 µg/mL. GENTAG, Inc., USA [35] together with MacroArray Technologies, LLC, USA have introduced a CP-based urine analysis platform and a disposable IA to detect prostate cancer diagnostic marker 1. The researchers have also demonstrated a CP-based electrochemical sensing platform [36] that is integrated with a disposable capillary flow microfluidic chip.

The researchers have also demonstrated a compact CP-based electrochemical (EC) detection system [36] for LOC-based POC IAs. The system comprises of a small embedded circuit for signal processing and data analysis, a disposable SIM card-size microfluidic chip for fluidic handling and sensing, a sample loading capillary, and processing and pumping (Fig. 6.5). It was employed for the detection of *Plasmodium falciparum* histidine-rich protein 2 (*Pf*HRP2) using a custom smart application that provides step-by-step instructions on the CP's screen.

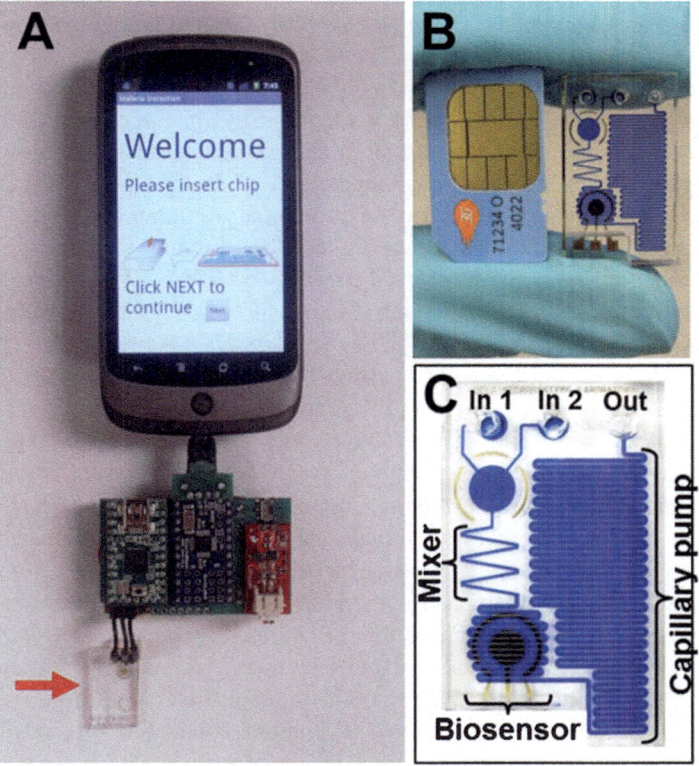

Fig. 6.5 (**a**) A CP-based electrochemical sensor with the microfluidic chip [36]. (**b**) Comparison of the size of a microfluidic chip with the CP SIM card. (**c**) Magnified view of a dye-filled microfluidic chip with labeled components. Reproduced with permission from the Royal Society of Chemistry

6.2.3 Paper

Paper-based IAs (PIAs) have been envisioned as the most cost-effective and easy-to-use assay format for the developing nations due to their cost-effectiveness, ease of manufacture, and simple operation. The colorimetric PIA is quantitatively visualized by comparing its colorimetric signal against a predetermined score chart by naked eyes [37]. However, the colorimetric signal of the PIA can be precisely quantified by employing cameras, scanners, commercial test strip readers, or handheld colorimeters. The most recent is the cost-effective highly-precise quantification of the colorimetric signal by CP-based image analysis [27, 29]. CPs are the ideal POC readers for the detection of colorimetric signals generated in PIAs.

Lateral flow IAs (LFIAs), dipstick IAs, and microfluidic paper-based analytical devices (µPADs) are the most used PIAs [38, 39]. The most used substrates for PIAs are the filter paper, chromatography paper, nitrocellulose membrane, and paper/polymer or paper/nanomaterial composites [40]. The immunodiagnostic applications of paper substrates are strongly dependent on their porosity, surface chemistry, and optical properties [41]. The nitrocellulose membranes available commercially have various pore sizes (0.05–12 µm), while polyethylene has controlled pore sizes [42]. LFIA employ nitrocellulose test strips along which the sample dispensed on to a sample pad flows laterally over a conjugate pad, where the analyte molecules bind to the gold nanoparticles (AuNPs) due to the capillary action provided by the absorbent pad (Fig. 6.6a). The home pregnancy test detecting human chorionic gonadotropin (hCG) in urine is the most used paper-based LFIA. LFIAs have also been developed for many other clinical analytes, such as primary hepatic carcinoma biomarkers [46] and HIV diagnosis [47].

Many PIAs have been developed using two- (2D) or three-dimensional (3D) µPADs [44, 48] (Fig. 6.6b). The 3D µPADs are obtained by stacking layers of a 2D patterned paper [45] or using other strategies such as spray adhesives [49], thermal adhesives (toner) [50], cutting and lamination [51], and origami [52]. Various bioanalytical applications have been demonstrated for PIAs on µPADs, such as sandwich ELISAs [53, 54] and microfluidic paper-based electrochemical devices (µPEDs) prepared by printing electrodes on paper [55, 56].

The main limitations of the conventional PIAs are the lack in desired analytical sensitivity and specificity of conventional PIAs for POCT. The sensitivity can be improved via signal enhancement using enzymes [57] and nanomaterials, e.g., AuNPs [58] or NP composites. The sensitivity can also be improved using plasmonic NP conjugation or aggregation [59], thermal contrasting methods [60], and optimization of test strip dimensions [61]. On the other hand, the non-specific binding on paper substrates can be decreased by employing customized blocking solutions and various surface functionalization chemistries. The current efforts are dedicated to the development of multiplex PIAs [62, 63] and fully-integrated LOC platforms capable of sample pretreatment and separation [64]. The PIAs have been discussed in more depth in the previous chapter of this book.

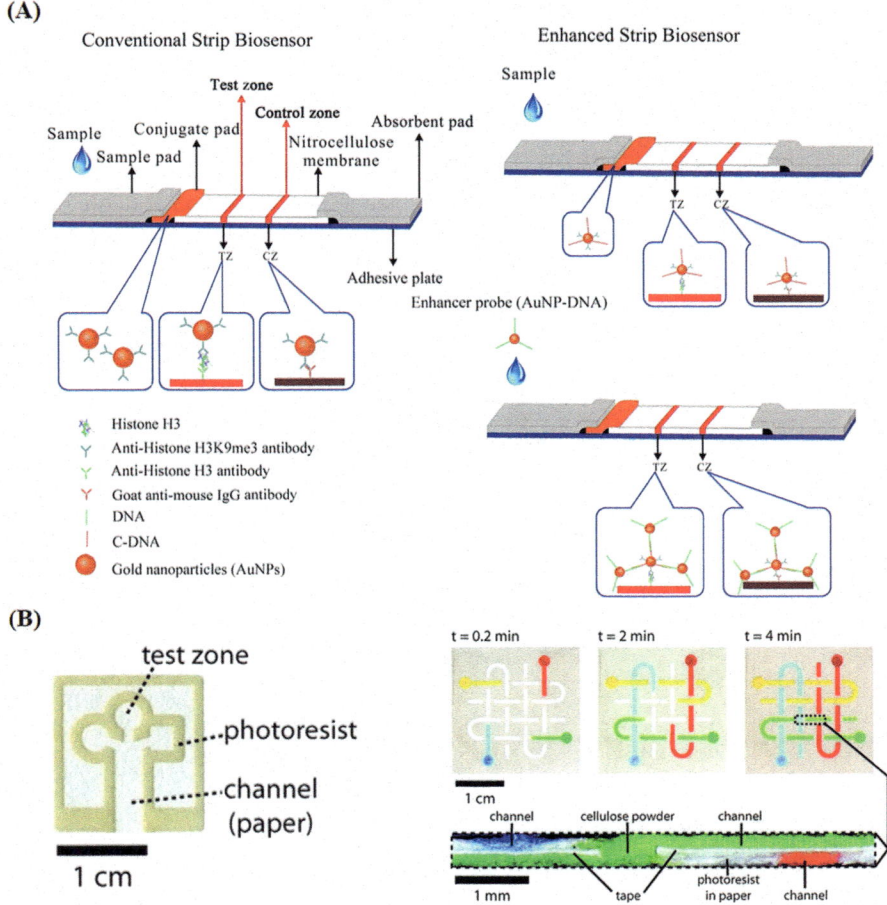

Fig. 6.6 (a) Conventional and enhanced LFIA for the visual detection of trimethylated lysine 9 of histone H3 (H3K9me3) in 20 ng of histone extract from HeLa cells within 15 min [43]. (b) A typical 2D [44] (left) and 3D [45] (right) microfluidic paper-based analytical device (µPAD). Reproduced with permission from the American Chemical Society

6.2.4 Immunoassay Formats

Several novel wash-free IA formats have been recently developed by researchers that would results in simple and rapid LOC-based POC IAs in the coming years. The most prospective IA formats are AlphaLISA® from Perkin Elmer, electrochemiluminescent ELISA from Meso Scale Diagnostics LLC, and metal-enhanced fluorescence IA from Fianostics GmbH. Meso Scale Diagnostics LLC's electrochemiluminescent ELISA [65] enables the high-throughput multiplex detection of analytes in a microwell. The highly-sensitive wash-free sandwich IA procedure on carbon electrodes in a microwell plate and SULFO-TAG™ label-bound detection Ab are employed for the detection of analytes, which result in the emission of chemiluminescent signal upon electrochemical stimulation (Fig. 6.7). On the other hand, AlphaLISA® [66] is based on the interactions between streptavidin-coated Alpha donor beads and anti-analyte Ab-conjugated AlphaLISA® acceptor beads, which results in the formation of sandwich immune complexes and generation of chemiluminescence signal in the presence of analyte. The excitation of donor beads at 680 nm in the presence of two bound beads in proximity generates singlet oxygen molecules that trigger a series of chemical reactions in the acceptor beads, resulting

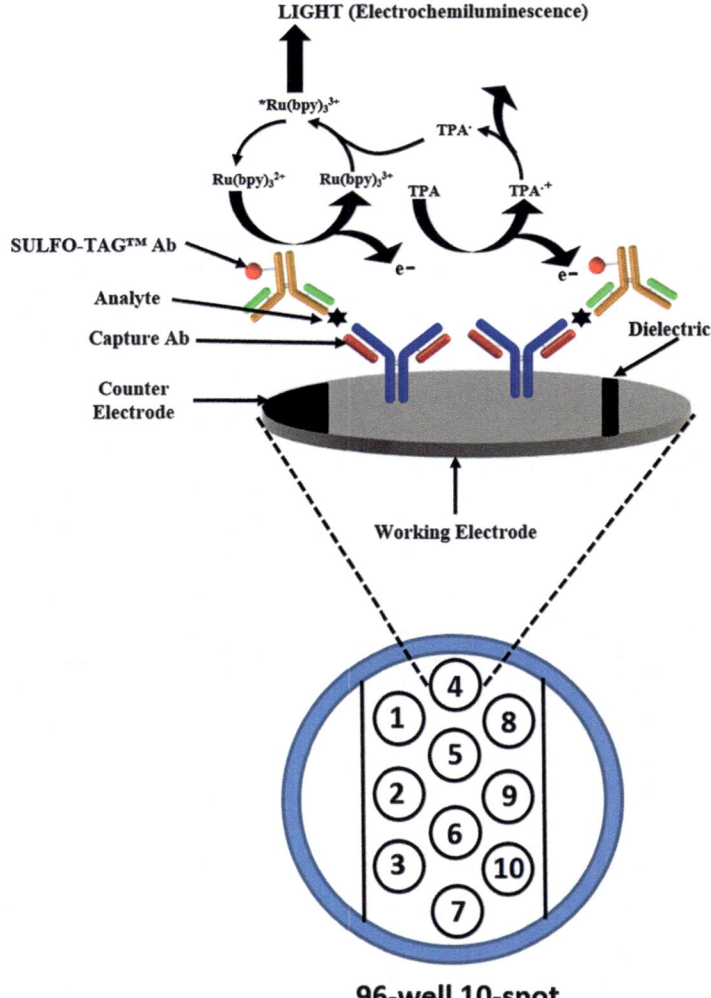

Fig. 6.7 Electrochemiluminescent ELISA-based wash-free sandwich IA from Meso Scale Diagnostics LLC for the highly-sensitive multiplex detection of analytes

in a sharp emission peak at 615 nm (Fig. 6.8). Of interest is the recently developed metal-enhanced fluorescence IA format developed by Fianostics GmbH [67]. It employs the standard 96-well MTP that has metallic nanostructures on its surface, which greatly enhance the fluorescence of molecules that are close to the nanostructures, i.e., less than 50 nm. The molecules further away, i.e., more than 50 nm, from the nanostructures do not increase in emission. Therefore, the developed IA format enables the effective discrimination between bound and unbound fluorescent molecules, which enables the detection of analytes in the bulk solution without any requirement for multiple washings (Fig. 6.9).

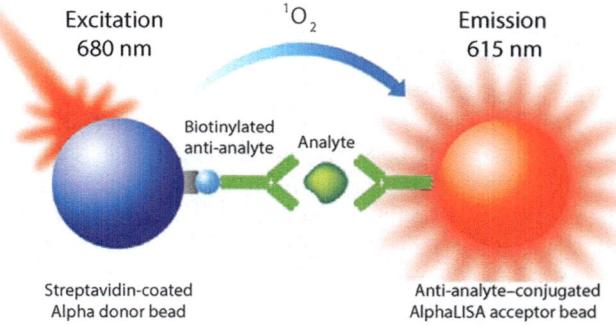

Fig. 6.8 AlphaLISA®, a wash-free IA, developed by Perkin Elmer. Reproduced with permission from the Nature Publishing Group [66]

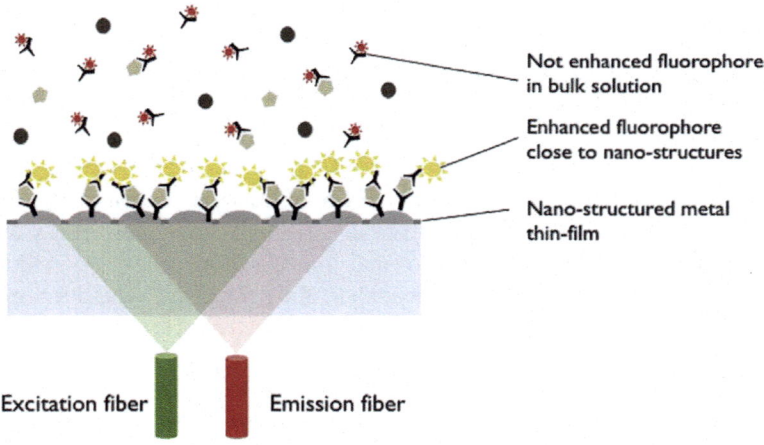

Fig. 6.9 Metal-enhanced fluorescence immunoassay format developed by Fianostics GmbH [67]. Reproduced with permission from Elsevier B.V

6.3   Critiques and Outlook

There is a need for rapid and simple IA procedures for the development of commercially- and clinically-viable LOC-based POC IAs. Apart from the novel IA formats discussed in the previous section, several innovative IA formats have been developed recently by researchers. An important advance is the EasyELISA platforms for colorimetric IAs, where the colorimetry signal is captured and analyzed by the SP's camera using an advanced image analysis algorithm [68]. EasyELISA is a very simple IA format for rapid LOC-based POC IAs as it involves the most highly simplified IA procedure in a conventional 96-well MTP and its colorimetric readout after the IA via the SP's camera using a dark hood and a simple mechanical attachment [68]. The recently developed one-step kinetics-based IA formats would be the most appropriate to develop LOC-based POC IAs that enable the detection of analytes in less than 30 min [69, 70].

The analytical performance of LOC-based POC IAs can be significantly enhanced by the use of optimal antibody immobilization chemistries, surface modification and bioconjugation strategies, signal enhancement procedures, and signal transduction or biosensing schemes [71]. Moreover, researchers are also looking into the development of novel biorecognition elements, such as aptamers, molecular imprinted polymers, and antibody fragments, which would have higher affinity for the target analyte than the conventional Ab in addition to improved stability, sensitivity, and specificity.

The prolonged storage of assay components is critical for most LOC-based POC IAs and is usually done using stabilizers, sugars, sugar alcohols, freeze drying, reagent pouches, or encapsulation in natural polysaccharides [72]. An innovative approach is the use of pullulan, a non-ionic natural polysaccharide, which enables the prolonged storage of biomolecules in their native three-dimensional form at room temperature. Pullulan forms an oxygen-tight solid tablet upon drying, which is water-soluble and does not interfere with the IA after solubilization as it is transparent. The IA reagents stored in pullulan are immediately released in aqueous solution after solubilization [72]. Similarly, trehalose, sugars with transition metal ions, and sugar alcohols with cationic polymers or zinc ions have also been employed for the long-term storage of reagents in LOC-based POC IAs. Another most widely used storage strategy is the use of lyophilized IA reagents. In another approach, the researchers demonstrated the prolonged storage of horseradish peroxidase-labeled Ab and its substrate (diaminobenzidine) by drying them onto a glass fiber pad [73].

There is a need for stringent validation and clinical testing to develop a clinically-viable LOC IA that has the desired bioanalytical performance. The developed IA should correlate well with the predicate device in clinical diagnostics and should not incur interference from potential interfering and cross-reacting substances [74, 75]. Moreover, the developed LOC-based POC IA must be robust and reproducible, which is a concern for PIAs due to their batch-to-batch variability and lack in quality controls [76, 77]. The analytical sensitivity of IAs could be improved by employing nanomaterials and nanocomposites as they provide greater surface area for the higher biomolecular binding. However, it is essential to fully characterize the physi-cochemical properties and behavior of these materials in different solutions and sample matrices. Similarly, the LOC-based POC IAs require the realization of microfluidic operational protocols to enable all the process steps in the IAs. The recent trend is strongly inclined toward the development of fully-integrated LOC-based POC IAs, which could be used at any place and time without any requirement for skilled analysts, specialized infrastructure, and expensive instruments. The auto-mated analyzer-based IAs cater to the need of high-throughput clinical POCT.

There are several challenges to be tackled in case of CP-based POC IAs to make them clinically-viable [4, 27, 78], the major ones being the hygiene aspects, dis-posal, and contamination of CP-based devices. The changing technical specifica-tions of CPs, especially the CP's camera, are posing a serious hurdle to their ubiquitous applications and regulatory compliance. This has led to the most recent trend toward the development of stand-alone smart devices with highly-reproducible imaging via the use of a fixed camera, which can be interfaced or attached to the CP [4]. It is essential for smart device manufacturers to employ advanced encryption algorithms for securing the patients' personal health records and tackling the grow-ing concerns about data security and ownership.

The economic feasibility is another factor that determines the commercialization and the adoption of LOC-based POC IAs. The low-cost LOC platforms, simple IA procedures, and inexpensive readers are critical to develop prospective commercially-viable LOC-based POC IAs. The use of complex platforms, IA procedures, and readers would increase the costs of LOC-based POC IAs considerably; they will require trained analysts, costly instruments, and decreased throughput. The health insurances play a critical role in the adoption of POC IAs as they are responsible for the reimbursement of healthcare costs in the developed countries. Therefore, they should be involved at a very early stage to steer the development of LOC-based POC IAs to develop medical value and commercially-viable IAs. The cost, utility, ease-of-use, and mass production of the IA are taken into consideration by the insurances together with the clinical relevance of the IA and its contribution to healthcare monitoring and management.

6.4 Conclusions

A wide range of LOC-based POC IAs have been developed employing various LOC platforms, rapid IA procedures, microfluidic operations, automated process steps, and low-cost readers. The developments in the complementary technologies, such as mobile healthcare, Cloud computing, smart applications, telemedicine, wireless communications, Internet, and RFID, are paving way to next-generation POCT. There is a strong international trend toward personalized mobile healthcare and empowerment of general population, which emphasizes the universal need for LOC-based POC IAs that could be used for the detection of analytes at any place and time. They would considerably improve the healthcare monitoring and management and enable personalized and preventive healthcare. The breakthroughs in LOC platforms, IA formats, biosensor concepts, and CP technologies, and continuous advances in complementary technologies would lead to novel LOC-based POC IAs.

References

1. Luppa PB, Müller C, Schlichtiger A, Schlebusch H. Point-of-care testing (POCT): current techniques and future perspectives. Trends Anal Chem. 2011;30(6):887–98.
2. mHealth solutions market. http://www.marketsandmarkets.com/PressReleases/mhealth-apps-and-solutions.asp (2017).
3. Point-of-care diagnostics market. http://www.marketsandmarkets.com/PressReleases/point-of-care-diagnostic.asp (2016).
4. Vashist SK, Luppa PB, Yeo LY, Ozcan A, Luong JHT. Emerging technologies for next-generation point-of-care testing. Trends Biotechnol. 2015;33(11):692–705.
5. Chin CD, Linder V, Sia SK. Commercialization of microfluidic point-of-care diagnostic devices. Lab Chip. 2012;12(12):2118–34.
6. Turner AP. Biosensors: sense and sensibility. Chem Soc Rev. 2013;42(8):3184–96.
7. Piccolo Xpress. http://www.abaxis.com/medical/piccolo-xpress (2017).
8. Kai J, Puntambekar A, Santiago N, Lee SH, Sehy DW, Moore V, et al. A novel microfluidic microplate as the next generation assay platform for enzyme linked immunoassays (ELISA). Lab Chip. 2012;12(21):4257–62.
9. Gyrolab CDs. https://www.gyrosproteintechnologies.com/gyrolab-cds-automated-immunoassays
10. Gyrolab xPlore. http://www.gyros.com/products/systems/gyrolab-xplore/.
11. Gorkin R, Park J, Siegrist J, Amasia M, Lee BS, Park JM, et al. Centrifugal microfluidics for biomedical applications. Lab Chip. 2010;10(14):1758–73.
12. Czilwik G, Vashist SK, Klein V, Buderer A, Roth G, von Stetten F, et al. Magnetic chemiluminescent immunoassay for human C-reactive protein on the centrifugal microfluidics platform. RSC Adv. 2015;5(76):61906–12.
13. Vashist SK, van Oordt T, Schneider EM, Zengerle R, von Stetten F, Luong JHT. A smartphone-based colorimetric reader for bioanalytical applications using the screen-based bottom illumination provided by gadgets. Biosens Bioelectron. 2015;67:248–55.
14. Coskun AF, Nagi R, Sadeghi K, Phillips S, Ozcan A. Albumin testing in urine using a smartphone. Lab Chip. 2013;13(21):4231–8.
15. Wei Q, Nagi R, Sadeghi K, Feng S, Yan E, Ki SJ, et al. Detection and spatial mapping of mercury contamination in water samples using a smart-phone. ACS Nano. 2014;8(2):1121–9.
16. Su K, Zou Q, Zhou J, Zou L, Li H, Wang T, et al. High-sensitive and high-efficient biochemical analysis method using a bionic electronic eye in combination with a smartphone-based colorimetric reader system. Sens Actuators B Chem. 2015;216:134–40.
17. Petryayeva E, Algar WR. Multiplexed homogeneous assays of proteolytic activity using a smartphone and quantum dots. Anal Chem. 2014;86(6):3195–202.
18. Yu H, Tan Y, Cunningham BT. Smartphone fluorescence spectroscopy. Anal Chem. 2014;86(17):8805–13.
19. Long KD, Yu H, Cunningham BT. Smartphone instrument for portable enzyme-linked immunosorbent assays. Biomed Opt Exp. 2014;5(11):3792–806.
20. Wang S, Zhao X, Khimji I, Akbas R, Qiu W, Edwards D, et al. Integration of cell phone imaging with microchip ELISA to detect ovarian cancer HE4 biomarker in urine at the point-of-care. Lab Chip. 2011;11(20):3411–8.

21. Venkatesh AG, van Oordt T, Schneider EM, Zengerle R, von Stetten F, Luong JHT, et al. A smartphone-based colorimetric reader for human C-reactive protein immunoassay. Methods Mol Biol. 2017;1571:343–56.
22. Coskun AF, Wong J, Khodadadi D, Nagi R, Tey A, Ozcan A. A personalized food allergen testing platform on a cellphone. Lab Chip. 2013;13(4):636–40.
23. Lee S, Oncescu V, Mancuso M, Mehta S, Erickson D. A smartphone platform for the quantification of vitamin D levels. Lab Chip. 2014;14(8):1437–42.
24. Oncescu V, Mancuso M, Erickson D. Cholesterol testing on a smartphone. Lab Chip. 2014;14(4):759–63.
25. Roda A, Michelini E, Cevenini L, Calabria D, Calabretta MM, Simoni P. Integrating bio-chemiluminescence detection on smartphones: mobile chemistry platform for point-of-need analysis. Anal Chem. 2014;86(15):7299–304.
26. Zangheri M, Cevenini L, Anfossi L, Baggiani C, Simoni P, Di Nardo F, et al. A simple and compact smartphone accessory for quantitative chemiluminescence-based lateral flow immunoassay for salivary cortisol detection. Biosens Bioelectron. 2015;64:63–8.
27. Vashist SK, Mudanyali O, Schneider EM, Zengerle R, Ozcan A. Cellphone-based devices for bioanalytical sciences. Anal Bioanal Chem. 2014;406(14):3263–77.
28. Ozcan A. Mobile phones democratize and cultivate next-generation imaging, diagnostics and measurement tools. Lab Chip. 2014;14(17):3187–94.
29. Mudanyali O, Dimitrov S, Sikora U, Padmanabhan S, Navruz I, Ozcan A. Integrated rapid-diagnostic-test reader platform on a cellphone. Lab Chip. 2012;12(15):2678–86.
30. Rapid assay reader. http://www.cellmic.com/content/rapid-test-readers/
31. Liu W, Cassano CL, Xu X, Fan ZH. Laminated paper-based analytical devices (LPAD) with origami-enabled chemiluminescence immunoassay for cotinine detection in mouse serum. Anal Chem. 2013;85(21):10270–6.
32. You DJ, Park TS, Yoon JY. Cell-phone-based measurement of TSH using Mie scatter optimized lateral flow assays. Biosens Bioelectron. 2013;40(1):180–5.
33. Zhu H, Sikora U, Ozcan A. Quantum dot enabled detection of Escherichia coli using a cell-phone. Analyst. 2012;137(11):2541–4.
34. Preechaburana P, Gonzalez MC, Suska A, Filippini D. Surface plasmon resonance chemical sensing on cell phones. Angew Chem Int Ed Engl. 2012;51(46):11585–8.
35. Santhiago M, Wydallis JB, Kubota LT, Henry CS. Construction and electrochemical characterization of microelectrodes for improved sensitivity in paper-based analytical devices. Anal Chem. 2013;85(10):5233–9.
36. Lillehoj PB, Huang MC, Truong N, Ho CM. Rapid electrochemical detection on a mobile phone. Lab Chip. 2013;13(15):2950–5.
37. Dineva MA, Candotti D, Fletcher-Brown F, Allain JP, Lee H. Simultaneous visual detection of multiple viral amplicons by dipstick assay. J Clin Microbiol. 2005;43(8):4015–21.
38. Mao X, Huang TJ. Microfluidic diagnostics for the developing world. Lab Chip. 2012;12(8):1412–6.
39. Li X, Ballerini DR, Shen W. A perspective on paper-based microfluidics: current status and future trends. Biomicrofluidics. 2012;6(1):11301–1130113.
40. Hu J, Wang S, Wang L, Li F, Pingguan-Murphy B, Lu TJ, et al. Advances in paper-based point-of-care diagnostics. Biosens Bioelectron. 2014;54:585–97.
41. Pelton R. Bioactive paper provides a low-cost platform for diagnostics. Trends Anal Chem. 2009;28(8):925–42.
42. Fernandez-Sanchez C, McNeil CJ, Rawson K, Nilsson O, Leung HY, Gnanapragasam V. One-step immunostrip test for the simultaneous detection of free and total prostate specific antigen in serum. J Immunol Methods. 2005;307(1–2):1–12.
43. Ge C, Yu L, Fang Z, Zeng L. An enhanced strip biosensor for rapid and sensitive detection of histone methylation. Anal Chem. 2013;85(19):9343–9.
44. Martinez AW, Phillips ST, Whitesides GM, Carrilho E. Diagnostics for the developing world: microfluidic paper-based analytical devices. Anal Chem. 2009;82(1):3–10.

45. Martinez AW, Phillips ST, Whitesides GM. Three-dimensional microfluidic devices fabricated in layered paper and tape. Proc Natl Acad Sci. 2008;105(50):19606–11.
46. Yang Q, Gong X, Song T, Yang J, Zhu S, Li Y, et al. Quantum dot-based immunochromatography test strip for rapid, quantitative and sensitive detection of alpha fetoprotein. Biosens Bioelectron. 2011;30(1):145–50.
47. van den Berk GE, Frissen PH, Regez RM, Rietra PJ. Evaluation of the rapid immunoassay determine HIV 1/2 for detection of antibodies to human immunodeficiency virus types 1 and 2. J Clin Microbiol. 2003;41(8):3868–9.
48. Nilghaz A, Wicaksono DH, Gustiono D, Majid FAA, Supriyanto E, Kadir MRA. Flexible microfluidic cloth-based analytical devices using a low-cost wax patterning technique. Lab Chip. 2012;12(1):209–18.
49. Lewis GG, DiTucci MJ, Baker MS, Phillips ST. High throughput method for prototyping three-dimensional, paper-based microfluidic devices. Lab Chip. 2012;12(15):2630–3.
50. Schilling KM, Jauregui D, Martinez AW. Paper and toner three-dimensional fluidic devices: programming fluid flow to improve point-of-care diagnostics. Lab Chip. 2013;13(4):628–31.
51. Cassano CL, Fan ZH. Laminated paper-based analytical devices (LPAD): fabrication, characterization, and assays. Microfluid Nanofluidics. 2013;15(2):173–81.
52. Liu H, Crooks RM. Three-dimensional paper microfluidic devices assembled using the principles of origami. J Am Chem Soc. 2011;133(44):17564–6.
53. Cheng CM, Martinez AW, Gong J, Mace CR, Phillips ST, Carrilho E, et al. Paper-based ELISA. Angew Chem Int Ed. 2010;49(28):4771–4.
54. Apilux A, Ukita Y, Chikae M, Chailapakul O, Takamura Y. Development of automated paper-based devices for sequential multistep sandwich enzyme-linked immunosorbent assays using inkjet printing. Lab Chip. 2013;13(1):126–35.
55. Nie Z, Deiss F, Liu X, Akbulut O, Whitesides GM. Integration of paper-based microfluidic devices with commercial electrochemical readers. Lab Chip. 2010;10(22):3163–9.
56. Lu J, Ge S, Ge L, Yan M, Yu J. Electrochemical DNA sensor based on three-dimensional folding paper device for specific and sensitive point-of-care testing. Electrochim Acta. 2012;80:334–41.
57. Parolo C, de la Escosura-Muniz A, Merkoci A. Enhanced lateral flow immunoassay using gold nanoparticles loaded with enzymes. Biosens Bioelectron. 2013;40(1):412–6.
58. Hu J, Wang L, Li F, Han YL, Lin M, Lu TJ, et al. Oligonucleotide-linked gold nanoparticle aggregates for enhanced sensitivity in lateral flow assays. Lab Chip. 2013;13(22):4352–7.
59. Choi DH, Lee SK, Oh YK, Bae BW, Lee SD, Kim S, et al. A dual gold nanoparticle conjugate-based lateral flow assay (LFA) method for the analysis of troponin I. Biosens Bioelectron. 2010;25(8):1999–2002.
60. Qin Z, Chan WC, Boulware DR, Akkin T, Butler EK, Bischof JC. Significantly improved analytical sensitivity of lateral flow immunoassays by using thermal contrast. Angew Chem Int Ed. 2012;124(18):4434–7.
61. Parolo C, Medina-Sanchez M, de la Escosura-Muniz A, Merkoci A. Simple paper architecture modifications lead to enhanced sensitivity in nanoparticle based lateral flow immunoassays. Lab Chip. 2013;13(3):386–90.
62. Vella SJ, Beattie P, Cademartiri R, Laromaine A, Martinez AW, Phillips ST, et al. Measuring markers of liver function using a micropatterned paper device designed for blood from a fingerstick. Anal Chem. 2012;84(6):2883–91.
63. Pollock NR, Rolland JP, Kumar S, Beattie PD, Jain S, Noubary F, et al. A paper-based multiplexed transaminase test for low-cost, point-of-care liver function testing. Sci Transl Med. 2012;4(152):152ra29.
64. Yang X, Forouzan O, Brown TP, Shevkoplyas SS. Integrated separation of blood plasma from whole blood for microfluidic paper-based analytical devices. Lab Chip. 2012;12(2):274–80.
65. MSD technology platform. https://www.mesoscale.com/~/media/files/brochures/techbrochure.pdf (2017).

66. Beaudet L, Rodriguez-Suarez R, Venne M-H, Caron M, Bédard J, Brechler V, et al. AlphaLISA immunoassays: the no-wash alternative to ELISAs for research and drug discovery. Nat Methods. 2008;5(12):A10–1.
67. Hawa G, Sonnleitner L, Missbichler A, Prinz A, Bauer G, Mauracher CJAB. Single step, direct fluorescence immunoassays based on metal enhanced fluorescence (MEF-FIA) applicable as micro plate-, array-, multiplexing-or point of care-format. Anal Biochem. 2018;549:39–44.
68. Vashist SK, Czilwik G, Alagarswamy GV. Elisa system and related methods. WIPO Patent Pub No WO/2014/198836.
69. Vashist SK, Czilwik G, van Oordt T, von Stetten F, Zengerle R, Marion Schneider E, et al. One-step kinetics-based immunoassay for the highly sensitive detection of C-reactive protein in less than 30min. Anal Biochem. 2014;456:32–7.
70. Vashist SK, Marion Schneider E, Zengerle R, von Stetten F, Luong JHT. Graphene-based rapid and highly-sensitive immunoassay for C-reactive protein using a smartphone-based colorimetric reader. Biosens Bioelectron. 2015;66(0):169–76.
71. Vashist SK, Lam E, Hrapovic S, Male KB, Luong JHT. Immobilization of antibodies and enzymes on 3-aminopropyltriethoxysilane-functionalized bioanalytical platforms for biosensors and diagnostics. Chem Rev. 2014;114(21):11083–130.
72. Jahanshahi-Anbuhi S, Pennings K, Leung V, Liu M, Carrasquilla C, Kannan B, et al. Pullulan encapsulation of labile biomolecules to give stable bioassay tablets. Angew Chem Int Ed. 2014;53(24):6155–8.
73. Ramachandran S, Fu E, Lutz B, Yager P. Long-term dry storage of an enzyme-based reagent system for ELISA in point-of-care devices. Analyst. 2014;139(6):1456–62.
74. Guidance for industry – Bioanalytical method validation. https://www.fda.gov/downloads/Drugs/Guidances/ucm070107.pdf (2001).
75. Guideline on bioanalytical method validation. http://www.emaeuropa.eu/docs/en_GB/document_library/Scientific_guideline/2011/08/WC500109686.pdf (2011).
76. Abe K, Kotera K, Suzuki K, Citterio D. Inkjet-printed paperfluidic immuno-chemical sensing device. Anal Bioanal Chem. 2010;398(2):885–93.
77. Li CZ, Vandenberg K, Prabhulkar S, Zhu X, Schneper L, Methee K, et al. Paper based point-of-care testing disc for multiplex whole cell bacteria analysis. Biosens Bioelectron. 2011;26(11):4342–8.
78. Vashist SK, Schneider EM, Luong JHT. Commercial smartphone-based devices and smart applications for personalized healthcare monitoring and management. Diagnostics. 2014;4(3):104–28.

Chapter 7
Multiplex Immunoassays

Sandeep Kumar Vashist

Contents

7.1   Introduction

The simultaneous detection of multiple analytes is desired in healthcare for the diagnosis, monitoring, and management of complex diseases. Therefore, there is a dire need of cost-effective, robust, and simple multiplex IAs that can reliably detect all the desired analytes from a single sample. Multiplex IAs would enable early and accurate diagnosis of complex diseases, which would give the desired opportunity to doctors to start the treatment at the earliest possible and lead to positive health outcomes for the patient. The rapid clinical diagnosis and the immediate start of treatment are crucial in emergencies and intensive care units, which require instant clinical decisions, such as patients with stroke [1]. In contrast, in cases of complex diseases such as sepsis, the clinical diagnosis cannot be made just based on the quantitative analysis of a single biomarker as there is a need to quantify multiple

© Springer Nature Switzerland AG 2019
S. K. Vashist, J. H. T. Luong, *Point-of-Care Technologies Enabling
Next-Generation Healthcare Monitoring and Management*,
https://doi.org/10.1007/978-3-030-11416-9_7

biomarkers to determine the various types of sepsis and analyze the efficacy of the treatment regimen.

The recent years have witnessed tremendous advances in multiplex IAs, which have shown significant promise for clinical diagnostics and point-of-care testing (POCT) [2]. Many prospective multiplex IA technologies and products would make their way to the market in the coming years. Apparently, the clinical diagnostics would be the foremost priority for multiplex IAs, however, rapid POC multiplex IAs at the point-of-need would also be of greater utility in environmental testing, food safety, veterinary sciences, and other bioanalytical applications [3]. Another emerging need for multiplex IAs would be for personalized healthcare monitoring and management as many smart healthcare devices are making their way to the market [4].

Various commercial devices are available for the multiplex detection of clinical analytes and parameters, such as Abaxis Piccolo Xpress and Abbott i-STAT system. They could perform multiplex detection of a limited but appropriate number of analytes. However, they employ expensive and bulky analyzer-based benchtop systems. Similarly, mass spectrometry (MS) [5], such as matrix-assisted laser desorption/ionization (MALDI)-MS, is widely used in healthcare for the rapid detection of pathogens and clinical analytes. But MS instruments are also costly, bulky, and require skilled analysts. Therefore, there is a need to develop rapid and cost-effective POC platform-based multiplex IAs and portable readers, which could be used for multiplex analyte detection at any place and time by users having basic operational skills. There is a strong emerging trend toward smart healthcare and diagnostic devices equipped with mobile healthcare and other advanced features. It substantiates the need for smart multiplex IA formats and smart readers, which could pave the way to personalized healthcare monitoring and management. The smartphone (SP)-based diagnostic readers and IAs, which have been widely demonstrated for the detection of numerous analytes, are providing an impetus to develop prospective SP-based multiplex IAs [4, 6–8].

7.2 Overview of Multiplex Immunoassay Formats

A wide range of multiplex IA formats has been developed based on the use of various strategies. The most prominent approach for multiplex IAs is the use of multiple spots on a solid substrate, where each spot can detect a separate analyte. The strategy has been employed by many companies and researchers for the development of various IAs. However, the preparation of such spotted substrates requires complex fabrication procedure and expensive instrument with precise control of spotted volume. The realization of the IA is also complicated as most of the IA procedures employ the same conventional and prolonged multistep ELISA procedure. There is a significant risk of misinterpretation, especially when nitrocellulose or nylon membranes are used for spotting as the background signal from a non-spotted substrate can vary a lot. Additionally, the imaging readout needs to be highly precise and accurate, where the specific assay signal should come only from the spots and should not be impacted by the background. As the morphology of the spots after the IA varies considerably, it is essential to take into account the signal from a fixed area within the spots. Some limitations of the approach are the limited number of multiplex IAs, increased complexity in imaging as the number of spots in the spotted array increases, and cross talk between the different assays as the assay components from a spot can diffuse to all adjacent spots [9–11]. The recent developments are specifically targeted at improving all these limitations. However, it remains to be seen whether such multiplex platforms could compete with clinically established predicate IAs in terms of desired bioanalytical performance.

A prospective strategy for multiplex detection is the use of different microchannels or various regions of a channel for the detection of multiple analytes. Similarly, various electrode arrays and lateral flow strips have also been employed for the multiple analytes. Of interest is the use of various beads and labels (such as dyes) for multiplex detection. Although colorimetry, fluorescence, chemiluminescence, and electrochemical signals are the most common signals that are employed for the readout of multiplex IAs [9, 12], the continuous developments in biosensors and IA formats are leading to innovative multiplex IAs.

Table 7.1 provides an overview of all major commercially-available multiplex IA technologies. The recent advances and ongoing efforts in POC and complementary technologies, such as microfluidic operations, lab-on-a-chip platforms, novel biosensor strategies, and prolonged reagent storage concepts, will pave the way to the significant improvements in multiplex IAs in the coming years [11, 41, 42].

7.3 Multiplex Immunoassays

Various commercial multiplex IAs developed to date by different companies are described here in detail together with the technical details, applications, main characteristics, and concerns.

7.3.1 Bead-Based Multiplex Immunoassays

A wide range of beads is used in diverse bioanalytical applications. They are available in various sizes [13], composition, and surface functionalities [2, 9] and could be bound to different enzymes, metal ions [43], quantum dots [44–46], and redox tags [47]. Moreover, they could be magnetic and nonmagnetic. Although the magnetic beads are the basis of nearly all clinical analyzer-based high-throughput immunodiagnostic assays, the non-magnetic beads are used for multiplex detection. Multiplexing can be achieved by employing beads of varying size/color, labeling them with different labels [43–47], or employing them for IAs in separate microchannels or chambers [48, 49].

Table 7.1 An overview of the major commercially available multiplex IAs

Multiplex IA type	Company	Main features	Refs.
Beads-based (xMAP® technology)	Luminex Corp., USA	• Can detect up to 100 analytes in a single 96-well microtiter plate (MTP) well using about 500 distinctly colored micron-sized polystyrene beads and a fluorescence IA • Assays could be performed using the flow cytometry-based analyzers developed by the company	[13–18]
Electrochemical ELISA	Meso Scale Diagnostics LLC, USA	• Wash-free electrochemical IA that could detect multiple analytes in complex sample matrices using carbon electrode surface-based microwell plates • Simple and easy-to-operate	[19–22]
Paper-based	Euroimmun, Germany	• Provides EUROLINE membrane test strips, i.e., line blots, based multiplex IA for the simultaneous detection of multiple antibodies in a sample • Provides EUROLineScan for the quantitative evaluation of EUROLINE membrane test strips using a flatbed scanner	[23, 24]
	Quidel Corporation, USA	• Provides Triage platform-based quantitative multiplex fluorescence LFIAs for the detection of cardiac biomarkers and drug screening in whole blood, plasma, or urine • Provides Triage® MeterPro to deliver rapid POC diagnostics results in three easy steps	[25, 26]
Array-based	Scienion, Germany	• Provides the complete technology solution for the development of multiplex IAs • Technologies include high-throughput sciFLEXARRAYER for printing arrays; sciPOLY3D polymer-based surface functionalization; sciBUFFER; assay protocols; sciREADER and software for fast readout of arrays in 96-well MTP in just 2 min; and customized solutions for multiplex IAs	[27–29]
	R-Biopharm AG, Germany	• Provides SeraSpot® microspot array for multiplex IA in 96-well MTP format • Provides SeraSight® strip • Provides SeraSpot® test kit-based ready-to-use reagents with the universal protocol for multiplex IA • Provides common ELISA processor for automated IAs • Provides SeraSight® plate mono instrument for image acquisition and interpretation of entire 96-well MTP • Provides SeraSight® strip instrument for image acquisition and interpretation of 8-well strip • Includes intelligent IA design with inbuilt reference spots for the reference curve, up to five controls for quality assurance, and a well-position marker, which is color-coded 0• Developed SpotSight® scanner and software for the image capture and interpretation-based readout of arrays in all 96 wells of MTP in 7 min 0• Provides a variety of tests for the detection of autoimmune and infectious diseases	[30]

(continued)

Table 7.1 (continued)

Multiplex IA type	Company	Main features	Refs.
	Randox, UK	• Provides the biochip array technology (BAT) for various bioanalytical applications • Developed the proprietary surface functionalization procedure for biochip and many BAT-based assays • Developed fully automated analyzers from medium to very-high throughput, i.e., Evidence Evolution, Evidence, and Evidence Investigator, and Evidence MultiSTAT	[31, 32]
	BioVendor, Germany	• Developed array-based multiplex colorimetric and fluorescent IAs • Provides Array Reader C-series and F-series reader instruments for the readout of colorimetric and fluorescent multiplex IAs, respectively, in 96-well MTP format in just 2 min	[33]
	Pictor Diagnostics Ltd., New Zealand	• Provides PictArray™ platform for semiquantitative multiplex detection using a customized ELISA-based procedure • Provides a compact PictImager™ for image capture and analysis of PictArray™	[34]
	GENSPEED Biotech, Austria	• Developed CE-certified IVD multiplex IA on a micro-ELISA chip for the detection of up to eight biomarkers for hospital-acquired infections and periodontitis in just 15 min using an array spotted using the Scienion's sciFLEXARRAYER, sciDROP, and sciPOLY 3D technologies	[35]
MF-based	Gyros Protein Technologies AB, Sweden	• Provides centrifugal MF-based Gyrolab Bioaffy CDs, i.e., a LabDisk platform with pre-integrated reagents for automated fluorescent IAs • Provides Gyrolab instrument (Gyrolab xPlore™) for running a single CD-based IA • Provides Gyrolab™ xP workstation for running up to five CDs simultaneously	[36, 37]
	Abaxis, Inc., USA	• Provides POC Piccolo Xpress™ whole blood chemistry analyzer for automated centrifugal MF-based assays • Provides several clinical laboratory improvement amendments (CLIA) waived tests for multiple analytes, biomarkers, toxins, nucleic acid, pathogens, etc. • Analyzer can perform up to 14 different tests on a LabDisk platform with pre-stored reagents	[38, 39]
	Samsung, South Korea	• Provides a handheld POC analyzer called Samsung LABGEO IB10 and centrifugal MF LabDisk platform-based fully automated IAs that detect multiple analytes in just 20 min • Detects up to three analytes in a single run	[40]

The xMAP® technology by Luminex Corp., USA [13] is the most widely used technology to develop bead-based multiplex IAs [14–16]. It can detect a large number of analytes just in a single 96-well microtiter plate's (MTP) well using the 500 distinctly colored bead sets that have been developed by Luminex Corp. The xMAP®-based multiplex IAs are cost-effective, rapid, reproducible, accurate, high-throughput, and require less analyst's time. The IA detects the analyte in the sample by binding to capture Ab-bound color-coded micro-sized polystyrene beads known as microspheres followed by the subsequent detection by binding to biotinylated detection antibody (Ab) and streptavidin-labeled fluorescent dye (Fig. 7.1). The readout of multiplex IA in the MTP wells is performed by an analyzer having multiple lasers or LEDs and high-speed digital-signal processors. The analyzer measures the fluorescent signals from each individual microsphere particle in the well and provides the results of the multiplex IA. The excitation of the microsphere's internal dyes by the laser or LED identifies the specific microsphere set, while a second laser or LED excites the fluorescent dye on the detection Ab. After that, high-speed digital signal processors identify each individual microsphere and provide quantified results for multiple analytes after the readout of fluorescent signals from them. Recently, the company has also offered an option to employ magnetic beads, which would be very useful to diagnostic companies for the development of automated IAs as it would enable easy and rapid separation just by using a magnetic separator. The company developed two flow cytometry-based analyzers, Luminex® 100/200™, with integrated fluidics, optics, lasers, and high-speed digital signal processors, which enable the development of multiplex IAs for the detection of up to 100 analytes in a single MTP well. However, the xMAP® technology-based multiplex IAs require expensive readout and analyzer instruments [17, 18]. They also need to be rapider so that they could be employed for POCT. The ongoing research efforts are focused on the development of low-cost lab-on-c-chip (LOC)-based flow cytometers for POCT [50, 51].

7.3.2 Multiplex Electrochemiluminescent ELISA

Meso Scale Diagnostics LLC has developed an innovative wash-free and high-throughput electrochemiluminescent ELISA for multiplex detection [19]. It is a highly-sensitive IA that detects multiple analytes in complex sample matrices using carbon electrode surface-based microwell plates and a wash-free sandwich IA procedure using SULFO-TAG-labeled detection Ab, which emits light upon electrochemical stimulation (Fig. 7.2). Being wash-free, it is simple to operate and avoids numerous unnecessary and labor-intensive wash steps. It has good analytical performance that is comparable to that of Luminex xMAP® multiplex IA [20–22].

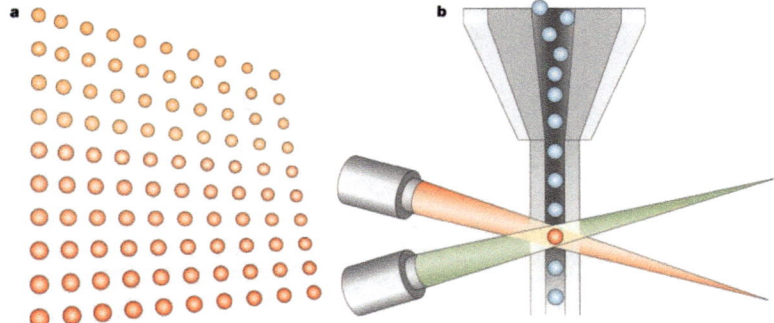

Fig. 7.1 Luminex *x*MAP® multiplex IA technology. (**a**) Polystyrene beads are internally colored with two different fluorescent dyes: red and infrared with up to 100 distinct bead regions generated by using different concentrations of red and infrared dyes. Each bead region, bound to a different capture Ab, detects its particular analyte, followed by the subsequent binding of a biotinylated detection Ab and streptavidin-conjugated phycoerythrin (reporter dye). (**b**) The beads are identified individually in a rapidly flowing fluid stream that passes by two laser beams: red classification laser (635 nm) or LED reveals the color code of the bead region, and green reporter laser (532 nm) or LED determines the analyte concentration by measuring the reporter fluorescence intensity [16]. Reproduced with permission from Elsevier B.V [16]

7.3.3   Paper-Based Multiplex Immunoassays

Several paper-based multiplex IAs have been demonstrated and are commercially-available. Lateral flow IAs (LFIAs) are the most simple, rapid, and cost-effective IA formats for POCT at homes, remote settings, decentralized laboratories, and point-of-need. LFIAs are described in depth in a separate chapter of this book. The conventional LFIA has been modified recently into multiplex formats by many companies [53]. Most multiplexed LFIAs are based on the detection of an optical signal [54–57], while a few also employ electrochemical detection [58, 59].

A prospective multiplex IA has been developed by Euroimmun, Germany, which involves the use of EUROLINE membrane test strips for the simultaneous detection of multiple antibodies in a sample [23]. A flatbed scanner and imaging system-based EUROLineScan [24] has been developed for the quantitative evaluation of EUROLINE membrane test strips. The company has developed several multiplex IA products for the diagnosis of several diseases, such as autoimmune liver diseases, antinuclear antibody (ANA), myositis, TORCH syndrome, extractable nuclear antigens (ENA), etc.

Quidel Corporation, USA, has developed the Triage platform-based quantitative multiplex fluorescence LFIAs for the detection of cardiac biomarkers and drugs in complex sample matrices of whole blood, plasma, or urine [25, 26, 60]. The multiplex IA provides quantitative results in just 20 min using a portable fluorometer called Triage® MeterPro [60], which delivers rapid POC diagnostic results in three easy steps.

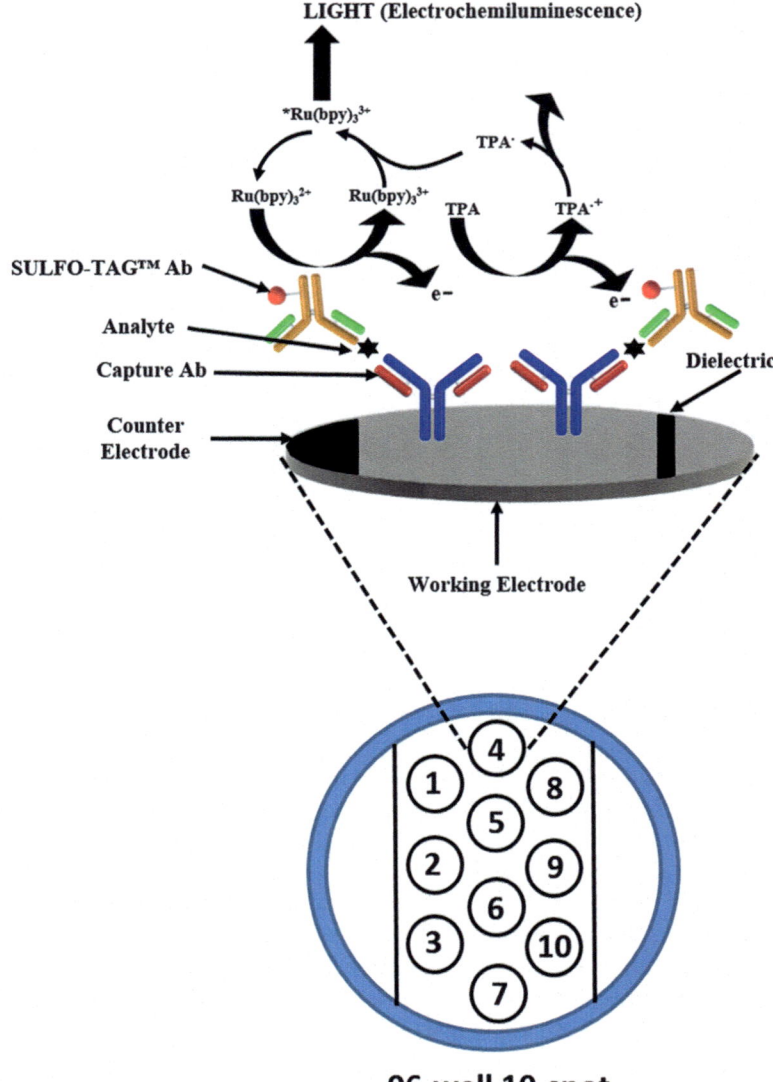

Fig. 7.2 Electrochemiluminescent ELISA-based wash-free sandwich IA for the highly sensitive detection of analytes in complex sample matrices. Upon electrochemical stimulation, light is emitted from the carbon electrode surface-based microwell plates with specific SULFO-TAG™ labels on the detection antibody. Reproduced with permission from Elsevier B.V [52]

During recent years, many innovative smart LFIA readers have been developed by several companies that have led to quantitative LFIAs. The smart readers, equipped with mobile healthcare tools and Cloud computing, have significantly increased the functionality of LFIAs. Some important examples are the smart LFIA readers developed by Cellmic, USA and BBI Solutions, UK, which are described in detail in another chapter of this book.

7.3.4 Multiplex IAs Using Microfluidic Paper-Based Analytical Devices

The use of microfluidic paper-based analytical devices (MF-PADs) has increased considerably during the last decade due to their low-cost, rapid fabrication, ability to manipulate liquids at a high level, adaptation of various microfluidic operations (such as mixing, splitting, separation, and filtration), improved assay performance, and flexibility [61–63]. They are ideal for multiplex IAs in the developing countries that have limited resources, healthcare infrastructure, and professionals. However, the MF-PAD format has not been a commercial success, which is mainly due to the increased fabrication efforts required for mass production, concerns about the reproducibility and performance of IAs, and need for the simplified operational procedure. The conventional MF-PAD-based IA, based on colorimetric detection via naked eyes, is mainly qualitative or semi-quantitative. The recent advances in the development of smart readers are paving the way to quantitative MF-PAD-based multiplex IAs.

An exciting development is the MF-PAD for on-site liver function testing by determining the levels of aspartate aminotransferase and alanine aminotransferase in whole blood using a colorimetric IA procedure that takes just 15 min [64]. The fabrication procedure and process steps of the multiplex IA are illustrated schematically in Fig. 7.3. In another approach, the electrochemical MF-PADs were used for the multiplex detection of glucose, lactate, and uric acid in human serum using the respective oxidase enzymes [66]. The SU-8 photolithography was used to pattern the microfluidics on the device, followed by the patterning of screen-printed electrodes on the filter paper. Of interest is the electrochemiluminescent MF-PAD for the multiplex detection of four tumor markers in human plasma [67]. There have been numerous developments in electrochemical MF-PADs [68–72], which might lead to critical diagnostic applications in the near future.

7.3.5 Array-Based Multiplex Immunoassays

The most popular high-throughput multiplex IA format is based on the formation of an array of spots, where each spot detects a specific analyte. Several companies, such as Scienion, R-Biopharma, BioVendor, Pictor, Randox, etc., have developed

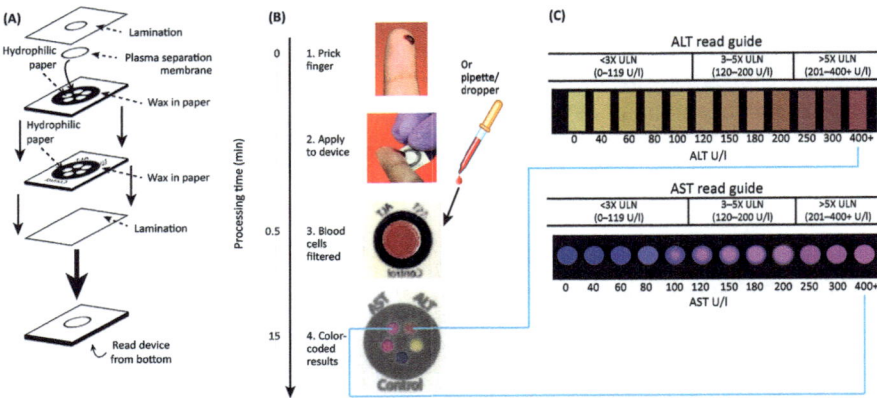

Fig. 7.3 Multiplex IA for on-site liver function testing using the microfluidic paper-based analytical device (MF-PAD). (**a**) Fabrication procedure for MF-PAD. (**b**) IA procedure. (**c**) Colorimetric readout guides for the quantitative determination of liver function enzymes. Reproduced with permission from AAAS [65]. ALT and AST stand for alanine aminotransferase and aspartate aminotransferase, respectively

the array format-based platforms for the detection of multiple analytes and the readers to determine the detection signals from each spot in the array. The main features of the products and technologies developed by various major companies are mentioned in detail in Table 7.1. The surface functionalization and immobilization of biomolecules play a prominent role in array-based multiplex IAs. One of the most widely used surface functionalization strategies is the use of silanized substrates [73] as reported by Randox and Scienion. The signal readout in case of such array platforms is mainly done by optical or electrochemical means [74]. The optical readout systems measure the fluorescence [75] or chemiluminescence [76] signals from the spots due to the binding of fluorescent- or chemiluminescent-labeled biomolecules. It is realized by image capture using a scanning charge-coupled device (CCD) or complementary metal oxide semiconductor (CMOS) camera. Some label-free microfluidic biosensor platforms have also been demonstrated employing array spots and localized surface plasmon resonance (LSPR) detection using metallic nanoparticles [77–79]. However, these are expensive as they employ complex manufacturing and process steps.

Another prospective development is the microelectrode array-based electrochemical detection of multiple analytes [80–82] by immobilizing the biorecognition elements on the microelectrodes. Various electrode materials, such as semiconductors, metals, or carbon-based materials, have been used for POC electrochemical detection [83]. Therefore, it is important to screen an optimal microelectrode material that would results in higher bioanalytical performance of an assay [84]. The ElectraSense platform from Custom Array Inc., USA is an excellent system that enables the electrochemical detection of multiple analytes on a CMOS-based Custom-Array chip with platinum microelectrodes. The signal, i.e., fluorescent or electrochemical, is measured using a handheld reader via multimodal signal read-out in less than 1 min [85, 86]. The chip can be reused for up to four times, while the biorecognition elements, i.e., DNAs and antibodies, are bound to the chip's surface via oligonucleotide hybridization. However, the chip is inappropriate for clinical diagnostics as their production is expensive and complex.

7.3.6 Microfluidics-Based Multiplex Immunoassays

Microfluidics (MF)-based multiplex IAs have been widely used for the simultaneous detection of different analytes, where each microfluidic channel is used for the quantitative analysis of a separate analyte [87]. They require an optimal MF array and design and the manipulation of fluids by a number of pneumatic valves integrated into polydimethylsiloxane (PDMS)-based devices [88–90]. An innovative MF-based multiplex IA, comprising of a disposable MF cartridge with preloaded reagents, and a handheld automated analyzer [91], detects HIV antigen, syphilis antigen, BSA, and Ab to goat IgG in each MF channel (Fig. 7.4). It can detect these four analytes in seven samples by employing four detection sites located in series in each MF channel. The multiplex IA could be performed manually or automatically by measuring the optical density signal obtained by the reduction of silver ions on the detection Ab tagged with gold nanoparticles (AuNPs). The signal is measured using a low-cost and compact reader that comprises of light-emitting diodes and photodetectors. The developed IA detects HIV and syphilis antigens in just 20 min using only 1 ml of finger-pricked whole blood. The results agreed well with those obtained by an established clinical laboratory reference test. Another prospective format is the paper-based MF device, i.e., DxBox, for the multiplex detection of malaria pfHRPII antigen and IgM antibodies to *Salmonella typhi* within 30 min in whole blood [57] (Fig. 7.5). The multiplex IA involves the delivery of sample and dried on-chip stored reagents over the multiple detection sites on the paper device via pneumatic actuation and performing the quantitative detection of analytes by imaging each spot via a flatbed scanner and determining its intensity. However, these MF-based multiplex IA formats are limited in terms of multiplexing and do not have the desired flexibility for various IA procedures.

   Another emerging format is the centrifugal MF (CMF)-based multiplex IA, which employs the compact lab-on-a-disc platform, where the various IA steps are performed by MF operations by navigating the fluids through the microchannels using centrifugal forces. The most widely used CMF-based multiplex IA formats are those from Gyros Protein Technologies AB, Sweden; Abaxis, Inc., USA; and Samsung, South Korea. The automated IAs are performed in a portable analyzer, where the signal from each IA is read by optical readout. The main advantages of the CMF format are the low sample requirement, rapid sample-to-answer time, and automated operations. But there are still considerable improvements required in terms of multiplexing, robustness, and IA formats.

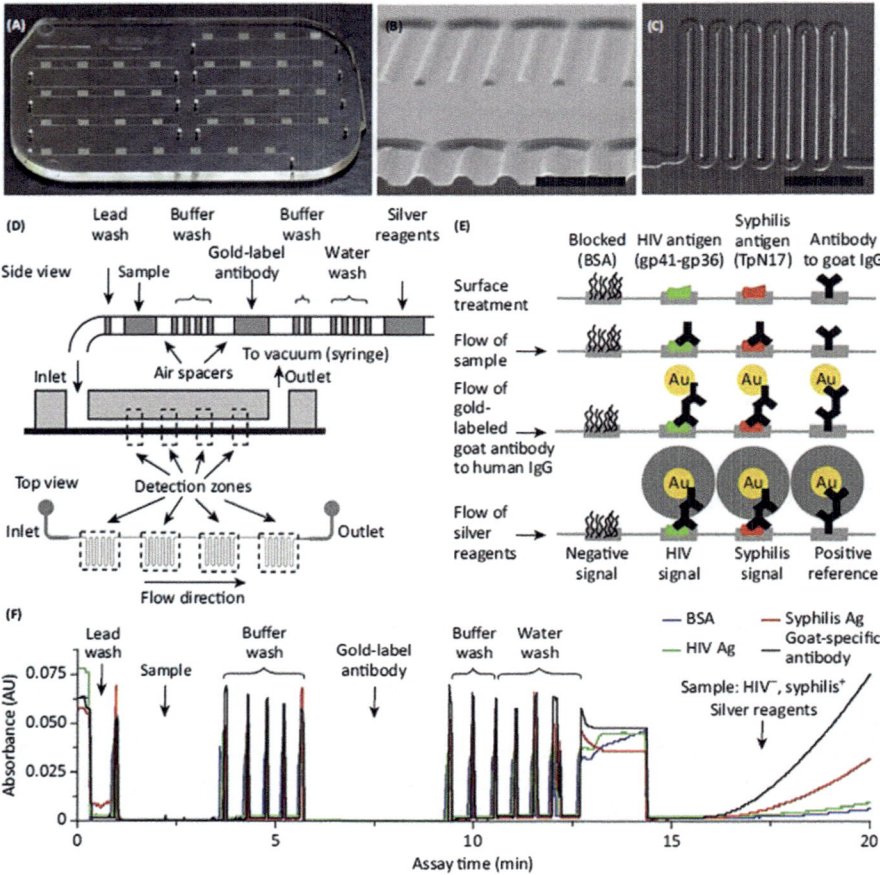

Fig. 7.4 Microfluidics (MF)-based multiplex IA platform. (**a**) MF polystyrene cassette with seven measurement units. (**b**) Scanning electron microscope image of channel cross section (scale bar: 500 mm). (**c**) Transmitted light micrograph of a single detection site (scale bar: 1 mm). (**d**) Passive delivery of a preloaded sequence of different reagents. (**e**) Schematic of assay reactions on different detection sites at various process steps. The signal detection occurs by the reduction of silver ions on detection Ab tagged with AuNPs. (**f**) Measurement of optical density signal in the developed multiplex IA for HIV and syphilis. Reproduced with permission from the Macmillan Publishers Ltd. [91]

Abaxis Inc., USA has developed a POC Piccolo Xpress™ whole blood chemistry analyzer [38] (Fig. 7.6a) that can perform automated IAs on a centrifugal MF-based LabDisk (CML) platform. The analyzer processes up to 14 different tests on a single barcoded LabDisk that has all the prestored reagents. The company has developed several clinical laboratory improvement amendments (CLIA) waived multi-analyte tests and other tests for biomarkers, toxins, nucleic acid, pathogens, and other analytes [39]. Similarly, Gyros Protein Technologies, Sweden has developed Gyrolab instrument (Gyrolab xPlore™ or Gyrolab™ xP workstation) [36] and

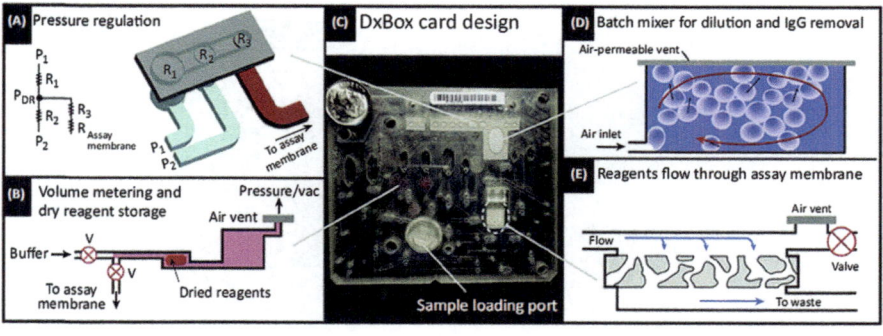

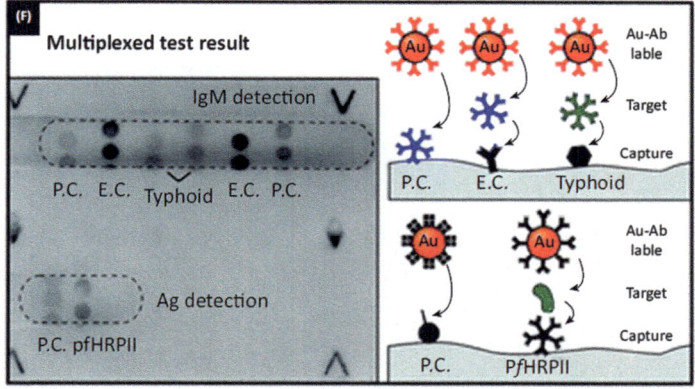

Fig. 7.5 DxBox Integrated Microfluidics (MF)-based paper card device for multiplex IAs. (**a**) Pneumatic regulation for the fluid manipulation. (**b**) On-card volume metering and freeze-dried storage of reagents. (**c**) Integrated MF cartridge. (**d**) Bath mixer for sample dilution and IgG removal. (**e**) Incubation procedure on the assay membrane. The application of an air vent and a valve removes the air between reagent deliveries and the reagents itself between different incubation steps. (**f**) Multiplex detection of IgM antibodies against typhoid infection and malaria pfHRPII antigen from human plasma. Reproduced with permission from the Royal Society of Chemistry [92]. E.C. and P.C. stand for endogenous control and process control, respectively

centrifugal MF-based Gyrolab Bioaffy CDs [37] (Fig. 7.6b). Gyrolab xPlore™ can perform a single IA on a CML platform, while Gyrolab™ xP workstation can simultaneously run up to five CML platforms. The company has also developed several IAs using a fluorescent IA procedure that involves the binding of the SA-coated bead to biotinylated capture Ab, followed by the binding of analyte and its detection via fluorescent-labeled detection Ab. Of interest is the handheld POC analyzer from Samsung, i.e., Samsung LABGEO IB10 [40], which employs CML platform-based fully automated IA for the rapid detection of multiple analytes in just 20 min. The analyzer has several advanced features, such as smart mobile healthcare tools, and can detect up to three different analytes in a single run. The CML platform contains all the prestored reagents for the IAs that are stable at room

(A)

(B)

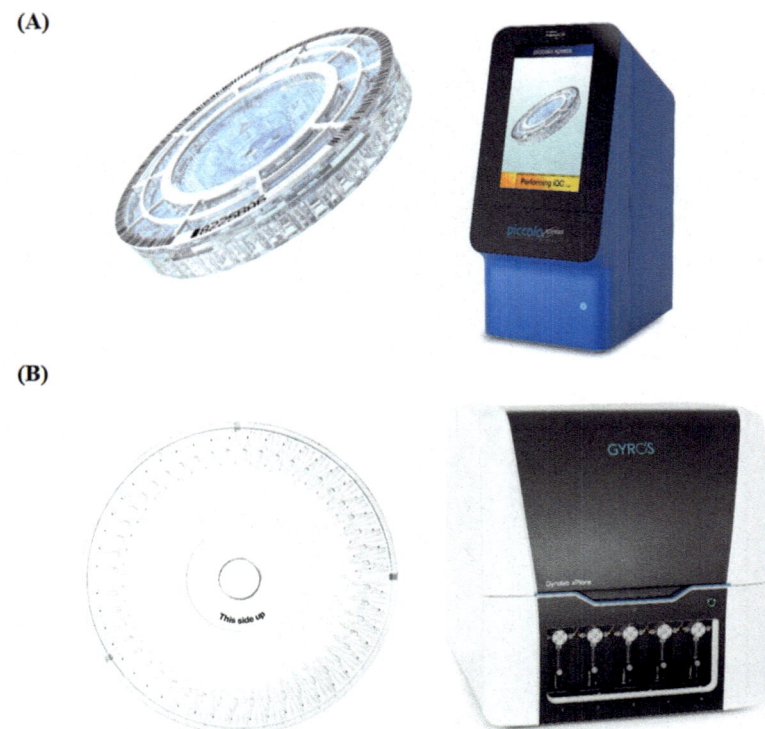

Fig. 7.6 (**a**) (left) Centrifugal microfluidics platform, i.e., LabDisk, for multiplex detection and (right) Piccolo Xpress chemistry analyzer for fully automated IA. (**b**) (left) LabDisk platform for fully automated IA and (right) Gyrolab xPlore™ system enabling fully automated IA. Reproduced with permission from Elsevier B.V [6, 52]

temperature for a month. The company has developed IAs for troponin I, myoglobin, CK-MB, thyroid-stimulating hormone, procalcitonin, and other analytes.

Further, the electrochemical detection-based microfluidic multiplex IAs could lead to rapid analyte detection and compact devices. An interesting development was the "MultiLab" platform-based MF electrochemical biosensor for multiplex detection of up to eight analytes [93], which employs a microfluidic channel network with eight separate immobilization sections in parallel that are combined with a single electrochemical measurement cell comprising multiple working electrodes. It was employed for the rapid quantitative detection of two antibiotics in human plasma in 15 min. The IA format was cost-effective and simple and required less sample and reagents, but it lacked an automated operational procedure via a portable analyzer.

7.4 Critiques and Outlook

The simultaneous detection of multiple analytes is an essential requirement for the clinical diagnosis of many complex diseases and differentiating among the similar ones. Moreover, the existing trend toward the use of clinical score, determined by assigning specific weightage to each biomarker in the multiplex panel, as a real-time and easy-to-use visual indicator of patient health for a particular disease emphasizes the need for multiplex IAs. The last decade has witnessed many multiplex IAs-based IVD products in the market from various companies, such as Luminex Corp., Meso Scale Diagnostics LLC, Gyrolab, Abaxis, Randox, R-Biopharm, BioVendor, TestLine, Scienion, Pictor, etc. Although the multiplex IAs from Gyrolab, Abaxis, Randox, and Luminex Corp. are among the most widely used, the other companies are also looking into increasing their multiplex IAs' portfolio. Further, a wide range of researchers is continuously developing innovative multiplex IAs employing the latest advances in lab-on-a-chip, microfluidic technologies, POC platforms, novel biosensors, new IA formats (such as wash-free IAs), system integration, smart system technologies, smart applications, and mobile healthcare. The cost-effectiveness, simplicity, robustness, analytical performance, ease of manufacture, and the clinical utility will be the critical factors for any multiplex IA format to be commercially- and clinically-viable. Doubtlessly, the use of multiplex IAs will be increasingly growing in clinical diagnostics and healthcare.

However, it remains to be seen whether the multiplex IAs could fulfill all the rigorous bioanalytical requirements as required by the regulatory and healthcare authorities for the clinical diagnostics [94]. The bioanalytical performances of all the IAs for the various biomarkers in the multiple IA should align well with the established predicate IAs for each biomarker. Therefore, there is a need for rigorous clinical validation of multiplex IAs. If a single biomarker in the multiplex IA format does not meet the desired bioanalytical performance, the whole multiplex IA will fail due to nonalignment with the predicate. In addition, there are several limitations in selected multiplex IA formats, which will impact the clinical analysis. As an example, most array-based multiplex IAs employ the controls and calibration spots, which is different from that of clinical analyzer-based assays that use calibrators, reference standards, and controls as samples. The spotted calibrators and controls doesn't simulate the actual IA procedure. Therefore, there is a need for critically investigating the IA format for its analytical performance.

The multiplex IAs would be very useful for physician office labs (POLs), remote settings, developing nations, and personalized healthcare monitoring. The multiplex IAs should have the desired precision, accuracy, sensitivity, specificity, reproducibility, robustness, and stability. Moreover, they should be rapid, simple to operate, low-cost, and easy to mass-manufacture. The multiplex IA kits should have prolonged storage stability for realistic applications. The array- and bead-based multiplex IAs have limitations as they require complex and expensive manufacturing and readout systems. On the other hand, the MF- and paper-based multiplex IAs are limited in terms of multiplexing. The realization and implementation of MF operations in multiplex IAs have simplified the IA format and led to the development of fully integrated MF cartridges for IAs, which obviate any manual fluid handling by the users. The advances in the system integration, engineering, and software have further led to advanced readers for multiplex IAs.

The current international trend is firmly focused on the use of smartphones (SP) as POC diagnostic readers [95]. Several companies have developed the rapid diagnostic test readers for LFIAs, which can be used at the point-of-need without any need for continuous electricity as they are equipped with rechargeable batteries. These inexpensive smart readers have tremendously increased the outreach of clinical diagnostics as they can be used at any place at any time. Further, they have turned the qualitative LFIAs into semi- or fully quantitative LFIAs. Apart from LFIAs, SP-based readers have been developed for a wide range of IA formats and bioanalytical applications [96]. However, there is a stringent requirement to ensure the safety of patient's data in accordance with the regulatory guidelines.

7.5 Conclusions

A wide range of multiplex IAs has been developed based on various IA formats. Although the most used formats are based on the use of various beads, an array of spots, and LFIA, there is an emerging trend toward POC, PADs, and MF-based multiplex IAs. However, despite several companies that have developed and are commercializing the multiplex IA-based IVD kits, the multiplex IA is still in the nascent stages in terms of technology development. The bioanalytical performance, costs, manufacturability, automation, and data analysis will play a key role in the market penetration and acceptance of multiplex IAs. There is no doubt that multiplex detection would be highly useful for the clinical diagnosis of complex diseases and would enable differentiation between closely related diseases. However, there is a need for stringent clinical validation of multiplex IAs and their alignment with established clinically accredited IAs. The coming years will witness numerous multiplex IAs making their way into the market. They would be based on novel IA formats and advances in complementary assisting technologies. The improvements in the technology would pave the way to regulatory-compliant and robust multiplex IAs, which would play a key role in healthcare monitoring and management.

References

1. Jung W, Han J, Choi J-W, Ahn CH. Point-of-care testing (POCT) diagnostic systems using microfluidic lab-on-a-chip technologies. Microelectron Eng. 2015;132:46–57.
2. Spindel S, Sapsford K. Evaluation of optical detection platforms for multiplexed detection of proteins and the need for point-of-care biosensors for clinical use. Sensors. 2014;14(12):22313–41.
3. Luppa PB, Bietenbeck A, Beaudoin C, Giannetti A. Clinically relevant analytical techniques, organizational concepts for application and future perspectives of point-of-care testing. Biotechnol Adv. 2016;34(3):139–60.
4. Vashist SK, Schneider EM, Luong JHT. Commercial smartphone-based devices and smart applications for personalized healthcare monitoring and management. Diagnostics. 2014;4(3):104–28.
5. Peacock PM, Zhang WJ, Trimpin S. Advances in ionization for mass spectrometry. Anal Chem. 2017;89(1):372–88.
6. Vashist SK, Luppa PB, Yeo LY, Ozcan A, Luong JHT. Emerging technologies for next-generation point-of-care testing. Trends Biotechnol. 2015;33(11):692–705.
7. Gauglitz G. Point-of-care platforms. Annu Rev Anal Chem. 2014;7:297–315.
8. Vashist SK, Mudanyali O, Schneider EM, Zengerle R, Ozcan A. Cellphone-based devices for bioanalytical sciences. Anal Bioanal Chem. 2014;406(14):3263–77.
9. Araz MK, Tentori AM, Herr AE. Microfluidic multiplexing in bioanalyses. J Lab Autom. 2013;18(5):350–66.
10. Gordon J, Michel G. Discerning trends in multiplex immunoassay technology with potential for resource-limited settings. Clin Chem. 2012;58(4):690–8.
11. Chin CD, Linder V, Sia SK. Commercialization of microfluidic point-of-care diagnostic devices. Lab Chip. 2012;12(12):2118–34.
12. Rusling JF. Multiplexed electrochemical protein detection and translation to personalized cancer diagnostics. Anal Chem. 2013;85(11):5304–10.
13. Dunbar SA. Applications of Luminex® xMAP™ technology for rapid, high-throughput multiplexed nucleic acid detection. Clin Chim Acta. 2006;363(1):71–82.
14. Skogstrand K, Thorsen P, Norgaard-Pedersen B, Schendel DE, Sorensen LC, Hougaard DM. Simultaneous measurement of 25 inflammatory markers and neurotrophins in neonatal dried blood spots by immunoassay with xMAP technology. Clin Chem. 2005;51(10):1854–66.
15. Kofoed K, Schneider UV, Scheel T, Andersen O, Eugen-Olsen J. Development and validation of a multiplex add-on assay for sepsis biomarkers using xMAP technology. Clin Chem. 2006;52(7):1284–93.
16. Braeckmans K, De Smedt SC, Leblans M, Pauwels R, Demeester J. Encoding microcarriers: present and future technologies. Nat Rev Drug Discov. 2002;1(6):447–56.
17. Ateya DA, Erickson JS, Howell PB Jr, Hilliard LR, Golden JP, Ligler FS. The good, the bad, and the tiny: a review of microflow cytometry. Anal Bioanal Chem. 2008;391(5):1485–98.
18. Godin J, Chen CH, Cho SH, Qiao W, Tsai F, Lo YH. Microfluidics and photonics for bio-system-on-a-Chip: a review of advancements in technology towards a microfluidic flow cytometry chip. J Biophotonics. 2008;1(5):355–76.
19. MSD Technology Platform. 2017. https://www.mesoscale.com/~/media/files/brochures/tech-brochure.pdf
20. Chowdhury F, Williams A, Johnson P. Validation and comparison of two multiplex technologies, Luminex® and Mesoscale discovery, for human cytokine profiling. J Immunol Methods. 2009;340(1):55–64.
21. Fu Q, Zhu J, Van Eyk JE. Comparison of multiplex immunoassay platforms. Clin Chem. 2010;56(2):314–8.
22. Breen EC, Reynolds SM, Cox C, Jacobson LP, Magpantay L, Mulder CB, et al. Multisite comparison of high-sensitivity multiplex cytokine assays. Clin Vaccine Immunol. 2011;18(8):1229–42.

23. The EUROLINE: a new technique for extensive antibody profiles. 2017. https://www.euroimmun.com/products/techniken/euroline/euroline-beschreibung.html
24. EUROLineScan. 2017. https://www.euroimmun.com/products/produkte-geraete-software/automatisierung-software/eurolinescan.html
25. Triage. 2018. https://www.quidel.com/immunoassays/triage-test-kits
26. Clark TJ, McPherson PH, Buechler KF. The triage cardiac panel: cardiac markers for the triage system. Point of Care. 2002;1(1):42–6.
27. sciFLEXARRAYER. 2018. https://www.scienion.com/products/sciflexarrayers/.
28. sciREADER. 2018. https://www.scienion.com/products/scireaders/.
29. sciCONSUMABLEs. 2018. https://www.scienion.com/products/sciconsumables/.
30. Array. 2018. https://clinical.r-biopharm.com/technologies/array/.
31. Biochip immunoassays. 2018. https://www.randox.com/biochip-immunoassays/.
32. Multiplex testing. 2018. https://www.randox.com/multiplex-testing/.
33. Multiplex assays. 2018. https://www.biovendor.com/multiplex-assays
34. PictArray™. 2018. https://www.pictordx.com/technology
35. Technology. 2018. https://www.genspeed-biotech.com/genspeed-biotech.com/technology/2/181/.
36. Gyrolab xPlore. 2018. http://www.gyros.com/products/systems/gyrolab-xplore/.
37. Gyrolab CDs. 2018. http://www.gyrosproteintechnologies.com/gyrolab-cds-automated-immunoassays
38. Piccolo Xpress. 2017. http://www.abaxis.com/medical/piccolo-xpress
39. Gorkin R, Park J, Siegrist J, Amasia M, Lee BS, Park JM, et al. Centrifugal microfluidics for biomedical applications. Lab Chip. 2010;10(14):1758–73.
40. Samsung LABGEO IB10. 2017. http://www.samsung.com/global/business/healthcare/healthcare/in-vitro-diagnostics/BCA-IB10/DE
41. Sackmann EK, Fulton AL, Beebe DJ. The present and future role of microfluidics in biomedical research. Nature. 2014;507(7491):181–9.
42. Robinson T, Dittrich PS. Microfluidic technology for molecular diagnostics. Adv Biochem Eng Biotechnol. 2013;133:89–114.
43. Feng LN, Bian ZP, Peng J, Jiang F, Yang GH, Zhu YD, et al. Ultrasensitive multianalyte electrochemical immunoassay based on metal ion functionalized titanium phosphate nanospheres. Anal Chem. 2012;84(18):7810–5.
44. Kong F-Y, Xu B-Y, Xu J-J, Chen HY. Simultaneous electrochemical immunoassay using CdS/DNA and PbS/DNA nanochains as labels. Biosens Bioelectron. 2012;39(1):177–82.
45. Wang J, Liu G, Merkoci A. Electrochemical coding technology for simultaneous detection of multiple DNA targets. J Am Chem Soc. 2003;125(11):3214–5.
46. Tang D, Hou L, Niessner R, Xu M, Gao Z, Knopp DJB, et al. Multiplexed electrochemical immunoassay of biomarkers using metal sulfide quantum dot nanolabels and trifunctionalized magnetic beads. Biosens Bioelectron. 2013;46:37–43.
47. Tang J, Tang D, Niessner R, Chen G, Knopp D. Magneto-controlled graphene immunosensing platform for simultaneous multiplexed electrochemical immunoassay using distinguishable signal tags. Anal Chem. 2011;83(13):5407–14.
48. Sato K, Yamanaka M, Takahashi H, Tokeshi M, Kimura H, Kitamori T. Microchip-based immunoassay system with branching multichannels for simultaneous determination of interferon-gamma. Electrophoresis. 2002;23(5):734–9.
49. Ko YJ, Maeng JH, Ahn Y, Hwang SY, Cho NG, Lee SH. Microchip-based multiplex electro-immunosensing system for the detection of cancer biomarkers. Electrophoresis. 2008;29(16):3466–76.
50. Shriver-Lake LC, Golden J, Bracaglia L, Ligler FS. Simultaneous assay for ten bacteria and toxins in spiked clinical samples using a microflow cytometer. Anal Bioanal Chem. 2013;405(16):5611–4.
51. Hashemi N, Erickson JS, Golden JP, Ligler FS. Optofluidic characterization of marine algae using a microflow cytometer. Biomicrofluidics. 2011;5(3):032009.

52. Vashist SK, Luong JHT. Handbook of immunoassay technologies: approaches, performances, and applications. London: Academic Press; 2018.
53. Li J, Macdonald J. Multiplexed lateral flow biosensors: technological advances for radically improving point-of-care diagnoses. Biosens Bioelectron. 2016;83:177–92.
54. Li J, Macdonald J. Multiplex lateral flow detection and binary encoding enables a molecular colorimetric 7-segment display. Lab Chip. 2016;16(2):242–5.
55. Song S, Liu N, Zhao Z, Njumbe Ediage E, Wu S, Sun C, et al. Multiplex lateral flow immunoassay for mycotoxin determination. Anal Chem. 2014;86(10):4995–5001.
56. Taranova N, Berlina A, Zherdev A, Dzantiev BJB. 'Traffic light'immunochromatographic test based on multicolor quantum dots for the simultaneous detection of several antibiotics in milk. Biosens Bioelectron. 2015;63:255–61.
57. Lafleur LK, Bishop JD, Heiniger EK, Gallagher RP, Wheeler MD, Kauffman P, et al. A rapid, instrument-free, sample-to-result nucleic acid amplification test. Lab Chip. 2016;16(19):3777–87.
58. Mao X, Baloda M, Gurung AS, Lin Y, Liu G. Multiplex electrochemical immunoassay using gold nanoparticle probes and immunochromatographic strips. Electrochem Commun. 2008;10(10):1636–40.
59. Mao X, Wang W, Du T-E. Rapid quantitative immunochromatographic strip for multiple proteins test. Sens Actuators B: Chemical. 2013;186:315–20.
60. Triage MeterPro. 2018. https://www.quidel.com/immunoassays/triage-test-kits/triage-meterpro
61. Ahmed S, Bui MP, Abbas A. Paper-based chemical and biological sensors: engineering aspects. Biosens Bioelectron. 2016;77:249–63.
62. Rolland JP, Mourey DA. Paper as a novel material platform for devices. MRS Bull. 2013;38(4):299–305.
63. Yang Y, Noviana E, Nguyen MP, Geiss BJ, Dandy DS, Henry CS. Paper-based microfluidic devices: emerging themes and applications. Anal Chem. 2017;89(1):71–91.
64. Vella SJ, Beattie P, Cademartiri R, Laromaine A, Martinez AW, Phillips ST, et al. Measuring markers of liver function using a micropatterned paper device designed for blood from a fingerstick. Anal Chem. 2012;84(6):2883–91.
65. Pollock NR, Rolland JP, Kumar S, Beattie PD, Jain S, Noubary F, et al. A paper-based multiplexed transaminase test for low-cost, point-of-care liver function testing. Sci Transl Med. 2012;4(152):152ra29.
66. Dungchai W, Chailapakul O, Henry CS. Electrochemical detection for paper-based microfluidics. Anal Chem. 2009;81(14):5821–6.
67. Ge L, Yan J, Song X, Yan M, Ge S, Yu J. Three-dimensional paper-based electrochemiluminescence immunodevice for multiplexed measurement of biomarkers and point-of-care testing. Biomaterials. 2012;33(4):1024–31.
68. Li X, Liu X. A microfluidic paper-based origami nanobiosensor for label-free, ultrasensitive immunoassays. Adv Healthc Mater. 2016;5(11):1326–35.
69. Li W, Li L, Ge S, Song X, Ge L, Yan M, et al. Multiplex electrochemical origami immunodevice based on cuboid silver-paper electrode and metal ions tagged nanoporous silver–chitosan. Biosens Bioelectron. 2014;56:167–73.
70. Wu Y, Xue P, Hui KM, Kang Y. A paper-based microfluidic electrochemical immunodevice integrated with amplification-by-polymerization for the ultrasensitive multiplexed detection of cancer biomarkers. Biosens Bioelectron. 2014;52:180–7.
71. Wu Y, Xue P, Kang Y, Hui KM. Paper-based microfluidic electrochemical immunodevice integrated with nanobioprobes onto graphene film for ultrasensitive multiplexed detection of cancer biomarkers. Anal Chem. 2013;85(18):8661–8.
72. Zang D, Ge L, Yan M, Song X, Yu J. Electrochemical immunoassay on a 3D microfluidic paper-based device. Chem Commun. 2012;48(39):4683–5.
73. Vashist SK, Lam E, Hrapovic S, Male KB, Luong JHT. Immobilization of antibodies and enzymes on 3-aminopropyltriethoxysilane-functionalized bioanalytical platforms for biosensors and diagnostics. Chem Rev. 2014;114(21):11083–130.

74. Ling MM, Ricks C, Lea P. Multiplexing molecular diagnostics and immunoassays using emerging microarray technologies. Expert Rev Mol Diagn. 2007;7(1):87–98.
75. Chandra PE, Sokolove J, Hipp BG, Lindstrom TM, Elder JT, Reveille JD, et al. Novel multiplex technology for diagnostic characterization of rheumatoid arthritis. Arthritis Res Ther. 2011;13(3):R102.
76. Kadimisetty K, Malla S, Sardesai NP, Joshi AA, Faria RC, Lee NH, et al. Automated multiplexed ECL Immunoarrays for cancer biomarker proteins. Anal Chem. 2015;87(8):4472–8.
77. Chen P, Chung MT, McHugh W, Nidetz R, Li Y, Fu J, et al. Multiplex serum cytokine immunoassay using nanoplasmonic biosensor microarrays. ACS Nano. 2015;9(4):4173–81.
78. Masson JF. Surface plasmon resonance clinical biosensors for medical diagnostics. ACS Sens. 2017;2(1):16–30.
79. Acimovic SS, Ortega MA, Sanz V, Berthelot J, Garcia-Cordero JL, Renger J, et al. LSPR chip for parallel, rapid, and sensitive detection of cancer markers in serum. Nano Lett. 2014;14(5):2636–41.
80. Schumacher S, Nestler J, Otto T, Wegener M, Ehrentreich-Forster E, Michel D, et al. Highly-integrated lab-on-chip system for point-of-care multiparameter analysis. Lab Chip. 2012;12(3):464–73.
81. Otieno BA, Krause CE, Jones AL, Kremer RB, Rusling JF. Cancer diagnostics via ultrasensitive multiplexed detection of parathyroid hormone-related peptides with a microfluidic immunoarray. Anal Chem. 2016;88(18):9269–75.
82. Wilson MS, Nie W. Multiplex measurement of seven tumor markers using an electrochemical protein chip. Anal Chem. 2006;78(18):6476–83.
83. Wan Y, Su Y, Zhu X, Liu G, Fan C. Development of electrochemical immunosensors towards point of care diagnostics. Biosens Bioelectron. 2013;47:1–11.
84. Díaz-González M, Muñoz-Berbel X, Jiménez-Jorquera C, Baldi A, Fernández-Sánchez C. Diagnostics using multiplexed electrochemical readout devices. Electroanalysis. 2014;26(6):1154–70.
85. Ghindilis AL, Smith MW, Schwarzkopf KR, Roth KM, Peyvan K, Munro SB, et al. CombiMatrix oligonucleotide arrays: genotyping and gene expression assays employing electrochemical detection. Biosens Bioelectron. 2007;22(9–10):1853–60.
86. Roth KM, Peyvan K, Schwarzkopf KR, Ghindilis A. Electrochemical detection of short DNA oligomer hybridization using the CombiMatrix ElectraSense microarray reader. Electroanalysis. 2006;18(19–20):1982–8.
87. Karle M, Vashist SK, Zengerle R, von Stetten F. Microfluidic solutions enabling continuous processing and monitoring of biological samples: a review. Anal Chim Acta. 2016;929:1–22.
88. Duncan PN, Ahrar S, Hui EE. Scaling of pneumatic digital logic circuits. Lab Chip. 2015;15(5):1360–5.
89. Araci IE, Brisk P. Recent developments in microfluidic large scale integration. Curr Opin Biotechnol. 2014;25:60–8.
90. Shao H, Chung J, Lee K, Balaj L, Min C, Carter BS, et al. Chip-based analysis of exosomal mRNA mediating drug resistance in glioblastoma. Nat Commun. 2015;6:6999.
91. Chin CD, Laksanasopin T, Cheung YK, Steinmiller D, Linder V, Parsa H, et al. Microfluidics-based diagnostics of infectious diseases in the developing world. Nat Med. 2011;17(8):1015–9.
92. Lafleur L, Stevens D, McKenzie K, Ramachandran S, Spicar-Mihalic P, Singhal M, et al. Progress toward multiplexed sample-to-result detection in low resource settings using microfluidic immunoassay cards. Lab Chip. 2012;12(6):1119–27.
93. Kling A, Chatelle C, Armbrecht L, Qelibari E, Kieninger J, Dincer C, et al. Multianalyte antibiotic detection on an electrochemical microfluidic platform. Anal Chem. 2016;88(20):10036–43.
94. Vashist SK, Luong JHT. Bioanalytical requirements and regulatory guidelines for immunoassays. In: Handbook of immunoassay technologies. London: Elsevier; 2018. p. 81–95.
95. Vashist SK, Luong JHT. Trends in *in vitro* diagnostics and mobile healthcare. Biotechnol Adv. 2016;34(3):137–8.
96. Contreras-Naranjo JC, Wei Q, Ozcan A. Mobile phone-based microscopy, sensing, and diagnostics. IEEE J Sel Top Quantum Electron. 2016;22(3):1–14.

Chapter 8
Bioanalytical Parameters in Immunoassays and Their Determination

Sandeep Kumar Vashist and John H. T. Luong

Contents

8.1 Introduction

The implementation of high-quality IAs is important in response to growing health concerns and increasingly stringent requirements for clinical testing. Essential bioanalytical parameters encompass precision, accuracy, selectivity, sensitivity, reproducibility, and stability. Therefore, the IVD manufacturers need to adopt an appropriate design and developmental plan with stringent quality control procedures to renovate and manufacture commercial IVD and POCT kits [1–4]. During the last decade, many commercial IAs for clinical testing have shown conflicting results, thereby signifying the need for even more stringent bioanalytical guidelines and regulatory requirements [5, 6]. Thus, all aspects of bioanalytical testing must be addressed while drafting appropriate regulatory guidelines for IVD. The continuously increasing number of IA formats and technologies [7], the emergence of novel technologies [8], improved healthcare monitoring and management procedures, and

© Springer Nature Switzerland AG 2019
S. K. Vashist, J. H. T. Luong, *Point-of-Care Technologies Enabling Next-Generation Healthcare Monitoring and Management*,
https://doi.org/10.1007/978-3-030-11416-9_8

new healthcare delivery concepts [9, 10] are posing a great challenge to the development of globally harmonized IVD guidelines.

The increased bioanalytical requirements for high-quality IAs are evident from the evolving IVD guidelines, normally associated with a high cost. In addition, significant improvements in IAs can be achieved by considering the feedback from the end-users and analysts. This chapter provides a comprehensive view of the bioanalytical parameters and performance of IAs together with the trends in bioanalytical testing/validation and technical challenges.

8.2 Bioanalytical Parameters of an Immunoassay

8.2.1 Precision and Accuracy

The IA precision indicates the nearness of individual test results for repeated analysis of an analyte concentration in multiple aliquots of a single homogeneous volume of the biological matrix. The IA precision for various analyte concentrations within its detection range should be <15% of the coefficient of variation (CV). In addition, its precision for the analyte concentration at the lower limit of quantification (LLOQ) should be within 20% of the CV. The "within-run (intra-batch)" precision is derived from a single analytical run, whereas the "between-run (inter-batch)" precision is obtained from multiple analytical runs over time.

The IA accuracy shows how close its mean test results are w.r.t. the actual target concentration, i.e., the nominal value. The mean value is within 15% of the nominal value for the entire detection range, whereas the mean LLOQ is within 20% of the nominal value. The IA accuracy is determined by replicate analysis of quality controls (QCs) using known analyte concentrations.

8.2.2 Sensitivity and Specificity

The IA sensitivity *is* the lowest detectable analyte concentration (LLOQ), with acceptable accuracy and precision. The IA selectivity is its ability to differentiate and quantify a target analyte from native samples in the presence of various endogenous interfering substances including physiological and pharmacological substances. The selectivity should be ensured at LLOQ and evaluated for each analyte in case of multiplex IA.

8.2.3   Calibration Curve

A calibration curve or plot is required for the determination of analyte concentration in an IA from the signal response. The signal response-analyte concentration relationship must be highly reproducible, and the calibration plot must be generated for each analyte in the sample in case of multiplex IA. The calibration standards are prepared by spiking known analyte concentrations in the native biological sample matrix. They cover the wide concentration range of an IA. However, substitute matrices could be used in case of special biological matrices, e.g., cerebrospinal fluid, which is difficult to obtain. The calibration curve is generated by employing a blank sample (no analyte or internal standard), a zero sample (no analyte but contains internal standard), and at least six analyte samples at varied analyte concentrations to cover the range of IA including LLOQ (with the analyte and the internal standard). The calibration standards are within 15% of nominal analyte concentrations for all concentrations above the LLOQ. At LLOQ, it should be within 20% of the nominal concentration.

8.2.4   Stability

Stability of IA reagents reflects their ability to retain the original performance and properties when stored under the defined conditions for a specified duration. The stability of an analyte should be determined for the specified duration in a matrix and container system. The real-time stability is determined by storing the IA reagents at 4 °C, while the accelerated stability is determined by storing them at 25 °C or 37 °C. The accelerated stability at such temperatures provides an estimate of the stability of IA reagents at 4 °C (Table 8.1). These determined values are based on the temperature coefficient Q_{10}, the increased reaction rate at a temperature increase of 10 °C. The freezing/thawing stability of the samples must be analyzed for up to three cycles of freezing/thawing, and this step should be performed in

Table 8.1 Evaluating the stability of IA kit at 4 °C from the determined accelerated stability at 37 or 25 °C

No. of days of testing	Estimate of days of stability of an IA kit at 4 °C based on testing at	
	37 °C	25 °C
7	68	30
14	137	60
21	207	90
28	276	120
35	345	150
42	414	180
49	483	210
56	552	240

similar experimental conditions as prevalent at the analytical lab. Another consideration is the stability of IA reagents during sample collection, handling, and transport. For automated IAs, the stability of IA reagents once they are opened and stored onboard the instrument must also be evaluated. Similarly, the "in-use" stability of IA reagents after opening and storage as per the instructions for use (IFU) must be addressed. Another issue is the sample stability during multiple freezing and thawing cycles. The stability analysis should employ samples prepared from a freshly prepared stock solution of analyte in a suitable biological matrix that does not contain any specific analytes and interferences.

8.2.5 Reproducibility and Recovery

The reproducibility is obtained by the replicate determinations of analyte concentrations in an IA using the desired QCs and samples. The recovery of an analyte in an IA is a measure of its analyte extraction efficiency. It is calculated using the detection signal obtained from the analyte concentration added to the biological matrix in comparison to the detection signal obtained for the same analyte concentration in a solvent. The desired percentage of recovery should be in the range of 90–110, although the values between 80 and 100 are still acceptable. The sample recovery experiments are conducted for each sample matrix if the IA is intended for multiple matrices. Such experiments determine the presence and extent of the matrix effect for a sample type.

8.2.6 Bioanalytical Performance Parameters

8.2.6.1 Limit of Blank (LOB), Limit of Detection (LOD), and Limit of Quantification (LOQ)

LOB is the highest measurement result, which is likely to be observed with a stated probability, usually at 95% certainty, for a blank native sample that does not contain any analyte (Fig. 8.1) [11]. The blank native samples must be real sample matrix instead of a clean buffer matrix. LOB is calculated as

$$\text{LOB} = \text{Mean of blank samples} + 1.645 \text{ standard deviation (SD)} \\ \text{of blank samples} \qquad (8.1)$$

LOD is the lowest analyte concentration in a sample that can be consistently detected with a stated probability, usually at 95% certainty [11]. The LOD, determined by Eq. (8.2), is based on the replicate analysis of real samples with very low analyte concentrations.

Fig. 8.1 The results for the blank sample having no analyte (left curve) should have 95% of the measurement results below the LOB (taking $\alpha = 0.05$). The results for the positive analyte sample having low analyte concentration at the LOD should have 95% of the results above the LOB (taking $\beta = 0.05$)

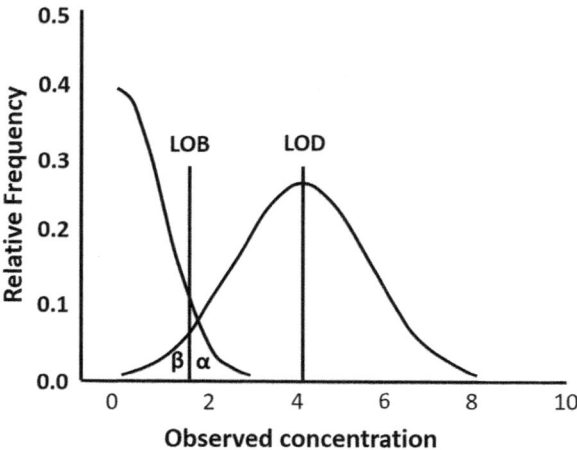

$$LOD = LOB + 1.645 \text{ SD of samples with low analyte concentration} \quad (8.2)$$

LOQ is the lowest analyte concentration that can be quantitatively detected with a stated accuracy and precision [11], which are set by the IA developers based on the predefined acceptance criteria, performance requirements, and end-user application. The lower LOQ (LLOQ) is the lowest calibration standard on the calibration curve where the detection signal for the analyte should be at least five times more than that of the blank sample. The precision of the determined analyte concentration should be within 20% of the CV, while its accuracy should be within 20% of the nominal analyte concentration. The upper LOQ (ULOQ) is the highest calibration standard on the calibration curve, where the analyte response is reproducible, the precision is within 15% of the CV, and the accuracy is within 15% of the nominal concentration.

The calibration curve should only be used between the LLOQ and the ULOQ for determining the analyte concentration in unknown samples. The practice of extrapolation below the LLOQ or above the ULOQ for the quantification of an analyte in samples is not recommended. The samples with analyte concentrations higher than the ULOQ must be diluted using the same matrix as the "real-world" sample. The samples with analyte concentrations below the LLOQ are reported as the zero concentration.

8.2.6.2 Lower Limit of the Linear Interval (LLLI) and Lower Limit of the Measuring Interval (LLMI)

LLLI is the lowest analyte concentration at which the detection signal shows a linear relationship with the analyte concentration. LLMI is the lowest analyte concentration at which all the specified performance characteristics of an IA, such as linearity, bias, and imprecision, are all met.

8.2.6.3 Linear Range and Analytical Measurement Range

The IA linear range is the analyte concentration range on the calibration curve, where the detection signal shows linearity with the analyte concentration in the sample. The linearity studies should be performed for each sample matrix of the analyte based on the intended use of the IA. The analytical measurement range of an IA is the analyte concentration range that an IA can determine in the sample without any sample pretreatment including dilution or pre-concentration.

8.2.6.4 Carryover and Errors

The carryover is defined as the error in the determination of analyte concentration in a sample when very concentrated samples are run before very low analyte concentration samples. The amount of analyte carried by the measuring system from a particular IA into subsequent IAs often introduces a significant error in the analyte determination [12]. It is calculated as the mean of the High-Low results minus the mean of the Low-Low results. The High-Low result is the result of low analyte concentration determination that immediately follows a high analyte concentration determination, whereas the Low-Low result is the result of a low analyte concentration determination that immediately follows a low analyte concentration determination.

The accuracy error is the deviation of the determined analyte concentration from the actual analyte concentration, defined as the sum of the random and systematic errors. The systematic error is the difference between the actual analyte concentration and the mean of an infinite number of analyte measurements carried out under repeatable conditions. The total analytical error is defined by Eq. (8.3) below, consisting of bias and imprecision based on a particular error model [13].

$$\text{Total analytical error} = \text{Bias} + 1.65 \ \text{Imprecision} \qquad (8.3)$$

8.2.6.5 Interference and Cross-Reactivity

The interference in an IA is the significant bias in the determined analyte concentration that may lead to imprecise results [14, 15]. It is due to the presence of nonspecific substances in a sample but could be tackled at the assay development stage by changing the formulation of IA reagents and/or the assay format [16–18]. However, if the interference from a nonspecific substance could not be obviated, this issue should be reported clearly in the instructions for use (IFU). The experimental procedure for the determination of such interferences in an IA involves the calculation of bias resulting from the addition of interfering substance. If the bias in an IA exceeds 10% after the addition of an interfering substance, it is important to determine the concentration of the interfering substances at which less than 10% bias is achieved to establish the interference threshold. The interference thresholds of interfering substances should be mentioned clearly in the IFU.

The cross-reactivity, defined as the percentage of the measured concentration of cross-reactant over its absolute concentration, is an indicator of the nonspecific reaction between an antibody and a nonspecific structural analog like the specific analyte of an IA. The IA should not have any cross-reactivity to the substances that are mentioned in the product design specifications (PDS) of an IA. But if there is cross-reactivity against a substance that cannot be obviated, it should be reported clearly in the IFU.

8.2.6.6 Bias and Method Comparison

The bias is the difference between the actual analyte concentration determined in a sample (accepted reference value) and the expected analyte concentration. It is measured by determining the analyte concentration in a sample at the beginning and the end of a long series of IAs when the same IA components are used under the same ambient conditions.

The method comparison is an essential requirement of all regulatory submissions to demonstrate the alignment of the developed IA with the predicate IA. It is determined by the measurement of correlation and bias between the developed IA and the established IA based on the testing of real samples. Most IA developers employ the method comparison results for their product flyers, marketing literature, and technology claims. The method comparison guidelines recommend taking real samples covering the reference range of an IA along with samples that are lower and higher than the reference range. Only pristine samples, not subjected to heat, pH, stripping, or filter treatment, should be used with about half of the samples above the reference range, while others should be within and below the reference range. The use of a large number of samples improves the statistical confidence of method comparison, while samples stored for more than 12 months should not be used.

8.2.6.7 The Hook Effect and Quality Controls (QCs)

The hook effect is observed in case of sandwich IA at very high analyte concentrations [19], when the increased number of analyte molecules could bind to both the capture and the detection Ab and prevent them from forming the sandwich immune complexes. This could result in the decrease in detection signal at extremely high concentrations, which could fall to the detection signal corresponding to lower analyte concentration within the calibration curve range. It could lead to a misleading lower analyte concentration, while the actual analyte concentration would be much higher. Therefore, the Hook effect must be critically evaluated in case of sandwich IAs, and the highest analyte detection range of such assays should be restricted to a high analyte concentration where there is no hook effect.

The QC samples play an important role in IAs as they are responsible for the acceptance or rejection of an IA run. At least three concentrations of QCs should be taken in duplicate for an IA. The low QC should be within three times the LLOQ of an IA, while the middle QC should be in the mid concentration range of an IA, and the high QC should be in the high concentration range of an IA. If at least 67% of QCs and 50% of QCs at each level are within 15% of their nominal concentrations, the IA run is bioanalytically successful. The calibration standards and QCs are prepared from separate stock solutions, but they can be prepared from same spiking stock solutions if the stock solution is verified as stable and accurate.

8.3   Critiques and Outlook

The developed IAs must be precise, accurate, sensitive, selective, and reproducible for the reliable detection of clinical analytes in healthcare and bioanalytical settings. The variability in IA results is one of the critical issues that is often observed with the end-users. Consequently, the IVD developers must consider all the factors that could lead to variability in IAs during the developmental stage. All desired measures must be taken to obviate the variability, including the testing of IAs with several potential end-users via alpha and beta site clinical trials during development. The various factors that are usually responsible for IA variability are instrument, reagent lot, calibration lot, calibration cycle, operator, consumables, laboratory, and environment.

LOD as the basis of IA improvements has been often exaggerated. Indeed, there is a need to critically assess the bioanalytical performance of an IA based on all the parameters and the intended use. The improved LOD is not an indicator of improved analyte detection; despite a low LOD, the IA linear range could remain the same. The IA linear range should cover the entire analytically relevant analyte concentration range, where the cutoff value (minimum analyte concentration that could be present in the patient's sample) is much above the LLOQ of the IA to enable reliable analyte detection.

Sandwich IAs are prone to the hook effect [19], resulting in a falsely low analyte concentration, while the actual analyte concentration is very high. Therefore, the Hook effect must be investigated and set IA linearity accordingly. For automated IAs, "the carryover" by the instrument should be obviated as it could lead to erroneous results, i.e., falsely elevated analyte concentrations for patient samples with low analyte concentrations. The intended use of an IA must be mentioned clearly in the IFU so that the end-users only use the IA for analyte detection in the specified sample matrix. The IVD manufacturers must provide to the end-users the detailed instructions, the IA protocol, and the application note to avoid any errors in analysis. The calibration of an IA plays a prominent role in automated IAs, which makes it obligatory for the users to follow the calibration procedure provided by the manufacturer at the start of the measurement and periodically thereafter at the specified frequency. Additionally, the manufacturers have to critically evaluate the quality of raw materials as their variability can affect the IA performance, leading to imprecision [20, 21]. Such materials must be specified to ensure their high quality and consistency.

The end-user scenario and conditions also play an important role in the development and validation of IA. As most IAs are developed in the standard bioanalytical labs under controlled ambient conditions, there is a lack of understanding of their performance in the end-user setting. The automated IAs must have random access capability as the running of a particular IA on an instrument should not impact the performance of subsequent IAs [22, 23]. All possible interferences for a particular IA must be scrutinized [14, 15, 24] and evaluated. The relevant and updated CLSI guidelines must be monitored as the list and concentrations of interfering substances may vary from time to time. A regulatory pre-submission at an early stage is needed to confirm the effects of all plausible interferences and their concentrations. If an IA has confirmed interference with some interfering substances, these must be clearly specified on the IFU. The selection of high concentrations of cross-reacting substances to be used for IA is often problematical as the regulatory authorities only recommend the use of sufficiently high concentrations of cross-reacting substances but not their exact concentrations. Thus, the use of varying high concentrations of cross-reacting substances by different IVD developers is often encountered. In general, there is a significant decrease in the error cases of IA during the last two decades, but the pre- and post-analytical steps still account for some significant errors [25, 26] that needs to be effectively tackled [27].

There are growing concerns about the conflicting results obtained from various IAs developed by different companies for the same analyte. Most IAs align well with the predicate IA that is specified by the regulatory authorities or selected by the developer based on the market intelligence. However, the developers are not considering if their developed IAs provide the same results as other most widely used commercial IAs. Therefore, to avoid discrepancy in results, the developers should evaluate the correlation of results obtained by their developed IA with those obtained by the predicate IA and the widely used IAs in healthcare. The developers should participate in external quality assessment and assurance schemes [28–30] and perform the validation of IA stringently as per the bioanalytical guidelines provided by the regulatory authorities [31].

The IA developers should know the end-user's scenario, i.e., analysis procedures, decision-making, sampling, etc. so that they could develop an IA that is well-suited to the intended bioanalytical application. They should monitor the performance of the developed IA using many real samples at the various clinical and bioanalytical settings available to the end-users. Moreover, they must keep themselves abreast of the bioanalytical guidelines and requirements, international standards, and trends in the field. If the international standard for an analyte is changed, the IA should employ the recent international standard only to avoid any discrepancy in results [32, 33]. The instruments must be well maintained, calibrated, and operating in stable conditions with stringent quality control during the entire course of IA development. Further, it is essential to check the integrity of data obtained by the instrument periodically. The persons involved in IA development and its use should be fully trained in all aspects of IA, instrumentation, and data analysis. In case of automated IA, the IA system must be verified periodically for any defect that adversely impacts the analysis. Moreover, it is important for IVD manufacturers to continuously monitor the performance of their IAs in the market. The manufacturing lots of IA that demonstrate inadequate bioanalytical performances should be recalled immediately to prevent any adverse events and detrimental consequences. The new IA systems as the automated IAs developed on the old IA system may not show the same analytical performance on the new IA system. Thus, it is obligatory for the manufacturer to validate the IAs on the new IA system before launch. There have been several instances where the same IA from the same manufacturer demonstrated significant variations on several IA systems developed by the manufacturer [34].

8.4 Conclusion

There is a constant and increasing need for critically improved IAs to have the desired optimal bioanalytical performance for clinical analytes. To date, some conflicting results still exist among various commercial IAs for the same analyte in interrogation. The IA developers need to follow a design and developmental plan to conform to the most updated regulatory bioanalytical guidelines. The IA bioanalytical performance must be established by determining all analytical parameters and performing statistical analysis in accordance with the established CLSI guidelines. The intended use of the IA must also be evaluated critically via independent end-user trials during the development. IVDmanufacturers must have a complete control over the development of IA, including the lot-to-lot consistency of manufacturing lots and raw materials. The regulatory authorities should keep track of the evolving technologies to update the bioanalytical guidelines.

References

1. Trullols E, Ruisanchez I, Rius FX. Validation of qualitative analytical methods. Trends Anal Chem. 2004;23(2):137–45.
2. Ellison SLR, Fearn T. Characterising the performance of qualitative analytical methods: statistics and terminology. Trends Anal Chem. 2005;24(6):468–76.
3. Stenman UH. Immunoassay standardization: is it possible, who is responsible, who is capable? Clin Chem. 2001;47(5):815–20.
4. Valentin MA, Ma S, Zhao A, Legay F, Avrameas A. Validation of immunoassay for protein biomarkers: bioanalytical study plan implementation to support pre-clinical and clinical studies. J Pharm Biomed Anal. 2011;55(5):869–77.
5. Guidance for industry – bioanalytical method validation. 2013. https://www.fda.gov/downloads/Drugs/Guidances/ucm368107.pdf
6. Guideline on bioanalytical method validation. 2011. http://www.ema.europa.eu/docs/en_GB/document_library/Scientific_guideline/2011/08/WC500109686.pdf

7. Marquette CA, Blum LJ. State of the art and recent advances in immunoanalytical systems. Biosens Bioelectron. 2006;21(8):1424–33.
8. Vashist SK, Luppa PB, Yeo LY, Ozcan A, Luong JHT. Emerging technologies for next-generation point-of-care testing. Trends Biotechnol. 2015;33(11):692–705.
9. Strandberg-Larsen M, Krasnik A. Measurement of integrated healthcare delivery: a systematic review of methods and future research directions. Int J Integr Care. 2009;9(1):e01.
10. Varkey P, Reller MK, Resar RK. Basics of quality improvement in health care. Mayo Clin Proc. 2007;82:735–9.
11. Armbruster DA, Pry T. Limit of blank, limit of detection and limit of quantitation. Clin Biochem Rev. 2008;29(Suppl 1):S49–52.
12. Armbruster DA, Alexander DB. Sample to sample carryover: a source of analytical laboratory error and its relevance to integrated clinical chemistry/immunoassay systems. Clin Chim Acta. 2006;373(1–2):37–43.
13. Krouwer JS. Setting performance goals and evaluating total analytical error for diagnostic assays. Clin Chem. 2002;48(6.1):919–27.
14. Kricka LJ. Interferences in immunoassay—still a threat. Clin Chem. 2000;46(8):1037–8.
15. Tate J, Ward G. Interferences in immunoassay. Clin Biochem Rev. 2004;25(2):105–20.
16. Ismail AAA. A radical approach is needed to eliminate interference from endogenous antibodies in immunoassays. Clin Chem. 2005;51(1):25–6.
17. Bjerner J, Nustad K, Norum LF, Olsen KH, Bormer OP. Immunometric assay interference: incidence and prevention. Clin Chem. 2002;48(4):613–21.
18. Niu H, Klem T, Yang J, Qiu Y, Pan L. A biotin-drug extraction and acid dissociation (BEAD) procedure to eliminate matrix and drug interference in a protein complex anti-drug antibody (ADA) isotype specific assay. J Immunol Methods. 2017;446:30–6.
19. Fernando SA, Wilson GS. Studies of the 'hook' effect in the one-step sandwich immunoassay. J Immunol Methods. 1992;151(1–2):47–66.
20. Class 2 Device Recall CoatACount Direct Androstenedione. 2014. https://www.accessdata.fda.gov/scripts/cdrh/cfdocs/cfRES/res.cfm?id=128287
21. Class 2 Device Recall IMMULITE/IMMULITE 1000 Systems Androstenedione. 2014. https://www.accessdata.fda.gov/scripts/cdrh/cfdocs/cfRes/res.cfm?id=124991
22. Carey G, Lewis SC. Method of handling reagents in a random access protocol. United States Patent, US6498037B1.
23. Gebrian PL, Evers TP. Random access reagent delivery system for use in an automatic clinical analyzer. United States Patent, US7169356B2.
24. Ismail AAA, Walker PL, Cawood ML, Barth JH. Interference in immunoassay is an underestimated problem. Ann Clin Biochem. 2002;39(4):366–73.
25. Carraro P, Plebani M. Errors in a stat laboratory: types and frequencies 10 years later. Clin Chem. 2007;53(7):1338–42.
26. Ismail Y, Ismail AA, Ismail AAA. Erroneous laboratory results: what clinicians need to know. Clin Med. 2007;7(4):357–61.
27. Plebani M. The detection and prevention of errors in laboratory medicine. Ann Clin Biochem. 2010;47(Pt 2):101–10.
28. Ceriotti F. The role of external quality assessment schemes in monitoring and improving the standardization process. Clin Chim Acta. 2014;432:77–81.
29. Perich C, Ricós C, Alvarez V, Biosca C, Boned B, Cava F, et al. External quality assurance programs as a tool for verifying standardization of measurement procedures: pilot collaboration in Europe. Clin Chim Acta. 2014;432:82–9.
30. Taverniers I, De Loose M, Van Bockstaele E. Trends in quality in the analytical laboratory. II. Analytical method validation and quality assurance. Trends Anal Chem. 2004;23(8):535–52.
31. Findlay JW, Smith WC, Lee JW, Nordblom GD, Das I, DeSilva BS, et al. Validation of immunoassays for bioanalysis: a pharmaceutical industry perspective. J Pharm Biomed Anal. 2000;21(6):1249–73.

32. Thaler M, Muller C, Schlichtiger A, Grundler K, Moore M, Luppa PB. Steroid binding properties of the 2nd WHO international standard for sex hormone-binding globulin. Clin Chem Lab Med. 2011;49(5):869–72.
33. Jin M, Wener MH, Bankson DD. Evaluation of automated sex hormone binding globulin immunoassays. Clin Biochem. 2006;39(1):91–4.
34. http://www.bernardmgross.com/sites/default/files/cases/2014/05/filed-complt-122.pdf (2010).

Chapter 9
Future Trends for the Next Generation of Personalized and Integrated Healthcare for Chronic Diseases

Sandeep Kumar Vashist, Lionel Gilles Guiffo Djoko, Stuart Blincko, and John H. T. Luong

Contents

9.1 Introduction

The recent years have witnessed tremendous developments in lab-on-a-chip (LOC) technologies, microfluidics, biosensors, rapid assay formats, prolonged reagents' storage, and complementary technologies [1]. These advanced technologies are paving the way for the development of the next-generation POCT technologies with many smart features. The potential benefits of these advances are large and, as yet, only partially realized. The potential is to move the testing out of the laboratory and for information to be directly available for the patient and the clinician. More than that, the ability to monitor in real time multiple parameters and to alert patients' clinicians of a crisis before the breakout is highly desired. The steps already made in glucose monitoring have paved the way but are remarkably a small part of the

© Springer Nature Switzerland AG 2019
S. K. Vashist, J. H. T. Luong, *Point-of-Care Technologies Enabling Next-Generation Healthcare Monitoring and Management*, https://doi.org/10.1007/978-3-030-11416-9_9

potential story. However, there are serious challenges to realizing this potential. These include the ability to manufacture multiplex assay systems. Specifically, it is very challenging to have, for example, 100 assays, all measuring reliably and passing quality control. Does a manufacturer issue for use a multiplex assay that only 95 out of 100 assays are under control, or does the manufacturer discard the multiplex and thus lose 95 working tests? The challenge of ensuring the tests being monitored by professional staff is significant.

As the major cause of death and disability worldwide, the incidence of chronic diseases has increased significantly during the last three decades [2, 3]. This is evident from the continuously increasing number of diabetics worldwide, which have surpassed all the estimates provided by the International Diabetes Federation (IDF) and World Health Organization (WHO) [4, 5]. Similarly, the increase in the sedentary behavior of the general population worldwide is responsible for the continuously increasing incidence of cancer, diabetes, depression, obesity, cardiovascular diseases (CVDs), and metabolic disorders [6]. This is apparent from numerous clinical studies during the last decade [7–9]. Therefore, the costs associated with the healthcare monitoring and management of these chronic diseases are substantially high and unsustainable [2]. This substantiates the need for next-generation POCT technologies, which would enable the subjects to perform clinical diagnostic tests at custom settings, i.e., homes, offices, physician office laboratories (POLs), remote settings, and decentralized settings.

The SPs have emerged as the universal device of billions of people worldwide, with over 70% of users in the developing countries [1, 10–12]. Doubtlessly, the next-generation POCT would be interfaced or based on SP and smart gadgets to provide the extensive outreach and facilitate increased compliance of subjects to clinical and lifestyle interventions [11]. The development and use of dedicated smart applications for healthcare offer the much effective healthcare monitoring and management [13]. The trend in the healthcare data enables the doctors to provide more effective treatment or intervention for their patients. The use of telemedicine and communication tools within in the upcoming smart applications facilitates the doctor-patient communication to avoid the unnecessary patient visits. Consequently, the doctors can provide consultancy to treat, monitor, and manage the healthcare of their patients with significant cost savings.

mH is anticipated to play a critical role in the healthcare in the coming era [1]. The three IVD giants, Roche, Abbott, and Bayer, have already developed the smart applications for the clinical and POC analyzers based on diagnostic testing in central laboratories in hospitals. Similarly, other companies have developed smart applications for diabetes management [14]. The POCT technologies developed during the last decade have also demonstrated mH as the key technology component. The diagnostic test results gathered by the users of such innovative POC devices are transmitted securely via Cloud to the central server. Via the Internet, the information can be assessed at any time and place by the patients, doctors, and authorized healthcare professionals. The Global Data Protection Regulation (GDPR), adopted by all IVD, healthcare, and other companies in 2018, further strengthens the development of mH by protecting the data and privacy of all individuals [15]. The patient personal data must be stored by anonymizing it and using the highest-possible privacy settings. The use of mH tools has greatly facilitated the healthcare by providing the desired features and capabilities, resulting in the better healthcare delivery as well as more effective diagnosis, treatment, and management of diseases [1]. It has strongly improved the patient's compliance with medication, clinical treatment, diagnostic tests, and appointments with physicians. The increased patient involvement in their healthcare is making them more aware and attributed to long-term benefits and sustainable healthcare [16, 17].

The next generation of POC devices will be personalized and based on fully integrated diagnostic platforms with low cost, robustness, reliability, and ease of use. Several innovative LOC platforms with integrated microfluidic operations have already been demonstrated [11, 18]. Significant advances in smart readers, mH, and complementary technologies in the coming years would be used in the next-generation POC devices for personalized and integrated healthcare. Such devices are deployed at any place and time without the need for a continuous power supply and highly skilled analysts. This feature is very useful in case of emergencies, e.g., epidemics when a larger population needs to be tested.

9.2 Chronic Diseases

9.2.1 Diabetes

As the most common noncommunicable chronic disease, diabetes has been declared as a global epidemic by the International Diabetes Federation (IDF) and the World Health Organization (WHO). In 2004, WHO expected the number of diabetics increases from 171 million (M) in 2000 to 366 M by 2030 [5], whereas IDF estimated 425 M diabetics in 2017 (Fig. 9.1A) and 629 M by 2045 [4] (Fig. 9.1B). This alarming increase demands an urgent need for counteractive measures, perhaps, the topmost healthcare concern globally for effective diabetic management. Diabetes is a major cause of mortality in the age group of 20–79 years, which is prevalent in 8.8% of adults and responsible for about 4 million annual deaths. Moreover, there are about 212 M undiagnosed diabetic cases, i.e., one in two adults with diabetes, who are progressing toward lethal diabetic complications totally unaware. Additionally, about 352 M people with impaired glucose tolerance (IGT), characterized by high blood glucose, have a high risk of developing type 2 diabetes mellitus (T2DM). Indeed, most of the patients with diabetes had never been diagnosed with this disease in their early years. A strong message issued by the IDF Diabetes Atlas in 2017 clearly portrayed a dark picture of diabetes as a major threat to global development. This is a wake-up call for all nations to take strong initiatives and actions to tackle this most challenging health problem of the twenty-first century [4]. Diabetes carries an unsustainable economic burden in terms of persistently high healthcare costs [19], greater care and financial support desired from family members/carers, loss of workplace productivity, and disability. It caused 4 M deaths in

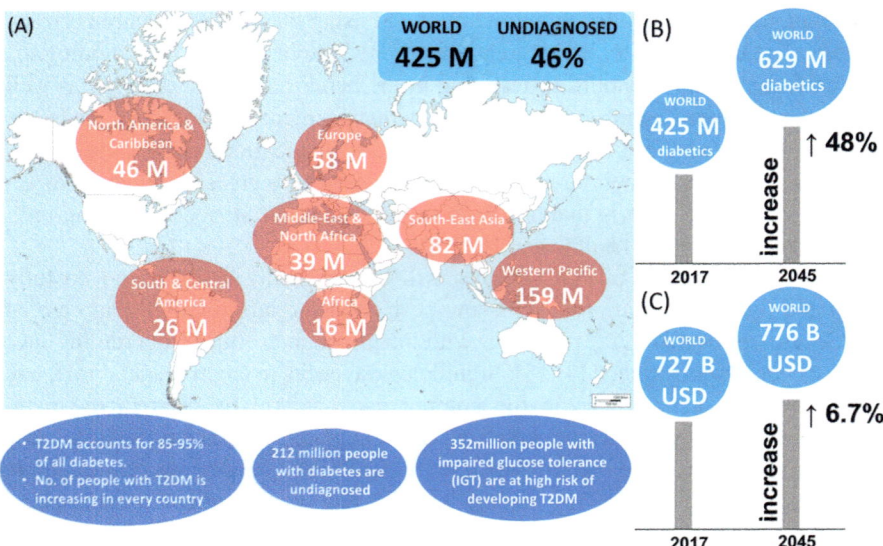

Fig. 9.1 (**A**) Prevalence of diabetes based on the IDF Diabetes Atlas, Eighth Edition [4]. IDF projections of (**B**) diabetics and (**C**) healthcare expenditure on diabetes for 2045

2017, which is similar in magnitude to the combined mortalities of HIV/AIDS, malaria, and tuberculosis. However, the precise mortality rate is difficult to access due to diabetic complications. It might account for 50% or more of deaths due to cardiovascular disease, a major diabetic complication. The health spending on diabetes in 2017 was US$727 billion and expected to reach US$776 billion in 2045 [4] (Fig. 9.1C). The top 10 countries that account for 60% of the number of diabetics and 69% of the global healthcare expenditure on diabetes are the United States, China, Germany, India, Brazil, Russian Federation, Mexico, Egypt, Indonesia, and Pakistan [4].

Type 2 diabetes accounts for 85–95% of all diabetes in high-income countries and even higher in low- and middle-income countries. The rapid cultural and social changes, increasing urbanization, change in diet, aging populations, reduced physical activities, and unhealthy behavior have contributed to this substantial increase. About 80% of people with diabetes live in low- and middle-income countries, and almost half of all adults with diabetes are in the age group of 40–59 years. A person with T2DM can live for several years without showing any symptoms, resulting in silent body damage and development of diabetic complications. In fact, several undiagnosed diabetics already acquired diabetic complications such as retinopathy, nephropathy, chronic kidney disease, and heart failure.

9.2.2 *Depression*

The modern lifestyle, environment, and social structures of communities have led to a significant increase in the stress levels of human beings. The acute psychological stress leads to depression, which has been recognized as a hidden burden by the World Health Organization (WHO) in 2013 [20]. There are at least 322 million people living with depression, and this is the leading cause of disability worldwide on top of 450 million people with mental disorders due to psychological stress. The incidence of depression stands at nearly the same level as diabetes, 382 million diabetics in 2013 [21]. Besides the affected patients, there are significantly impacts on their families and the society due to difficulties in relationships and social contacts. It carries a huge burden regarding treatment costs, the mental anguish on families and carers, and the reduced workplace productivity. Depression accounts for ~12% total years lived with disability [22] in an affected individual, causing tremendous reduced workforce productivity. The extreme form of the depression leads to suicide as attested by ~1 million suicidal cases each year among over 20 million attempted cases. Despite the availability of effective treatments, most people with depression do not receive sufficient healthcare and support due to the lack of access to treatment and the lingering social stigma attached to mental disorders.

The most severe form of stress-related depression is observed in patients with post-traumatic stress disorders (PTSD) following a sexual assault, major tissue injury and sepsis, war veterans, and the experience of other kinds of disasters. Stress can also affect the next generation as the epigenetic mechanisms shape short- and long-term responses to stress [23]. WHO started the Mental Health Gap Action Programme (mhGAP) [24], which aims at creating options for the management and treatment of depressed people. This alarming incidence of depression worldwide is a wake-up call to find solutions to address this rapidly growing global epidemic. The diabetics often have coexisting depression, associated with significantly increased morbidity, mortality, and healthcare costs [25]. Therefore, the number of diabetics, 425 million in 2017 and 629 million in 2045 [4], will also lead to a substantial increase in the number of diabetics with coexisting depression. The practice guidelines from the International Diabetes Federation (IDF) indicate this trend. Thus, there is a strong requirement of periodic assessment and monitoring of depression and other mental health conditions for effective diabetes management [26, 27].

About 60–80% of persons afflicted with depression can be treated by antidepressants and structured physiological therapies. However, fewer than 25% of these are receiving such treatments due to the lack of early-stage stress monitoring procedures [28]. Physicians in the primary care settings are seldom trained to distinguish depression from other medical conditions with the same symptoms [25].

Depression is the third leading cause of burden of disease in 2004, which will rise to the first place by 2030 as estimated by WHO (Table 9.1). Depression accounts for approx. 12% total years lived with disability [20]. "The global burden of disease (GBD): 2004 update" by WHO states that neuropsychiatric disorders cause one-third

Table 9.1 WHO estimates of ten leading causes of burden of disease, world, 2004 and 2030

2004 Disease or injury	As % of total Rank DALYs	Rank		Rank	As % of total Rank DALYs	2030 Disease or injury
Lower respiratory infections	6.2	1		1	6.2	Unipolar depressive disorders
Diarrhoeal diseases	4.8	2		2	5.5	Ischaemic heart disease
Unipolar depressive disorders	4.3	3		3	4.9	Road traffic accidents
Ischaemic heart disease	4.1	4		4	4.3	Cerebrovascular disease
HIV/AIDS	3.8	5		5	3.8	COPD
Cerebrovascular disease	3.1	6		6	3.2	Lower respiratory infections
Prematurity and low birth weight	2.9	7		7	2.9	Hearing loss, adult onset
Birth asphyxia and birth trauma	2.7	8		8	2.7	Refractive errors
Road traffic accidents	2.7	9		9	2.5	HIV/AIDS
Neonatal infections and other	2.7	10		10	2.3	Diabetes mellitus
COPD	2.0	13		11	1.9	Neonatal infections and other
Refractive errors	1.8	14		12	1.9	Prematurity and low birth weight
Hearing loss, adult onset	1.8	15		15	1.9	Birth asphyxia and birth trauma
Diabetes mellitus	1.3	19		18	1.6	Diarrhoeal diseases

DALYs is disability-adjusted life years [29]

of the years lost due to disability (YLD). The unipolar depressive disorders are the leading cause of disease burden for women in high-, low-, and medium-income countries (Fig. 9.2).

Depression is associated with a 60% increase of the type 2 diabetes [30]. Moreover, patients with diabetes and coexisting depression had 4.1-fold increased odds of disability compared with the 1.7-fold increase among adults with diabetes only and 1.3-fold increase among adults with depression alone [31]. Depression significantly deteriorates the quality of life of diabetics [32] and increases the all-cause mortality (Fig. 9.3). The total healthcare expenditures were 4.5 times greater among diabetics with depression than nondepressed counterparts [34]. Thus, the coexistence of depression in diabetics is associated with increased healthcare service utilization and costs.

The improved mental health in the workplace will lead to reduced employee sickness absence, better staff retention, and increased economic productivity and performance [35].

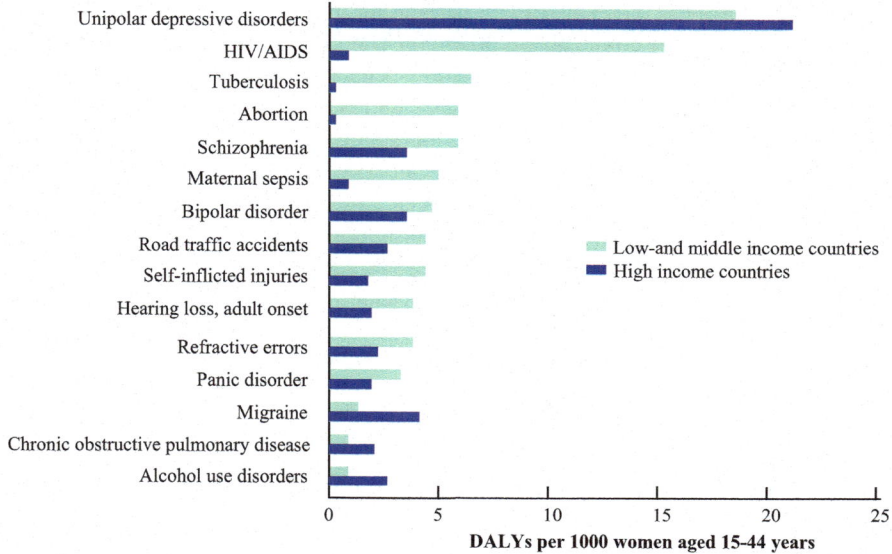

Fig. 9.2 Leading causes of disease burden for women aged 15–44 years in high-income countries and low- and middle-income countries, 2004. (Source: 'The global burden of disease: 2004 update' by WHO [29])

Fig. 9.3 Effect of depression on all-cause mortality in patients with diabetes [33]. Reproduced with permission from the American Diabetes Association

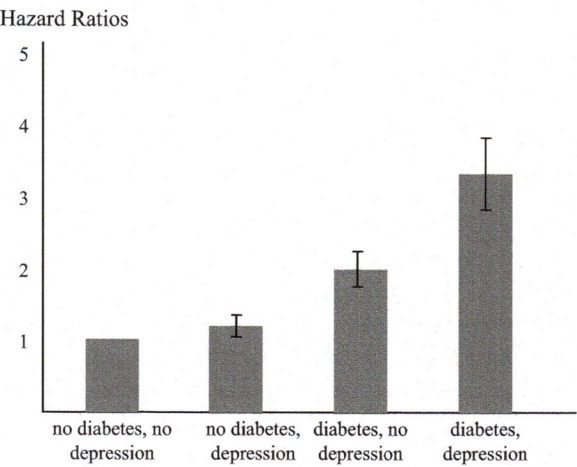

9.2.3   Obesity

Obesity is one of the major healthcare concerns worldwide but highest in the United States and Europe [36]. In the United States, more than 36.5% of the population is considered obese, and about 62% are overweight [37]. The incidence of obesity is significantly higher in women. It is higher among middle-aged adults between 40 and 59 years and older adults above 60 years. The global prevalence of obesity in men and women has doubled in the last three decades. Presently, more than half a billion adults worldwide are obese, a striking statistic.

The ideal mean body mass index (BMI) for healthy adults should be 21–23 kg/m^2, but 18.5–24.9 kg/m^2 is still acceptable and regarded as the goal of the healthy population. The individuals having BMI in the range of 25–29.9 are considered overweight, who are susceptible to increased risk of comorbidities. The individuals having BMI more than 30 are obese, which makes them more vulnerable to moderate to severe risk of comorbidities. The increased BMI is an important cause of chronic diseases such as type 2 diabetes, heart disease, stroke, and certain types of cancer [38]. In 2008, about \$147 billion of the healthcare costs was associated with obesity.

9.2.4 Cancer

Cancer is the second largest cause of death that accounted for more than 8.8 million cases worldwide in 2015 [39]. About 70% of deaths due to cancers occurred in low- and middle-income countries, where cancer-causing infections, such as hepatitis B–C viruses (HBV/HCV) and human papillomavirus (HPV), are responsible for up to 25% of all cancer cases [40]. The leading cancers in decreasing order of mortality are lung, liver, colorectal, stomach, and breast. Albeit the incidence of cancer rises with age, the consumption of tobacco and alcohol, physical inactivity, unhealthy diet, and high BMI are the major risk factors. Indeed, tobacco use is the major risk factor that accounts for about 22% of cancer-related deaths worldwide [41]. The late-stage presentation and inaccessible diagnosis and treatment of cancer are the major concerns in low-income countries.

Cancer accounts for substantial economic cost as the total healthcare costs, about US\$1.16 trillion in 2010 [42]. The development of POC technologies for the early-stage detection of cancer and management of cancer patients can significantly reduce the cancer burden as many cancers, such as breast, cervical, oral, and colorectal, have a high chance of cure if they are detected early and treated according to best practices. About one million cancer cases could be prevented each year by vaccinating the subjects against HBV and HPV [40].

9.2.5 Cardiovascular Diseases (CVDs)

CVDs are the leading cause of deaths worldwide, attributed to about 31% of all global deaths or about 17.7 million, in 2015 [43]. Coronary heart disease and stroke account for 7.4 million and 6.7 million deaths, respectively. The low- and middle-income countries account for more than 75% of the CVD deaths, plausibly due to the lack of early-stage detection technologies and treatment of people with CVD risk factors. The risk of CVDs increases with the population aging [44, 45], dependent upon the social, economic, and cultural factors, such as stress, poverty, hereditary factors, etc.

There is a need for POC technologies for the early-stage detection and management of CVDs so that the affected patients could be effectively treated. The general population must be educated to prevent CVDs by avoiding the aforementioned risk factors: physical inactivity, tobacco use, alcohol use, unhealthy diet, and obesity [46, 47]. CVDs place an unsustainably higher economic burden [48] on the economies of low- and middle-income countries and are draining a lot of healthcare costs globally.

9.2.6 Sexually Transmitted Infections (STIs)

There is an alarming increase in the number of persons acquiring STIs worldwide as the current estimate states over one million STIs are acquired every day [49]. About 357 million new STIs are acquired by persons every year for one of the four main STIs: gonorrhea, syphilis, chlamydia, and trichomoniasis [49]. Over 500 million people have genital infection with herpes simplex virus (HSV), while more than 290 million women have a human papillomavirus (HPV) infection [50]. The prevalence of HSV type 2 and syphilis in persons make them at an increased risk of HIV acquisition. The infection of pregnant women with syphilis could adversely affect the birth outcomes. This is evident from 350,000 adverse birth outcomes in more than 900,000 pregnant women in 2012 [51]. Gonorrhea and chlamydia are the major causes of pelvic inflammatory disease (PID) and infertility in women. HPV infection also leads to more than 0.5 million cervical cancer cases every year. Moreover, STIs could also adversely affect the reproductive health of persons, leading to infertility and transmission from mother to child. The detection of STIs is sometimes difficult as most of the STIs have no or only mild symptoms. The drug resistance is also posing a major limitation to decrease the incidence of STIs. Although most STIs spread majorly by sexual contact, some STIs can also spread via blood or blood products. STIs could also be transmitted from mother to child during pregnancy and childbirth.

9.2.7 Tuberculosis (TB)

This communicable disease caused by *Mycobacterium tuberculosis* affects most often the lungs and spreads from person to person through the air. About 25% of the world's population has latent TB, i.e., they are infected by *M. tuberculosis* but not ill with TB and thus cannot transmit it to others [52]. However, they carry a risk of 5–15% of developing active TB. In particular, people with compromised immune systems, such as those affected with HIV, diabetes, and malnutrition and who use tobacco, are more prone to developing active TB. HIV-positive people have 20–30 times higher risk of developing active TB in comparison with HIV-negative persons [53, 54]. HIV and TB form a deadly combination as each speeds the other's progress. TB is a leading killer of HIV-positive people as about 40% of the global HIV deaths were due to TB in 2016. There were 1.7 million deaths due to TB in 2016 out of which 0.4 million was deaths due to TB in HIV-positive people. The number of people who fell ill with TB was 10.4 million in 2016. Although the global TB incidence is falling at the rate of about 2% per year, the multidrug-resistant TB (MDR-TB) is a major threat to public health [55, 56]. About 0.6 million new TB patients have developed resistance to rifampicin, which is the most effective first-line drug for treating TB, while about 0.49 million of such patients had developed MDR-TB. TB is one of the top 10 leading causes of death worldwide, particularly in India [52]. About 64% of the global incidence of TB is accounted for by India, Indonesia, China, the Philippines, Pakistan, Nigeria, and South Africa. In 2016, about 45% of new TB cases occurred in Asia, while about 25% occurred in Africa. WHO initiated the "End TB strategy" that aims to reduce the deaths due to TB by 90% and to decrease new TB cases by 80% between 2015 and 2035 [57].

The WHO recommends the use of Xpert MTB/RIF® rapid 2-hour test for the simultaneous detection of TB and resistance to rifampicin, the most widely used TB medicine. The test is widely used globally as evident by the procurement of more than 6.9 million cartridges in 2016. However, the diagnosis of MDR-TB, as well as HIV-associated TB, is complex and expensive. Therefore, there is an extensive need for new POC tests for the rapid diagnosis of TB and identifying the resistance to rifampicin and multiple TB drugs.

9.2.8   Human Immunodeficiency Virus (HIV)/Acquired Immunodeficiency Syndrome (AIDS)

Human immunodeficiency virus (HIV) weakens the immune system of the infected patients, and they become more prone to infections, cancers, and other diseases due to the low CD cells [58, 59]. The acquired immunodeficiency syndrome (AIDS) is the most advanced stage of HIV infection, which takes many years (2–15 years) to manifestation based on the state of the infected individual. It is characterized by infections, cancers, and severe clinical conditions. WHO in 2016 estimated about 25.6 million HIV cases in Africa among 36.7 cases worldwide [60]. It is mainly prevalent in adults (about 34.5 million) in comparison with children (<15 years) (about 2.1 million). About 1.8 million people are newly infected with HIV in 2016, most of them being adults, i.e., 1.7 million. Similarly, there were about 1 million HIV-related deaths in 2016. However, there is a global decline in the number of newly HIV-infected people dying from HIV-related causes during the last decade. The WHO is targeting to reduce the number of newly HIV-infected people to less than 0.5 million and 0.2 million by 2020 and 2030, respectively. Further, it is aiming to reduce the number of people dying from HIV to less than 0.5 million and 0.4 million by 2020 and 2030, respectively. The increase in the number of people receiving antiretroviral treatment from 19.5 million in 2016 to about 30 million and 33 million, by 2020 and 2030, is a future target for WHO. However, there is no cure for HIV except the effective antiretroviral (ARV) drugs that can control the virus and prevent its transmission. Most of the HIV-positive persons are infected with TB, which is the main cause of death [61]. Therefore, TB preventive therapy and screening of TB must be provided to the HIV-positive patients.

9.3   Future Trends and Need for Personalized and Integrated Healthcare

There is an extensive and urgent need for personalized and integrated healthcare for chronic diseases to improve the health of the patients and cut down the healthcare costs. It would enable the healthcare professionals to provide more effective treatment and intervention to their patients. The current international focus is to empower the patients [16, 17] by developing personalized healthcare devices, enabling them to take charge of their health by monitoring their basic health parameters and follow personalized nutritional, physical activity, and lifestyle interventions to improve their health. This is evident from the exponentially growing use of wearable personalized devices such as smartwatches and SP- and smart gadgets-interfaced blood glucose monitors, pulse oximeters, electrocardiogram (ECG), blood pressure monitors, body analysis scales, etc. [13, 62]. Among many smart applications, iHealth Pro by iHealth Labs [14] enables the users to see the trends in their basic health parameters, correspond to their physicians, and notice the effect of their lifestyle/clinical/nutritional/activity-based intervention on their health. The most recent trend is the promotion of health in population by specific health-oriented games on virtual reality and game consoles (such as Xbox, PlayStation, Nintendo, etc.) [63–65]. Moreover, the next generation of POC diagnostics for a particular disease would be based on the multiplex detection of several biomarkers, which would provide an easy-to-use indicator as the clinical score for a particular disease. The trends in the clinical score for chronic diseases such as diabetes and depression would enable the patients and doctors to monitor and manage the disease more effectively.

During the last 5 years, a wide range of POC devices and assays based on SP [1, 11, 12] was developed along with the dedicated smart applications [13, 14], enabling the users to detect various clinically relevant analytes with good analytical performance. The spatiotemporal tagged data and Cloud would be very helpful in emergencies and epidemics. Similarly, mH is leading to new healthcare delivery concepts to minimize the unnecessary clinical visits to cut down healthcare costs but lead to better health outcomes by increasing patient's compliance, awareness, and communication. The evolving mH concepts would also pave the way to electronic health record (EHR) of the patient, which could be assessed by health professionals in various countries where the patient might be traveling. Therefore, the personalized health monitoring and management together with the integrated health concepts would significantly increase the outreach of healthcare, thereby leading to more effective therapy and health of patients. The increased awareness of patients and general population via dedicated smart applications and Internet has already contributed to significant improvement in their health. The frequent communication between doctors and patients via dedicated smart application enables the doctors to take care of their patients more effectively in addition to saving the time and costs.

The modern era of globalization and urbanization has introduced significant changes in the lifestyle of the general population [66, 67]. The current generation is more prone to sedentary behavior, unhealthy food habits, solitude, increased pressure on social media, and adapting to the rapidly changing technologies. All these factors are contributing to the increase in chronic diseases worldwide. Therefore, there is a tremendous need for global efforts to counteract these growing health concerns. In June 2018, WHO launched the "WHO Global action plan on physical activity and health 2018–2030: More active people for a healthier world" [68]. The main focus is to motivate the general population to have regular physical activity, which is the main factor in preventing and treating noncommunicable diseases. The action plan targets the reduction in physical inactivity in adults and adolescents by 15% by 2030. Physical inactivity is a critical health concern, which is estimated to cost US\$54 billion in direct healthcare. The public sector accounts for 57% of the cost, while lost productivity accounts for US\$14 billion. Similarly, WHO launched the "Global action plan for the prevention and control of noncommunicable diseases (NCDs) 2013–2020" in 2013, which aims for reducing the number of premature deaths from NCDs by 25% by 2025 [69].

The continuously increasing efforts in the development of POC devices, LOC platforms, mH, and smart technologies together with the evolving complementary technologies are aiding the development of personalized and integrated healthcare. The day is not far off when we will see a plethora of next-generation technologies making their way into the healthcare and transforming our lives.

9.4 Conclusions

Numerous technological advances have been made in the field of POC, smart systems, and personalized wearable devices, as evident from the continuously increasing number of commercial devices that are being used by millions of people. The last decade has brought transformational changes in healthcare due to the significant improvement in assays, bioanalytical platforms, LOC technologies, microfluidic operations, biomolecular recognition elements, biosensing concepts, readers, mH, automation technologies, miniaturization, and complementary technologies. The most prominent development is the multifarious SP-based as the POC diagnostic applications and devices that have been demonstrated for a wide range of analytes. Moreover, many SP-based devices for personalized and integrated healthcare monitoring and management have been successfully commercialized with wide-spread uses. The next generation of personalized and integrated healthcare devices would revolutionize the healthcare and cut down the healthcare costs by manyfolds.

References

1. Vashist SK, Luong JHT. Trends in *in vitro* diagnostics and mobile healthcare. Biotechnol Adv. 2016;34(3):137–8.
2. Abegunde DO, Mathers CD, Adam T, Ortegon M, Strong K. The burden and costs of chronic diseases in low-income and middle-income countries. Lancet. 2007;370(9603):1929–38.
3. Moussavi S, Chatterji S, Verdes E, Tandon A, Patel V, Ustun B. Depression, chronic diseases, and decrements in health: results from the world health surveys. Lancet. 2007;370(9590):851–8.
4. IDF Diabetes Atlas: 8th ed. http://diabetesatlas.org/resources/2017-atlas.html. Accessed 18 July 2018.
5. Wild S, Roglic G, Green A, Sicree R, King H. Global prevalence of diabetes: estimates for the year 2000 and projections for 2030. Diabetes Care. 2004;27(5):1047–53.
6. Vashist SK. Too much sitting: a potential health hazard and a global call to action. J Basic Appl Sci. 2015;11:131.
7. Healy GN, Wijndaele K, Dunstan DW, Shaw JE, Salmon J, Zimmet PZ, et al. Objectively measured sedentary time, physical activity, and metabolic risk: the Australian diabetes, obesity and lifestyle study (AusDiab). Diabetes Care. 2008;31(2):369–71.
8. Owen N, Sparling PB, Healy GN, Dunstan DW, Matthews CE. Sedentary behavior: emerging evidence for a new health risk. Mayo Clin Proc. 2010;85(12):1138–41.
9. Owen N, Healy GN, Matthews CE, Dunstan DW. Too much sitting: the population health science of sedentary behavior. Exerc Sport Sci Rev. 2010;38(3):105–13.
10. Vashist SK, Luong JHT. Smartphone-based immunoassays. In: Handbook of immunoassay technologies. Amsterdam: Elsevier; 2018. p. 433–53.
11. Vashist SK, Luppa PB, Yeo LY, Ozcan A, Luong JHT. Emerging technologies for next-generation point-of-care testing. Trends Biotechnol. 2015;33(11):692–705.
12. Vashist SK, Mudanyali O, Schneider EM, Zengerle R, Ozcan A. Cellphone-based devices for bioanalytical sciences. Anal Bioanal Chem. 2014;406(14):3263–77.
13. Vashist SK, Schneider EM, Luong JHT. Commercial smartphone-based devices and smart applications for personalized healthcare monitoring and management. Diagnostics (Basel). 2014;4(3):104–28.
14. Vashist SK, Luong JHT. Diabetes management software and smart applications. In: Point-of-care glucose detection for diabetic monitoring and management. Boca Raton: CRC Press; 2017. p. 135–54.
15. Data Protection. https://ec.europa.eu/info/law/law-topic/data-protection_en. Accessed 18 July 2018.
16. McAllister M, Dunn G, Payne K, Davies L, Todd C. Patient empowerment: the need to consider it as a measurable patient-reported outcome for chronic conditions. BMC Health Serv Res. 2012;12(1):157.
17. Househ M, Borycki E, Kushniruk A. Empowering patients through social media: the benefits and challenges. Health Informatics J. 2014;20(1):50–8.
18. Vashist SK, Luong JHT. Lab-on-a-chip (LOC) immunoassays. In: Handbook of immunoassay technologies. Amsterdam: Elsevier; 2018. p. 415–31.
19. van Susan D, Beulens JW, van der Schouw Yvonne T, Grobbee DE, Nealb B. The global burden of diabetes and its complications: an emerging pandemic. Eur J Cardiovasc Prev Rehabil. 2010;17(1_suppl):s3–8.

20. WHO Depression Global Burden. http://www.who.int/healthinfo/global_burden_disease/en/. Accessed 18 July 2018.
21. IDF World Diabetes Facts. http://www.idf.org/worlddiabetesday/toolkit/gp/facts-figures. Accessed 18 July 2018.
22. WHO Depression. http://www.who.int/mental_health/management/depression/en/. Accessed 18 July 2018.
23. Nestler EJ. Epigenetics: stress makes its molecular mark. Nature. 2012;490(7419):171–2.
24. Fleischmann A, Saxena S. Suicide prevention in the WHO mental health gap action programme (mhGAP). Crisis. 2013;34(5):295–6.
25. Pincus HA, Pettit AR. The societal costs of chronic major depression. J Clin Psychiatry. 2000;62:5–9.
26. IDF Clinical Guideline Task Force: Global guideline for Type 2 diabetes. http://www.idf.org/webdata/docs/IDF%20GGT2D.pdf. Accessed 18 July 2018.
27. IDF Clinical Guideline Task Force: Global guideline for Type 2 diabetes. http://www.idf.org/sites/default/files/IDF%20T2DM%20Guideline.pdf. Accessed 18 July 2018.
28. European Brain Council Depressive disorders in RU. http://www.europeanbraincouncil.org/pdfs/Documents/Depression%20fact%20sheet%20July%202011.pdf. Accessed 18 July 2018.
29. WHO Global Burden Disease. http://www.who.int/healthinfo/global_burden_disease/GBD_report_2004update_full.pdf. Accessed 18 July 2018.
30. Mezuk B, Eaton WW, Albrecht S, Golden SH. Depression and type 2 diabetes over the lifespan: a meta-analysis. Diabetes Care. 2008;31(12):2383–90.
31. Katon WJ, Russo JE, Von Korff M, Lin EH, Ludman E, Ciechanowski PS. Long-term effects on medical costs of improving depression outcomes in patients with depression and diabetes. Diabetes Care. 2008;31(6):1155–9.
32. Grandy S, Chapman R, Fox K. Quality of life and depression of people living with type 2 diabetes mellitus and those at low and high risk for type 2 diabetes: findings from the study to help improve early evaluation and management of risk factors leading to diabetes (SHIELD). Int J Clin Pract. 2008;62(4):562–8.
33. Egede LE, Nietert PJ, Zheng D. Depression and all-cause and coronary heart disease mortality among adults with and without diabetes. Diabetes Care. 2005;28(6):1339–45.
34. Egede LE, Zheng D, Simpson K. Comorbid depression is associated with increased health care use and expenditures in individuals with diabetes. Diabetes Care. 2002;25(3):464–70.
35. Improved Mental Health Will Dec the Losses. http://www.chex.org.uk/media/resources/mental_health/Mental%20Health%20Promotion%20-%20Building%20an%20Economic%20Case.pdf. Accessed 18 July 2018.
36. Obesity. http://www.who.int/gho/ncd/risk_factors/obesity_text/en/. Accessed 18 July 2018.
37. Adult Obesity Facts. https://www.cdc.gov/obesity/data/adult.html. Accessed 18 July 2018.
38. Zheng W, McLerran DF, Rolland B, Zhang X, Inoue M, Matsuo K, et al. Association between body-mass index and risk of death in more than 1 million Asians. N Engl J Med. 2011;364(8):719–29.
39. Cancer. http://www.who.int/news-room/fact-sheets/detail/cancer. Accessed 18 July 2018.
40. Plummer M, de Martel C, Vignat J, Ferlay J, Bray F, Franceschi S. Global burden of cancers attributable to infections in 2012: a synthetic analysis. Lancet Glob Health. 2016;4(9):e609–16.
41. Forouzanfar MH, Afshin A, Alexander LT, Anderson HR, Bhutta ZA, Biryukov S, et al. Global, regional, and national comparative risk assessment of 79 behavioural, environmental and occupational, and metabolic risks or clusters of risks, 1990–2015: a systematic analysis for the global burden of disease study 2015. Lancet. 2016;388(10053):1659–724.
42. Stewart B, Wild CP. World cancer report 2014. Health 2017.
43. Cardiovascular Diseases (CVDs). http://www.who.int/news-room/fact-sheets/detail/cardiovascular-diseases-(cvds). Accessed 18 July 2018.
44. Fyhrquist F, Saijonmaa O, Strandberg T. The roles of senescence and telomere shortening in cardiovascular disease. Nat Rev Cardiol. 2013;10(5):274–83.
45. Samani NJ, van der Harst P. Biological ageing and cardiovascular disease. Heart. 2008;94(5):537–9.

46. Luepker RV, Murray DM, Jacobs DR Jr, Mittelmark MB, Bracht N, Carlaw R, et al. Community education for cardiovascular disease prevention: risk factor changes in the Minnesota heart health program. Am J Public Health. 1994;84(9):1383–93.
47. Kahn R, Robertson RM, Smith R, Eddy D. The impact of prevention on reducing the burden of cardiovascular disease. Circulation. 2008;118(5):576–85.
48. Yusuf S, Reddy S, Ounpuu S, Anand S. Global burden of cardiovascular diseases: part I: general considerations, the epidemiologic transition, risk factors, and impact of urbanization. Circulation. 2001;104(22):2746–53.
49. Sexually Transmitted Infections (STIs). http://www.who.int/en/news-room/fact-sheets/detail/sexually-transmitted-infections-(stis). Accessed 18 July 2018.
50. de Sanjose S, Diaz M, Castellsague X, Clifford G, Bruni L, Munoz N, et al. Worldwide prevalence and genotype distribution of cervical human papillomavirus DNA in women with normal cytology: a meta-analysis. Lancet Infect Dis. 2007;7(7):453–9.
51. Newman L, Kamb M, Hawkes S, Gomez G, Say L, Seuc A, et al. Global estimates of syphilis in pregnancy and associated adverse outcomes: analysis of multinational antenatal surveillance data. PLoS Med. 2013;10(2):e1001396.
52. Tuberculosis. http://www.who.int/news-room/fact-sheets/detail/tuberculosis. Accessed 18 July 2018.
53. Corbett EL, Watt CJ, Walker N, Maher D, Williams BG, Raviglione MC, et al. The growing burden of tuberculosis: global trends and interactions with the HIV epidemic. Arch Intern Med. 2003;163(9):1009–21.
54. Dye C, Williams BG. The population dynamics and control of tuberculosis. Science. 2010;328(5980):856–61.
55. Millard J, Ugarte-Gil C, Moore DA. Multidrug resistant tuberculosis. BMJ. 2015;350:h882.
56. Zignol M, Hosseini MS, Wright A, Weezenbeek CL, Nunn P, Watt CJ, et al. Global incidence of multidrug-resistant tuberculosis. J Infect Dis. 2006;194(4):479–85.
57. The End TB Strategy. http://www.who.int/tb/strategy/en/. Accessed 18 July 2018.
58. Palella FJ Jr, Delaney KM, Moorman AC, Loveless MO, Fuhrer J, Satten GA, et al. Declining morbidity and mortality among patients with advanced human immunodeficiency virus infection. N Engl J Med. 1998;338(13):853–60.
59. Fauci AS. The human immunodeficiency virus: infectivity and mechanisms of pathogenesis. Science. 1988;239(4840):617–22.
60. HIV/AIDS. http://www.who.int/en/news-room/fact-sheets/detail/hiv-aids. Accessed 18 July 2018.
61. Daley CL, Small PM, Schecter GF, Schoolnik GK, McAdam RA, Jacobs WR Jr, et al. An outbreak of tuberculosis with accelerated progression among persons infected with the human immunodeficiency virus: an analysis using restriction-fragment length polymorphisms. N Engl J Med. 1992;326(4):231–5.
62. Son D, Lee J, Qiao S, Ghaffari R, Kim J, Lee JE, et al. Multifunctional wearable devices for diagnosis and therapy of movement disorders. Nat Nanotechnol. 2014;9(5):397–404.
63. Papastergiou M. Exploring the potential of computer and video games for health and physical education: a literature review. Comput Educ. 2009;53(3):603–22.
64. Peng W, Crouse JC, Lin J-H. Using active video games for physical activity promotion: a systematic review of the current state of research. Health Educ Behav. 2013;40(2):171–92.
65. Primack BA, Carroll MV, McNamara M, Klem ML, King B, Rich M, et al. Role of video games in improving health-related outcomes: a systematic review. Am J Prev Med. 2012;42(6):630–8.
66. Godfrey R, Julien M. Urbanisation and health. Clin Med (Lond). 2005;5(2):137–41.
67. Gong P, Liang S, Carlton EJ, Jiang Q, Wu J, Wang L, et al. Urbanisation and health in China. Lancet. 2012;379(9818):843–52.
68. WHO launches Global Action Plan on Physical Activity. http://www.who.int/news-room/detail/04-06-2018-who-launches-global-action-plan-on-physical-activity. Accessed 18 July 2018.
69. Global Action Plan for the Prevention and Control of NCDs 2013–2020. http://www.who.int/nmh/publications/ncd-action-plan/en/. Accessed 18 July 2018.

Index

© Springer Nature Switzerland AG 2019
S. K. Vashist, J. H. T. Luong, *Point-of-Care Technologies Enabling
Next-Generation Healthcare Monitoring and Management*,
https://doi.org/10.1007/978-3-030-11416-9

Printed by Printforce, the Netherlands